Andrew Stanway, MB, MRCP, worked on the Professorial Medical Unit at a London teaching hospital until 10 years ago. He now lectures, broadcasts, writes and makes films on medical topics both for the medical profession and for the public.

He has written many books including *The Boots Book of First Aid*; *Alternative Medicine – a Guide to Natural Therapies*; *Why Us?: a Common-sense Guide for the Childless*; *Taking the Rough with the Smooth*; and *Overcoming Depression*. *The Pears Encyclopaedia of Child Health* and *Breast is Best* (which has become a best seller) were written jointly with his wife Penny.

Dr Stanway has three children and lives in Surrey.

D1785254

# Dr Andrew Stanway

# A Dictionary of
# Operations

A PALADIN BOOK

**GRANADA**

London Toronto Sydney New York

Published by Granada Publishing Limited in 1981

ISBN 0 586 08368 5 (paperback)
ISBN 0 246 11644 7 (hardback)

A Granada Paperback Original
Copyright © Dr Andrew Stanway 1981

Granada Publishing Limited
Frogmore, St. Albans, Herts AL2 2NF
and
3 Upper James Street, London W1R 4BP
866 United Nations Plaza, New York, NY10017, USA
117 York Street, Sydney, NSW 2000, Australia
100 Skyway Avenue, Rexdale, Ontario M9W 3A6, Canada
PO Box 84165, Greenside, 2034 Johannesburg, South Africa
61 Beach Road, Auckland, New Zealand

Printed and bound in Great Britain by
Cox & Wyman Ltd, Reading

Set in Linotype Plantin

Granada ®
Granada Publishing ®

# Contents

# Acknowledgements

My thanks to:
Dame Elizabeth Ackroyd
Action on Smoking and Health
Adrian Allaway, MB, BS, FRCS
Nicholas Breach, FDS, FRCS
Austin Brown, FRCS
BUPA and PPP
Bernard Crymble, FRCS
Claude Eastes, MB, BS, FRCS
Janet Gooch, SRN, DN(Lond.), RCT
Neil Hodson, FRCS
The Hospital Secretary and staff of King's College Hospital
David Ingram, MA, MB, B.Chir., FRCS
The Librarian and staff of King's Fund Centre
The Librarian and staff of the Royal Society of Medicine
The Mastectomy Association
The National Association for the Welfare of Children in
    Hospital
The Patients' Association
Jean Robinson
Richard Vincent, MB, MRCP
John Williams, FRCP
Cyril Young, MRCOG
All the self-help groups listed on pages 427-431, who gave me
invaluable help, and all the many patients who have given me
their time and opinions so that I could write the book in a
way to help others.

My special thanks are due to Brian Hogbin, FRCS,
consultant surgeon to the Brighton Health District, whose
painstaking and sensitive comments on the final manuscript
have greatly enriched the book.

# Foreword
*By Brian Hogbin FRCS*

Some books are needed and wanted but are not written because the problems seem too great. That may well be why it has been necessary to wait until now for this book.

How can anyone hope to explain clearly and accurately the whole range of operations available when it can take a surgeon twelve years to train in just one field? Yet Dr Stanway has tackled it and has produced a most useful and comprehensive result. It would, of course, have been possible for a number of specialists each to write a section of such a book but this would have produced many problems for the reader. Dr Stanway has, I believe, managed to write a well-balanced book on the subject single-handed but has taken care to have each section checked by a specialist. This book describes the main lines of thought and practice at the present time in surgery.

We all know that there is more than one way to do most things and the treatment of illness is no exception. Often a given condition can be treated in a variety of ways, either because they all work equally well or because all have their own particular weaknesses. Sometimes the treatment will vary from patient to patient and it is certain that individual surgeons have their own favourite operations for specific conditions. This variety has led to special problems in writing the book for almost every sentence could be expanded, explained further or exceptions given. Every detail of modern surgery is discussed at length in the learned literature and at endless meetings around the world but this book has distilled the most common, important and generally agreed-upon courses of treatment and set them out clearly for the general public. If you, your condition or its management do not seem to fit into the description in the book, discuss the matter with your surgeon.

They say 'A little knowledge is a dangerous thing', but if used correctly as a basis for understanding what is happening then the reader's path to health should be smoothed.

# Introduction

Going into hospital is not much fun and having an operation is even more stressful. To many it is one of the most unpleasant episodes in their lives and to some even stands out as a life crisis.

Much of this is inevitable. Hospitals are strange places to most people and even for those who are used to working in and around hospitals, an admission for an operation puts them firmly on 'the other side of the fence'.

It is not only unfamiliarity (after all, most of us will on average only have one or two operations in a lifetime) but also the fear of the unknown that weighs heavily when we hear we have to have an operation. People going into hospitals for medical as opposed to surgical treatment know pretty well what they are in for. Usually, the 'worst' they have to fear are some strange investigations but otherwise they will be given tablets or other forms of treatment, some of which are unusual but certainly not invasive in the way that surgery is.

So, given that most of us are apprehensive at best and terrified at worst when we are to have an operation, why write a book about it? Is ignorance not the bliss it has been made out to be?

I'm afraid it is not. Repeatedly, surveys have shown that the commonest complaint surgical patients have is that they are not told enough. My personal research bears this out. 'Why can't they treat me like a human being?' 'It's my body.' 'More information would have given me much more peace of mind'. 'Whenever they told me nothing, I worried'. 'The doctors treated me as though I was stupid' and 'Why not tell people what any reasonably intelligent person could understand', are just some of the complaints I heard time and again when researching this book.

The answers are not simple and certainly do not mean that doctors and nurses are uncaring people who think the public should be kept in ignorance.

The greatest problem is the communication gap that crops up whenever anyone enters a potentially stressful situation. Most of us find we have not made ourselves clear or really understood what our GP has told us – and that is when we are dressed, sitting down comfortably and talking to someone we know in reasonably familiar surroundings. Even in these conditions it has been shown that people remember very badly what the doctor said even when questioned five minutes later.

How much worse then will effective communication be when you are in a strange setting and feeling very nervous? I know from personal experience that I have explained carefully and slowly a certain procedure to an intelligent person lying in his hospital bed, only to be told later that he had not got the message at all – even though at the time he (and I) thought he had. As soon as we enter the hospital's doors to have an operation a subtle change overcomes us. We become dependent and childlike within minutes and the condition lasts until we are discharged, and in some cases even after that.

So in this childlike state of dependence, when someone asks us if we have understood, we tend to say 'yes', simply because of our new state of mind and our new-found desire to please. Had we felt at ease, as when buying a new washing machine, for example, we wouldn't let so much go unquestioned and would certainly demand better answers to our questions than we get in hospital.

All this seems to point an accusing finger at the medical and nursing professions. But this is an unfair interpretation of the situation. Doctors and nurses are human beings as well as professionals. Recent research which looked at what surgical patients wanted to know from the nurses and what the nurses *thought* their patients wanted to know has shown that the two are very different. The nurses by and large told their patients what they felt competent to disclose, and most often the patients, feeling they had been told *something*, did not like to bother the nurses with the questions they *really* wanted answered. This means the onus may be on you to ask the questions which are important to you. You cannot expect the staff to read your mind and they will not mind you asking.

Many doctors in the UK and especially those working in the junior posts in hospitals do not have English as their first language, which is also unhelpful on many occasions. This is not their fault and the system would collapse without them but it still represents a communication problem to many, especially the elderly.

Add to this the general pressure of the average hospital doctor's work load and the fact that many doctors are not naturally good communicators and you have a situation which fast becomes more stressful than it need be for the person on the receiving end.

What I have tried to do in this book is to explain all the common and many of the not-so-common operations in a straightforward way so that someone about to have an operation can, in his own home and at his own pace, come to grips with what is going to happen to him.

Having said this though – a word of caution. Every surgeon is an individual and each will have his own way of dealing with any particular condition. This has made the book very difficult to write because surgery is a fast-moving science that is influenced by new drug discoveries just as it is by new ways of making surgery technically easier, safer or more successful. Each surgeon brings to his job (as does everybody else) his own approach to life. If he has a conservative old-fashioned approach, it will appeal to many. If he is a 'whizz-kid' surgeon who tries anything new and is always up with all the advances, he will please other patients. Surgery abounds with fashions and styles, both in actual operations and the way in which they are carried out. Most surgeons steer a middle course, trying to give their patients the best of the new combined with the best of the old, well-tried methods and this works well. It does, however, mean that your surgeon may well not treat you exactly as I have outlined in the book for any given condition. What the book should do, though, is to give you enough information to be able to ask the right questions. It should also give you the confidence to feel more 'at home' in a very unfamiliar setting.

# Introduction

'But do people really want to know?' is the question that many people asked me while I was writing this book. The answer is, as you would expect, 'yes' and 'no'. There is no doubt (and research has borne this out) that many people do not want to know much about their operations. This has been shown to be especially true of old people. Most though, certainly do want to know. We live in a much more open society today when institutions and givernment bodies are becoming more accessible to the public. The general mood is one of openness yet so many complain of an apparent veil of secrecy on a matter that deeply affects them – their body and its malfunction. Naturally, people's desire for information varies enormously. Even the same person under different circumstances will want to know very different things about his medical care. But there is only one way that this ingorance can be dispelled and that is by asking. Work out the questions you most want answered, even make a note of them to help you remember and then ensure that someone tells you what you want to know.

The other reason why many people feel they want to know more is that so many operations are relatively minor and the person is otherwise well. If you go into hospital with raging pneumonia or a heart attack you will not be in a condition to appreciate a lecture on your medical condition or want one either. Most people having an operation, on the contrary, are generally fit and very much want to know what is happening.

My aim in writing this book has been to give the reader enough information to enable him to participate intelligently in his hospital stay. That this is valuable and worthwhile has been shown in many studies. Those who have pre-operative knowledge and understanding fare rather better post-operatively than those who are told nothing. Not only do people who are informed fare better in measurable medical ways but they also recover faster and go home sooner after their operations than others who have had no pre-operative counselling.

Being a surgical patient should not be a passive state. We can all do so much to help the professionals make us well quicker. This book tells you how you can help yourself.

# Part I
# Having an Operation

# Introduction

Each year more than two and a half million operations are performed in the UK. Many of the people operated on have never been in hospital as in-patients so the experience is a new one. Most operations are not done as emergencies so there is usually a reasonable period of time in which one can get information about being in hospital as a surgical patient. Most people do not bother and then wonder why it all seems so strange when D-Day arrives.

This section of the book outlines briefly what it is like to be a surgical patient and takes you from the day you first think there is something wrong right through the operation and then until you are back home again. If you are on the waiting list for an operation, read this section so that if you are called in quickly (which often happens) you will be prepared.

In this section of the book, readers will note that there are many references to the National Health Service. In order to be really helpful to the British reader the book has been written with him or her in mind. In many overseas countries which have based their medical-care systems on the British NHS, readers will find a number of areas of common practice. Aside from practical details, the main concepts in this section are of course universal and will be helpful to readers in any country.

# GETTING INTO HOSPITAL

There are two ways of ending up in a hospital bed for a surgical procedure. The first is through the surgical out-patients' department and the second is as an emergency.

### Emergency admission

The story usually starts with you calling your general practitioner about a problem and he may come and see you at home. This might be because you have a severe pain, because you have vomited or passed blood or because of one of a host of other things that *you* feel count as an emergency. Very often such 'emergencies' in your eyes turn out to be nothing urgent but if your doctor feels you need a surgical opinion or even possibly admission to hospital, he will telephone the hospital (from your home if you have a telephone) and speak to the doctor or admissions officer on duty. Most larger hospitals have full-time admissions officers who know exactly what the state of the bed occupancy is at any time and can tell the doctor whether and where there is a bed available for you. In other hospitals this information is in the hands of the surgical team (see page 35) dealing with emergency admissions on that day.

In the biggest cities there is a centralized emergency bed service (EBS). These take calls from family doctors and then phone around the hospitals to find a bed. This naturally saves the doctor a lot of time, for the EBS system means that the doctor makes only one phone call and they do the rest. They also have the power to insist that a hospital take a patient if all the other local hospitals are full. A general practitioner cannot do this.

If you are severely ill your doctor will phone for a 999 ambulance but usually things are not this urgent so he will ask an ambulance on routine duty to pick you up from your home. If the need arises an ambulance can come within an hour but if your doctor has told the ambulance service that there is no emergency, your wait may be longer.

While you are waiting, unless you are very ill, your doctor will go to see other patients and this gives you and your relatives time to get a few things together. By definition you will not have been expecting this emergency admission so you will not have prepared anything. Get a small case or bag and pack the following (if you have them).

Pyjamas or nightdress
Slippers (type that stay on easily)
Towels
Dressing gown
Washing things (do not forget a razor)
A little money (including plenty of coins for the phone)
AND your front door key if you live alone

If you do not own a dressing gown, for example, do not buy one as the hospital will supply you with one.

If you have previously been to a hospital for anything (even if it was not an operation) take with you your appointments card or something else with a hospital reference number on. This will enable the hospital to find your notes or to contact another hospital for details of your medical past. If you are receiving any National Insurance payments and if you can find it easily, take your pension or allowance book.

Lastly, gather together any drugs you may be on. A knowledge of the drugs you are taking can be crucial to the anaesthetist if you have to have an operation. It is vital that you tell the hospital about anti-depressant drugs, steroids, anti-coagulants and the Pill. You may have a medallion that warns of your being on a particular drug. Wear it to hospital.

When the ambulance arrives, take all these things together with the letter that the doctor has written outlining your problem to the hospital surgeon and go to the hospital with a friend or relative if at all possible. Make sure that this friend has everything he or she needs to return home as the ambulance service has no obligation to take either you or your relative home. Switch off things around the house and lock up securely.

Once you arrive at the hospital you will be taken to a special receiving room or directly to a surgical ward. It is usual to be examined and asked a lot of questions by a junior doctor at this stage. Once he has completed this examination, he may arrange for some tests to be carried out and will then call a senior colleague who will come and ask a lot of the same questions all over again. This repetition has been found to be the best way to sort out problems and to avoid missing anything important.

The senior doctor decides whether an operation is necessary and if you have not eaten or drunk anything for four hours you may be operated on at once. If the situation is so urgent that an immediate operation seems to be needed even though you have recently had a meal, your stomach can be emptied using a nasogastric tube (see page 403). The reason surgeons worry so much about your having an anaesthetic with anything in your stomach is because during or after the operation you could vomit and inhale the fluid. This can be very dangerous. It makes sense not to eat or drink anything if your doctor tells you he thinks you might need an emergency operation. Unless you have to wait for a very long time for an ambulance to pick you up, this is no hardship. Incidentally, there is no law that says you have to arrive at hospital in an ambulance. You could ask a relative or friend to take you in if your doctor agrees this is advisable and if you live close to the hospital. This may be much more pleasant than waiting around a long time for an ambulance.

Under normal circumstances you will be asked to sign a consent form before any surgical procedure is carried out on you (for more details on consent forms see page 47). If the emergency renders you unconscious or incapable of signing a form, permission for the operation can be given by a relative. If the surgical team feels that waiting for this would harm you or make the operation less safe, they have the right to go ahead and operate without your consent. This is clearly in your best interests.

## Non-emergency admission

The vast majority of surgery is carried out 'cold' – that is after the patient has been through the hospital system, waited for some time and then been admitted to hospital in a controlled way, often at a time to suit him. Such an admission is initiated, as is an emergency admission, by your family doctor. If you see him about a symptom which he feels needs a surgeon's opinion, he will book an appointment in the surgical out-patients' department at a hospital (usually one local to you) where you will be seen by a specialist so that tests or investigations can be carried out and a diagnosis arrived at. Just because you find yourself in a surgical out-patients' department does not mean that you will necessarily end up having an operation. Even if an operation is necessary, many minor ones can be (and are increasingly being) carried out on an out-patient basis and you may never need to be admitted to hospital.

Consultations with specialists (consultants) are not directly available to the public but must be arranged by general practitioners. Even if you want to see a surgeon privately you will need a letter from your family doctor telling him the nature of your problem in medical terms. Many people are worried that if they suggest they would like a surgeon's opinion, their doctor may be offended or even refuse. The vast majority of doctors will not be upset and they are not allowed to refuse you access to a specialist opinion. Any reasonable request will be dealt with speedily and pleasantly, so do say if you feel your condition needs more specialist attention. It may be apparent that your doctor is doing all that can be done but if a visit to a consultant surgeon could put your mind at rest, it is worthwhile. Remember though that the more people who are referred just to be reassured, the less time the surgeon has to explain things to those who really do need operations.

Once you have a letter from your doctor (he may send it directly to the hospital), you can phone the surgical out-patients' department at the hospital to make an appointment. In some general practices the doctor or his receptionist will phone for an appointment for you. Your doctor may then give you a form to complete and send to the appointments office which then sends you an appointment card. Very often people are shocked when they see the appointment date because it is so far ahead. When your doctor arranges the appointment he will say if he thinks it is a matter of urgency that a consultant sees you soon. Your doctor will also know which surgeon (or even hospital if there is a choice) has the shortest waiting list and may refer you to him. However, your doctor may want an opinion from a particular surgeon in preference to the others at the hospital because he knows that that surgeon will be most appropriate for your problem. This man may be unavailable for weeks or months. It is at this stage that some people start to think of the private sector (see page 69).

If your doctor thinks you need seeing urgently, this will be arranged. If your condition deteriorates while awaiting either an out-patient consultation or admission, do tell your doctor who will arrange an earlier appointment. Also, it is only fair to point out that some people have very good non-medical reasons for wanting an early out-patient appointment (fear of dismissal from work because of poor attendance, for example). If you tell your family doctor about such problems, he will do all he can to help.

# THE OUT-PATIENTS' DEPARTMENT

When you get to the out-patients' department, go to the desk and hand over the letter from your doctor. The staff will take down your general details, if you have not sent them on before on a form provided by your doctor and if you have not been a patient in the hospital before. If you have, your file of records will be there. Hospital notes contain everything about your previous visits to hospital whether as an in- or out-patient and have all the test results arranged in chronological order for easy reference. These notes are usually kept for at least ten years since they were last used, but this varies from hospital to hospital.

The out-patients' department staff will usually give you a card with the address and telephone number of the hospital, the consultant's name, your name and spaces in which appointments can be entered. Keep this card and show it when you go to each out-patient appointment. You will soon realize that having the right piece of paper at the right time greatly eases your passage through the hospital system.

To your astonishment you will find that half of the town seems to have been booked in for an appointment at exactly the same time as you! This block booking, as it is called, is very popular with hospitals because it allows them to make the maximum use of the doctor's time. It would seem more reasonable to ask people to come along at regular intervals (and indeed some hospitals do this) but so many people arrive late (or even not at all) that the doctors could be kept waiting. This obviously is not in anybody's interest, which you will certainly understand if you have already waited weeks to see one of them. It is impossible to organize a perfect 'no-waiting' out-patient system because so many unforeseen circumstances can arise. A surgeon can get called away to an emergency; a difficult operation may overrun from the morning; another patient may pose a particularly difficult problem that cannot be dismissed in a few minutes and so on.

The answer is to go prepared to stay all afternoon or morning, as the case may be. If you go in the knowledge that it will be a half-day event, you will be much less upset by the whole thing. If you feel you may have been forgotten, ask the receptionist how things are progressing. Also, do not forget that the doctor may send you off for blood tests or other investigations or you may collect a prescription, and this will add to the time you spend in the hospital.

At the first visit you will probably see the consultant surgeon. (For what a consultant is, see page 35). The consultant tries to see each new patient. He may have junior doctors with him in the consulting room. There will usually be a nurse and there may be medical students. This may not make you feel at ease if you have come with a 'personal' problem but if you would rather not discuss certain parts of your story or complaint in front of other people, do say so and the consultant or one of the senior staff will see you alone.

The consultant will ask you lots of questions, most of which your own doctor will already have asked. This does not mean that he is ignoring your doctor's letter but rather that, with his specialist knowledge, he wants to sort out your problem in his own way. It is he who has to decide what to do and this means that he has to understand your condition clearly. So that he can do this, he may ask questions which seem strange to you, but there are bound to be good reasons for knowing the answers. If you do not understand the question, ask him to repeat it in another way.

After the question and answer session is over (and do not forget this is a time for you to ask questions too), the surgeon will ask you to go with a nurse to a cubicle where you can undress. While you are doing this he will see another patient. Many people feel uneasy about how much to take off but if you are not told anything specific, remove everything down to your underclothes. Some people do not like the idea of putting on the hospital dressing gown supplied and if you feel this way, put your coat or jacket on or cover yourself up with a blanket.

When the consultant returns, he will examine the part of you which seems to be giving the trouble and then he will examine other parts to give himself a general idea of your state of health. Do not worry if this latter examination seems to be rather perfunctory: it does not matter too much because he knows that you will be on the waiting list for some time, that your health could change during this time and that you will be thoroughly examined before your operation anyway. If you are a woman you will always have a nurse present if the doctor is a man. The surgeon may not only *feel* your body but he may also use instruments to examine various parts.

Once all this is completed you will be asked to dress and to see the consultant again. In the majority of cases his experience of similar problems will have told him exactly what should be done next and he may tell you then and there if he thinks an operation is necessary. Sometimes though he will be unable to be certain until particular tests have been done. Arrangements will be put in hand immediately and some may even be carried out the same day.

If the surgeon has been able to sort things out at the first appointment he will ask you about coming in for an operation. This is the time to ask any questions you may have and he will do his best to answer them. He will then put you on the waiting list (see below).

If, as is often the case, further tests are necessary, you will be asked to return to the hospital (possibly to several departments) on other occasions. This stage may take weeks or more to complete, depending on the complexity of your condition and the demands on the investigating departments at that time. Most people return only *once* more to the surgical out-patients' department to find out the results of the tests and to hear what the surgeon plans to do. On this second visit the first thing to do is 'register' with the receptionist that you have arrived. You may not see the consultant himself but his staff will deal with you along the lines laid down by him. He will almost certainly be in an adjoining room and can be consulted by the staff if they (or you) feel it necessary.

Just because you are in a surgical out-patients' department, do not *expect* the team to come up with surgery as the answer to your problems. They may suggest drugs, radiation therapy or even that nothing be done at all.

Once the decision on how to manage your problem has been taken, the surgeon will write a letter to your doctor explaining what he plans to do. This is not only a courtesy to the person who has to look after you on a day-to-day basis while you are awaiting further treatment but also enables the general practitioner to discuss the whole matter with you. After all, he knows your background and home circumstances better than the surgeon can hope to. This letter will take about a week to get to your doctor, so do not phone up the day after seeing the surgeon because your family doctor will be no wiser than you are. Telephone first to see if the hospital has contacted him and then arrange an appointment to discuss the matter if you feel you want to know more. And most people do. Sitting in a surgical out-patients' department half-naked does not make for easy communication, but back on your 'home' medical territory you should be more relaxed. This talk with your general practitioner is also helpful if you have any doubts as to the judgement of the surgeon. After all, you may not want an operation, yet do not know if one is essential. On the other side of the coin are those who feel that the 'wait-and-see' approach suggested by the surgeon is not what they want. In either case, now is the time to seek a second opinion, if you think one is necessary.

Having discussed the consultant's recommendation with your general practitioner you may still feel unhappy with the advice you have received and wish for a second opinion. There is no stigma attached to this and you can quite legitimately ask your general practitioner to send you to another consultant but do listen to what your own doctor says because you may be wasting everybody's time by trying to avoid an inevitable situation. Every 'second opinion' a surgeon gives means someone else has to wait longer for a first opinion. Most doctors readily agree to a second opinion, especially if you are not aggressive or unpleasant about it, and will tell the second surgeon that you have already seen the first. The two surgeons will sometimes confer on the subject of your illness in an effort to do the best for you and it is not at all uncommon today for a surgeon to refer you to another colleague with special knowledge of a particular subject, without being asked.

It is rarely necessary to 'do the rounds' of surgeons. With the vast majority of conditions seen by surgeons the answers are fairly straightforward and where they are not, you will probably be told.

# WAITING TO GO IN

With some hospitals, as soon as you are put on the waiting list for an operation you will be given a date to see if it is suitable for you. If it is not good, do say so there and then and do not leave it until a few days before they expect you to arrive. It is more normal though for your name to be put on a list from which people are chosen according to the urgency of their need; the demand on beds for emergency admissions; the speed at which any given surgeon discharges his patients from hospital; the normal working of the hospital (financial cuts or industrial action can revolutionize the best-planned waiting list); and a host of other factors.

Some people need considerable notice to arrange care for children or dependent relatives, for example, while others can go in at a moment's notice if a bed becomes vacant unexpectedly. If you can be ready for immediate admission, tell the admissions staff because in this way they can keep the beds filled (this is what running a hospital is all about) and you may well get your operation very much sooner than expected.

Organizing a waiting list for surgery is an almost impossible task as there are so many unforeseeable variables with the result that many people have to wait very long times indeed even for common minor operations. Everyone working in the hospital system knows this is not ideal but financial restrictions make it inevitable.

Waiting lists vary in length from hospital to hospital, from surgeon to surgeon and from area to area and are constantly readjusted every day within any one hospital. The hospital's aim, under normal circumstances, is to keep the surgical staff totally occupied and the beds full. The main bottle-neck facing surgeons today is effective theatre-time and there are many factors tending to reduce this. Staff and money shortages mean that operating theatres, which could theoretically be operational for 24 hours of the day, are in fact only used for a fraction of this time. This helps contribute to the length of waiting lists. Because there are so many variables, it may be impossible to give you more than an approximate idea of when you will be admitted but rest assured that if your admission is required urgently, you will be able to go in.

One way around the long waiting list for patients needing relatively minor operations is to operate on them as day cases. Several studies have shown that with careful patient selection, the post-operative problems are very few indeed and that the patients themselves very much like going into hospital for one day only. We have become used to accepted cultural 'norms' of 'being ill' and 'having an operation' but many people who need surgery simply have a technical hitch and do not need full hospital treatment. As people's (and surgeons') attitudes to surgery change, such day-case surgery will become even more popular. This system works well for investigative 'operations' such as cystoscopy and laparoscopy and sometimes is appropriate for hernias, varicose veins and some simple procedures on children, for example. Some patients are not suitable for treatment as 'day cases' though because of their general state of health.

When you go home from a day-case unit, your general practitioner and the local district nurse will look after you and you will return to see the surgeon at a later date, just like other in-patients. Only one in 100 people operated on as day cases have to be re-admitted to hospital because of problems.

Not only will you need good medical and nursing backup to be considered a suitable 'day case' but you will also need good domestic help too. You will need someone to come and collect you by car and your home will have to have enough facilities to be considered safe for your recovery. Unfortunately, there are fairly large numbers of people who cannot arrange domestic help or are otherwise unsuitable for day operations but for those who are suitable it is often an excellent alternative to a full hospital stay.

While awaiting admission you may be able to work or you may be too ill to work. If your condition is keeping you away from work you can claim sickness benefit (see page 73) and your doctor will try to hasten your admission. If you have any difficulty in arranging care for your family or dependent relatives, talk to the Social Services Department at the town hall. Should you decide for any reason not to have the operation (or if you have it done elsewhere, or privately) do remember to tell the admissions office at your hospital so that they can remove you from their list.

# GOING IN

One day you will receive a note from the hospital saying that they have a bed for you. Often this gives you very little notice, which seems amazing after such a long wait. I have explained why this happens and it really is unavoidable. If you cannot manage to go in when they suggest, do phone and say so: do not just let it drop or they will have an empty bed that someone else could have used. Do not worry that they will put you back at the bottom of the list: they will not, unless you keep turning down suggested dates. It does not matter to the hospital who they get in. If you are ill, have a cold or are having a period when they call for you, talk to your doctor and see what he suggests.

Some hospitals ask you to phone on the morning of admission, just to make sure that the bed is still empty, and has not been filled with an emergency in the night.

The admission note tells you when and where to go and what to take in. You may also be sent a booklet about the hospital you're going to. Read this fully because it will answer a lot of your questions. Some hospitals send a form to fill in to save time when you arrive. If they do, remember to take it with you.

## WHAT TO TAKE IN

Pyjamas or nightdress
Brush and comb
Toothbrush and paste
Slippers (that stay on)
Towel
Washing and shaving things
Dressing gown
Paper tissues
Hand mirror
Nail file and scissors
Cosmetics
Warm cardigan or bed jacket
Writing paper, envelopes and stamps
Stamped post cards
Pen
Books (not too many)
Glasses (for reading)
Bottle of your favourite fruit squash (in case water tastes unpleasant)

Transistor radio (only if it has an earpiece)

NHS medical card

National Insurance number if you are claiming benefit

Details of or papers relating to sickness insurance schemes

Pension, Supplementary Benefit or Family Income Supplement order books. The address of your social security office (to claim sickness benefit while in hospital).

Details of next-of-kin

Front door key (if you live alone)

A small amount of money

All the medicines you are taking

Do not take in anything very valuable because it is awkward for the ward staff who have to keep such things. Hospitals are not the most secure of places and you will be worried if you are not sure what has happened to your favourite ring or necklace, for example. Do not take a lot of money because you will not need it and can always get visitors to bring you more if needed.

When you arrive at the hospital go to the admissions office or direct to the ward, whichever you have been asked to do in the note you received through the post. You will probably be welcomed by the sister or senior nurse on duty but many hospitals now have a ward receptionist who greets each new patient and fills out all the necessary forms.

Once the paperwork has been completed you will be shown to your bed. You will probably be asked to undress straight away and get into bed, partly because there is nowhere else for you to go and also because the doctor may come at any time to examine you. The bed you are allotted may be yours for the duration of your stay or you may be moved if the sister considers it necessary.

A ward is a collection of beds organized by a nursing team. Old-style wards contain about thirty beds and have a couple of single rooms that are used for special patients. Sometimes these single rooms are used for really ill, disruptive or paying patients. The beds are arranged in two rows along each of the long walls and the nursing station is in the centre or in a small room known as the sister's office. Most modern wards are built with the beds in small groups (often of four or six) and provide more privacy as each four-bedded unit feels more like a room than a ward. Even in these smaller units the privacy is limited and many people feel happier on a big ward where there is more going on and where the general noise level means that not everything you say is overheard.

As soon as you are in bed a wrist band made of plastic will be put on so that you can be identified in the event of you being unable to say anything yourself. This has your name and hospital number and possibly the name of your surgeon and should not be removed until you are back home again. In some hospitals a card is placed by your bed with the name of the surgeon on it. It tells the nurses which patients are being looked after by which surgeons and this helps them on ward rounds (see below) and even in your clinical management as certain surgeons want specific routine things done to their patients. A drug chart and another chart on which pulse rate and temperature may be recorded are often clipped to the bottom of the bed.

While waiting for the doctor to come you may be allowed to walk around. Make the most of this opportunity as it enables you to meet the other patients and to get the feel of the ward. Use this opportunity to find out where the lavatories are; where the dayroom is (if there is one); how the radio and TV work; and generally to get the lie of the land. Most people are admitted only one day before their operation, so once the doctor comes to start you on the road to your operation you may not have much time or opportunity to look around.

## WHO'S WHO IN THE HOSPITAL

A modern hospital of any size is in reality a large hotel that provides medical facilities and as such the hotel staff vastly outnumber the medical staff. A major hospital has hundreds of employees from gardeners and engineers to cooks and cleaners. To all of these people the hospital is their workplace yet you will only come into contact with a fraction of them. The people you will meet in the ward are doctors, nurses, paramedical staff (such as physiotherapists, occupational therapists, and medical social workers), the ward receptionist or clerk, domestic staff and various others including voluntary staff and clergy. Of all of these the nurses are by far the most important because it is they who run the ward (and thereby your life) for 24 hours of every day. Doctors come and go and perform many of their duties elsewhere (in out-patients' departments and operating theatres, to mention but two places) and this makes them relatively remote.

The **DOCTORS** are a team headed by the consultant surgeon. People get very confused about what a consultant surgeon is. Quite simply he is a doctor who has specialized in surgery (or a specialized field of surgery such as eye surgery). He is fully trained in his field, a training which may have taken eight to twelve years to complete. He may have started off his specialist post-graduate training with a general surgical post or two and will then have spent several years in posts to give him experience around the subject he aims eventually to concentrate on. In this way, a consultant general surgeon may have held posts in urology, chest or other branches of surgery over a period of several years.

Consultant surgeons do not, contrary to popular belief, spend all day doing operations. They spend a lot of their time in the out-patients' department seeing new people and deciding what treatment they need; following up their patients after operations; training nurses and junior doctors; and sitting on committees to help make the hospital run. Some consultants have a contract with the National Health Service which allows them to do a fixed number of sessions of private surgery during each week. In addition to all these activities, many consultant surgeons work at more than one hospital, so it is hardly surprising that they are to be seen so rarely in any one place. This means in practice that you will see the consultant very little and his juniors much more. When you are under the care of a particular consultant, he or one of his team is responsible for your care and no other doctor will be involved unless invited.

Working directly under a consultant is a surgical registrar. In larger and teaching hospitals there will also be a senior registrar – a doctor who has nearly completed his specialist training and who will be a consultant himself very soon. The registrar is the doctor responsible for his consultant's patients on a day-to-day basis when his chief is not there. He will have been qualified for several years, will have committed himself to a career as a specialist surgeon and will have passed or will be working for post-graduate examinations in surgery.

Under the registrar is the house surgeon (houseman – who may be a woman!). He or she is a recently qualified doctor completing a six-month training period in surgery before being able to register as a fully qualified doctor. The vast majority of surgical housemen are *not* going to be surgeons and will end up as physicians, specialists in other fields, in general practice or in some other area of medicine.

The consultant will normally go around all his patients once a week to satisfy himself about their progress, to modify treatment, if necessary, and to decide when they should go home. The registrar will see every patient every day to deal with day-to-day problems. The houseman will be on hand to do all the routine medical work associated with his consultant's patients. It is housemen and registrars who work the long hours one hears so much about and you will see a lot of them both day and night.

In the UK it is a custom to address consultant surgeons and usually the registrars as 'Mister' X but they will not be offended if you call them 'Doctor'. All other staff wear badges with their names and titles and you will soon get used to addressing them appropriately.

If you are in a teaching hospital there will be students attached to the surgical team (often called a 'firm'). You will obviously know that the hospital is a teaching school before you are admitted but that does not necessarily mean that you are obliged to have students examining you or even present when you are examined by the consultant. The vast majority of people are not concerned by the presence of students or, if they are, realize that everyone has to learn and so quietly accept the situation. If you feel strongly about this, you have the right to object and are not bound to have students around you. If you object, you may have to wait longer until the consultant has finished teaching or he may get one of his other staff to see to you. To broaden their training medical students often spend time in district hospitals so they may be met almost anywhere, even outside teaching hospitals.

The **NURSES** are organized in a hierarchical structure like the doctors. Old titles (such as matron) have been replaced by numerical grades. The highest grade is a number 10 and is known as the chief nursing officer. She is in charge of the nursing service for a group of hospitals. Directly under her are a few number 9s (principal nursing officers), each responsible for a hospital within the group. Next in line come senior nursing officers (grade 8s) and nursing officers (grade 7s) who are responsible for several wards. The person that has most influence on ward life is the sister (a number 6) who is still called 'sister'. She and all those below her still wear uniforms that look like old-style nurses' uniforms whereas the nurses of higher grades wear plain (often green) suits or something similar. The ward sister is the highest grade of nurse that comes into daily direct contact with patients and the higher grades are by and large involved in administrative, organizational and teaching duties.

Working on the ward there are staff nurses (grade 5s) who are fully qualified nurses who take over from the sister when necessary. All staff nurses are state registered nurses (SRNs) and can apply for promotion to any level in the hierarchy. State enrolled nurses (SENs) have a two-year training course (as opposed to the SRNs' three-year one) and are more practically than theoretically trained. SENs cannot be promoted *higher* than to the level of staff nurse.

In most hospitals there are also nurses undergoing their training and nursing auxiliaries, women who do many of the straightforward, more domestic duties on the ward such as cleaning lockers, arranging flowers and bed making.

Each hospital has its own uniform that enables nursing grades to be distinguished one from another. Today, most nurses also wear name badges which greatly help. Sisters like to be called 'sister', staff nurses like to be called 'staff' but everyone else can be safely called 'nurse' without causing offence. Senior, non-uniformed nurses are called by their names and usual titles, for example Miss Jones.

Today's nurses are highly-trained and some even have degrees. The days of the nurse-skivvy have gone and they do not (like most of us) enjoy being talked down to, ordered around or treated like servants. If you develop a good relationship with the nurses you will enjoy your hospital stay much more.

The other **PARAMEDICAL** staff you will come across have functions which rapidly become apparent and will not be detailed here.

# A DAY ON THE WARD

Although research shows that many people do not read them, most hospitals' booklets about the hospital usually contain a section on ward routine. There has to be a pretty strict routine in any close-knit community, especially one in which a lot of work has to be done. Patients come and go a lot in surgical wards, for investigations, physiotherapy, occupational therapy, to operating theatres and so on. The surgical ward is a busy place and there has to be a routine if it is to function properly.

Having said this, life is much more relaxed in hospitals today than ever before and the days of lying to attention in bed as the consultant comes round have, thankfully, gone for good. Some older ward sisters still maintain some of the traditional ideas of ward discipline but most are relaxed and easy in their manner.

Each sister can theoretically organize her ward how she likes, as long as everything gets done. However, the hospital's work shifts for nurses tend to dictate the times of various activities and this is something the ward sister can do little about.

The day usually begins at about 6.30 am, although some wards in some hospitals let you sleep later than this. The day begins with a cup of tea. In fact ward life is punctuated by drinks. It is worth accepting all of them because you can easily become dehydrated, especially in the newer, air-conditioned wards. There is always a jug of water on each locker which is refilled regularly in case you are thirsty in between the formal drinks rounds. You can drink that at any time unless you need to be on restricted fluids.

Although the majority of our hospitals are old and were planned around bed-bound patients, the average surgical patient is up and about the day after the operation. This presents problems because most hospital wards have too few lavatories and first thing in the morning there are queues. If you cannot get out of bed, a bottle (for men) or a bedpan will be brought round. The curtains will be drawn around your bed while you are using a bedpan or bottle. If you find using a bedpan difficult ask the nurse if you could use a commode by the bedside. People who are bed-bound are brought water for washing and are helped if necessary. All your personal washing things are kept in the locker by your bed. If you are too ill to shave yourself the nurse may help or there may be a hospital barber who does the rounds.

The greatest complaints about hospital life involve washing and lavatory facilities. Every ward has a bathroom or two where there are cubicles for basins, baths and lavatories. If you find yourself getting constipated in hospital (and the food and lavatory facilities certainly do nothing to help), ask your visitors to bring in plenty of fresh fruit or even some bran to sprinkle on your breakfast. Ask sister first if this is all right. Because many hospital ward lavatories lack privacy to some degree and may have no locks (so that you can easily be retrieved if you collapse in the lavatory), it really does pay to prevent constipation.

Once all the washing and lavatory duties are out of the way, breakfast is served. All those who can, eat at one or more central tables or by their bedsides but if you are too ill or it is inappropriate for you to be up you will be given your food in bed or even fed, if necessary.

Mail comes round on a trolley and most wards have a postbox that is emptied at least once a day. Almost all wards have a telephone or two on trolleys. These can be plugged in at points along the ward so that they can reach every bed. Newspapers may be delivered on request. Books may be available from a library trolley run by volunteers. Television is not neglected either and some wards have a set in plain view of most of the beds but the sound turned down so that you are not troubled by it as others listen in on their headphones. Other wards have a set in a day room at one end where those who are up and about can sit, talk, play cards or watch TV.

Every bed has headphones, though they frequently do not work. It is best to take your own radio in with you and to use an earpiece. Some hospitals have a very good local radio station especially for the patients.

A trolley is brought round regularly by volunteers with useful toilet requisites, writing paper and a host of other items. Bigger hospitals have a shop with a wide range of things for sale. Hairdressing facilities are now very common: talk to the sister about these.

Although it may seem a strange time to have to make the superhuman effort of stopping smoking, this is exactly what you will have to do in some hospitals because many of them do not allow smoking. This leads to all kinds of clandestine practices reminiscent of school days, which can be dangerous because both before and after an operation it can be bad for you to smoke and may severely delay your return home if you sustain a chest infection (which is more likely if you smoke). Increasing numbers of hospitals allow smoking in certain areas, for example in the day room, but even when smoking is allowed you should be guided by what you are told by the medical or nursing staff. Whilst on the subject of vices, never take alcoholic drinks into hospital with you or allow visitors to bring any in. These may react with drugs you are having and make you very ill. Alcohol in your system could also interfere with the anaesthetic.

One of the commonest complaints about ward life is the boredom. All around you there is activity but within a day or two of your operation, you are feeling well enough to be up and about (except after a major procedure) yet not well enough to do anything constructive. Many people find that helping the nurses serve food each day and doing other chores is therapeutic for them and talking to bedridden patients or even feeding them helps both the other patient and the staff and gives you something to do.

Because, naturally, you easily tire in hospital, many wards have a quiet time or rest hour, usually in the early afternoon, during which there is minimal activity and patients can sleep for a while. This will be the only time you will be expected to be in bed during the daytime (unless, of course, the sister or your surgeon thinks you are too unwell to be up).

An evening meal is served around six o'clock and this is followed by washing and lavatory rounds so that the ward is ready to be handed over to the night nursing staff.

Medicines are given out by a nurse at regular intervals throughout the day and in theory the nurse should watch you actually consume them. This is to ensure that you are in fact getting the prescribed medication and that you are not hoarding any. If you ever think that the tablets seem wrong to you, do say so as mistakes can be made. Every evening the night nurse comes round with the drug trolley to give out sleeping tablets and pain-relieving drugs, if necessary. As the round takes some time it occasionally happens that people are actually asleep before the sleeping tablets come round. They are then woken to take their sleeping tablets, much to their amazement. There is a reason behind this. Many people sleep very badly in hospital. There are often snoring patients and those who call out, and even at night there is activity in the ward which keeps some people awake. Because of pain or these other reasons people who have never had sleeping tablets in their lives may take them whilst in hospital. When the nurse comes round the ward on the evening drug round she would rather you had your tablets so that you get a good night's sleep than that you wake at 2.00 am and remain sleepless for some time while she and her colleagues are dealing with an emergency on the ward. In a sense this is an example of the system being too rigid, but there is a method in the madness.

The ward day ends at about 10.30 or 11 pm when the main

lights are put out and you will be expected to go to sleep. Do not worry if you sleep badly but do not want to take sleeping tablets – most people are not in hospital for long with the average operation and you will soon catch up on lost sleep when you are back in your own bed. If you are in for a long time then a loss of sleep may become a real problem and you will then have to take sleeping tablets.

# WHAT IT IS LIKE BEING A SURGICAL PATIENT

From the moment you go into hospital you start being treated like a patient and soon begin to behave differently. This happens for several reasons. First, it is a nerve-racking experience going in for an operation and very few people are completely unemotional about it. Add to this the dislocation from one's friends, family and work; the unfamiliar restrictions and routines of ward life, and the boredom and it is not surprising that most people find going into hospital relatively unpleasant.

The way in which people react to being in hospital varies greatly according to their age, personality type, expectations, and the seriousness of the operation, but another important factor is the proposed duration of stay. If you are in for a day or two for a D and C or some minor procedure your attitude will be very different than if you know you will be in for weeks for a serious or life-threatening procedure.

The new hospital patient is placed in such an unusual world (to him) that he finds himself questioning nearly everything he had previously taken for granted. This comes about not only because he is naturally concerned for his own safety and well-being but also because he has been catapulted into a world that has different rules. It is this feeling of helplessness that strikes many people as being the over-whelming emotion on going into hospital. Patients are not only generally not in a position to do what needs to be done, but they do not know what needs to be done or even how to judge what needs to be done. Some people overcome this by 'leaving it all to the doctors' but with increasing levels of education and expectations, especially among the young and middle-aged, this attitude is less common than it was.

As soon as any one of us steps into a hospital bed we label ourselves as being in a crisis situation. It has been said that to a patient there is no such thing as a minor operation but there *are* levels of crisis, depending on many factors within or outside us. Crises produce fear and anxiety and because these are often confused and are almost universally experienced by surgical patients, let us look at them in more detail.

Fear can be defined as an emotional response to a known threat from outside. Anxiety is an emotional tension brought on by threatened danger or discomfort, the nature of which may be unknown. Clinically, fear and anxiety manifest themselves as a raised pulse rate and blood pressure; dryness of the mouth; sweating; an inability or unwillingness to look at a nurse or doctor while speaking; rapid or darting eye movements; clenching of the fists, nail or lip biting; and a host of other signs.

Considerable research has been done on people's emotions before and after operations and about half of those questioned say that they are scared or very frightened on the eve of their operation. Although it had been suggested by previous studies that older people might be less anxious than younger ones; that females might admit to more anxiety than males; that the fear of the unknown might play a big part so that those who have been in hospital before are less afraid; and that patients facing safe forms of surgery are less apprehensive of the whole procedure, recent research finds some of these concepts to be ill-founded.

There is no provable difference, for example, in the levels of anxiety experienced according to a person's age, but reports that women show higher levels of anxiety are based on fact. The proportion of women showing any given level of anxiety is greater than the proportion of men showing such levels. People having disfiguring or destructive surgery understandably feel more anxious than those undergoing less invasive procedures.

Repeated research has shown that good pre-operative

information and counselling helps people not only then and there (before the operation) but also after the operation. It helps someone about to have an operation to find out all he can so that his mind is as free as possible of anxieties and fears which are often based on ignorance. This raises the fascinating question of information and what people about to undergo surgery really want to know. Different people want to know different things but the person who wants to know most is not necessarily the one who asks most. A few people genuinely want to know nothing. They are mostly elderly and are prepared to 'leave it to the doctors'. But doctors and nurses may not know what to tell people. A significant piece of American research found that what patients wanted to know and what the nursing staff *thought* they wanted to know were often completely different. This led to the nurses feeling good because they thought they had been open and informative to the patients and the patients feeling anxious because they had been told things that were of little value to them and were left in the dark with their real fears unanswered.

This is just one example of the communication gap that is so prejudicial to the peace of mind of hospital patients. A lot of research shows that patients do not say what they want to know, yet this is something that can easily be overcome. In my research for this book I talked to many patients in the surgical wards of a large hospital. The vast majority of their fears and anxieties were over things that I knew would never in fact happen and many of the remainder were worries about the unknown (which I was often able to explain to their complete satisfaction in minutes). So the lesson must be that if you are worried about something, say so and ask someone to explain. The staff cannot read your mind and everyone's fears and anxieties are different, even though there are some anxieties that are common to many people.

A way around a lot of this anxiety is to get things sorted out in your mind before going into hospital at all. But it is because it is not easy to do this that I have written this book. Many general practitioners can be very helpful, but only if they know you are concerned. If, for example, you feel you might have a cancer, talk it over with your doctor, either before you go or when you arrive in hospital. Cancerophobia has not quite reached the level in the UK that it has in the US but many people worry quite unnecessarily about a cancer they do not have.

Let us assume that by carefully questioning the right people you can overcome your fears of the unknown this still leaves all the legitimately felt fears about the mechanics of undergoing surgery; the loss of privacy; the personal ministrations by strange people; the various onslaughts on our bodies in the form of enemas, injections and so on; the close physical contact with people we do not know; the fear of the diagnosis; the fear of disability; the fear of pain; and the dislocation from our normal environment. All of these are worrying and it is perfectly normal to be anxious and fearful before an operation. Having an operation rates as one of life's more stressful experiences and only so much can be done to alleviate certain elements of the stress. Pre-operative counselling helps enormously and is being carried out in increasing numbers of hospitals. Where it is done, post-operative progress is found to be improved, demands for pain-relieving drugs fewer and hospital stays shorter.

Let us assume now that the operation is over: what is it like then? The answer to this depends very much on how much pain you are in and how mobile you are. For more about post-operative pain, see page 52.

If you are in for a minor operation, you will probably be amazed how ill many of those around you are. This may make you feel 'strong' by comparison, so much so that you will enter into relationships and even friendships that you would never have considered in the outside world. You may also find that you are spending a lot of time with old people (nearly half of all surgical patients are over 65) which may also be unfamiliar to you.

Even the strongest of us with all our normal, protective barriers find that being ill in a ward is a great leveller. After all, with our clothes off we are all much of a muchness, especially when we are weak and insecure. Many discharged surgical patients say that they discovered something about humanity which changed their view of life; that they were filled with admiration at people's response to pain; that they actually learned a lot from people outside their normal social spheres; or that they realized, perhaps for the first time, something of the fragility of human life and the strength that there is in other people's friendship in a time of need. Being in a surgical ward brings out all these mixed feelings and can have a longstanding beneficial effect on a person. For most of us, though, the day we leave hospital the 'real' world takes us over again and the sworn friendships and deeply felt emotions of the time are all too soon forgotten.

## BEFORE THE OPERATION

Once you are established in the ward the preparation for your operation begins in earnest. A surgical houseman will come and take a full medical history from you and will want to know about any tablets or medicines you are taking. He will look at the tablets you have brought in (if you have not already given them to the sister) and will take them from you so that they can be dispensed at the appropriate time during drug rounds. Obviously, you should not take medicines of any kind unless the hospital staff say so. If you are aware that you have any drug sensitivities (allergies) tell the houseman so that he can mark your notes accordingly. Also, tell him if you are allergic to sticking plaster so that they can use something else in the operating theatre.

Once the history-taking is over the houseman will examine you all over – not just the part you have come into hospital about. Although this is mainly done to ensure that you are fit for the operation, he may also pick up things you were not aware of and suggest that some investigations or treatment be done before (but usually after) your operation. Obviously, if he detects a condition that would make your operation inadvisable, he will tell you there and then and will suggest what should be done. In practice, this rarely happens. In a teaching hospital a student may come with the houseman to learn how things should be done or, if he is more senior, he may come later to do another examination by himself.

Before the operation the registrar and/or the consultant may come to see you briefly but often the consultant relies on his junior staff's opinion of the situation and may not see you until the operation itself.

Any blood tests that need to be done are carried out at once, as are any X-rays that are considered necessary. The houseman will write up any drugs you might need post-operatively; will organize your pre-medication (pre-med); and will ensure that your drug chart is written up for sleeping tablets, if you feel you might need them. It is probably better to go along with this suggestion because although you may never have taken sleeping tablets in your life you may well find you will need them and as they can only be prescribed by a doctor you could be awake half of the night, while he is busy in the operating theatre, for example.

Before the houseman leaves he will discuss the operation with you. Now is your chance to ask any questions you have. Ask him to draw you a diagram of what is going to happen if you cannot visualize things clearly. While he is explaining the operation to you he will probably give you a consent form to sign, although a nurse may give you this later.

Technically speaking, no one can so much as touch you in a hospital without your permission or you could take legal action for assault. Each time a procedure or investigation is carried out on you the fact that you agree to have it done means you have implicitly given your permission in legal terms. When it comes to an operation though, the hospital staff will want to have had your consent in writing to perform the operation. This form also covers the administration of an anaesthetic. The form simply says that you, the patient, have had the operation explained to you and that you consent to it (and any further measures that may become necessary during the operation) being done. The form also states that no particular surgeon will perform the operation. You sign this form, as does the doctor who explained the operation to you. This is usually the houseman or, less commonly today, the anaesthetist. Never sign a blank form and be sure to read everything on it. Do not let anyone rush you. If there is anything you feel you cannot sign, simply cross out the phrase or sentence and then sign it. This may raise problems, but they will usually be overcome by discussion with the medical and nursing staff.

If the person to be operated on is under 16, a parent or guardian will have to sign the consent form on his behalf. In Scotland the parent's or guardian's consent has to be obtained for boys under 14 and girls under 12. For an operation which will make you sterile many hospitals insist on the consent of your spouse and some surgeons will not operate unless they have such consent.

For someone who is very ill, a consent form is not essential because the doctors will go ahead if life is threatened and operate anyway, especially if there is no next-of-kin to give permission. Consent forms are not legally essential but do show that consent was given.

Depending on your particular operation and your general state of health two other people may come to see you. The first is a physiotherapist. She will come the day before the operation to teach you about breathing and coughing post-operatively to help keep your lungs clear after the anaesthetic. She may explain about keeping your legs moving in bed so that the chances of developing a clot in the veins are reduced (see page 56). The physiotherapist will also try to convince you that you should not smoke before the operation. This is good advice because there is a far greater chance of developing a chest infection post-operatively if you smoke and coughing can be very unpleasant when you have a stitched wound, especially on the abdomen.

An anaesthetist used always to come around and see every patient the night before the operation but this is uncommon today. He will usually be guided by the house surgeon's notes if you are perfectly fit but will come and see you if you have a condition that might affect the anaesthetic, or if you have been ill recently. If the houseman is in any doubt about your ability to withstand an anaesthetic he will ask the anaesthetist to see you specially. Anything the anaesthetist is unhappy about will be investigated and treated first before he agrees to go ahead with the operation. It is always annoying to have an operation postponed but if it is for your safety, there really is no choice. When an operation and anaesthesia are undertaken less than three months after a heart attack, for example, more than a third of people have another heart attack post-operatively. If the operation is postponed until six months or more after the heart attack, the risk drops to 5 per cent.

As the time for the operation gets closer you will have special preparations which vary according to the procedure to be performed. You may have an enema but this is not routinely done except in those having bowel surgery. Any areas of special interest to the surgeon will be marked with a dye or felt-tip pen so that there is no possibility of the wrong side being operated on, for example.

The area around the operation site will be shaved, although some hospitals are now finding that depilatory creams used by the patient himself are more acceptable to the patient and produce just as clean a surface. Hair has to be removed because it gets caught in stitches and Elastoplast dressings stick to it. After this you will have a bath and get into a white, back-opening nightdress-type garment with or without a paper cap and woollen socks.

For four hours before the operation you must not eat or drink anything – not even water, though if your operation is in the afternoon you will be allowed to eat a small, light breakfast. This starvation is not a frill but is very serious. If you vomit during an anaesthetic (an uncommon event) you could inhale the vomit and choke to death if your stomach is full. This can be prevented by inserting a nasogastric tube (see page 403) up which stomach contents can be sucked, but this is not routine except for people having stomach or upper abdominal operations.

About an hour before the operation you will be given an injection containing your pre-medication (pre-med). This is supposed to calm you down and also dries up saliva and urine production. Some places give tablets instead of an injection. Once you have had your pre-med you will feel drowsy and may even sleep on and off. If your operation is delayed for any reason the pre-med may have nearly worn off by the time you get to the theatre. If this is the case tell a doctor or nurse.

You will be asked to remove any dentures, contact lenses, watches and jewellery but if you do not want to (or cannot) remove your wedding ring, for example, ask them to stick tape around it.

The next stage is to wait for a porter to take you to the operating theatre on a trolley. When you get there you will go straight to the anaesthetic room where the anaesthetist or his assistant will check from the band around your wrist that you are the right person for the planned operation. He will look through the notes briefly, then give you an injection to put you to sleep. This takes only a few seconds and is a pleasant feeling. Many people fear the black mask and the smell of anaesthetic gases but these are almost never used today to get people off to sleep. Some people fear having an anaesthetic more than anything else about an operation. Today this is unnecessary because modern anaesthetic drugs are safe and have very few, if any, side-effects. It is also a fact that fewer than one person in 15,000 dies as a result of having an anaesthetic.

# IN THE OPERATING THEATRE

An operating theatre, like a ward, is a busy working unit with its own life-style, rules and routines. All of these are aimed at providing the best possible environment in which to carry out several operations a day almost every day of the year.

Around the table there will be a surgeon (usually the consultant or his registrar) and a variable number of helpers. A minor operation needs only a surgeon and a nurse but a major procedure may call for a surgeon, his registrar and houseman and even a student, technicians and several nurses. At least one nurse is scrubbed up, that is, dressed in sterile kit and gloves like the surgeon, but there are usually one or two others who fetch and carry various necessities as and when they are needed.

The anaesthetist sits at the head end of the operating table with his anaesthetic machine which delivers gases to the patient to keep him anaesthetized. These gases are usually given down a tube inserted into the throat (after the original injection has taken effect) and this is why you may wake up with a slightly sore throat after an operation, even though the tube will have been removed by then.

The anaesthetist watches all the body's vital functions during the operation and finally reverses the effects of any drugs he has given so that you wake up feeling normal quite quickly.

Once the operation is completed you may be wheeled off into a recovery room where you wake up. (Some hospitals do not have recovery rooms, in which case you will wake up in a room adjoining the operating theatre). All such rooms are geared up for any emergencies that might occur and are staffed by highly trained nurses. The longer the operation, the longer it takes to wake up but with today's anaesthetics most people are awake enough to respond to instructions within a few minutes of the end of the operation. This does not mean you could sit up and do the *Times* crossword: it takes a lot longer to regain full consciousness. When you get back to the ward, the curtains are left drawn back so that the nurses can keep an eye on you as they go about their duties. Slowly you wake up and begin your recovery.

## AFTER THE OPERATION

Most people are returned to the ward after a short stay in a recovery room but if surgery has been extensive or has involved the heart, lungs or brain you will be sent to an intensive care unit. This is a specialized unit, manned by highly trained senior nurses who are used to looking after severely ill people. They will monitor your body functions and supervize specialized equipment, such as respirators, if necessary. Being in an intensive care unit is not at all like being in a normal ward because all the people there are bed-bound and often very ill. Continuous supervision 24 hours of the day is very exhausting for the patient and it is often difficult to relax or sleep properly because there is so much going on around you. It is not at all uncommon for patients in these units to become depressed on about the fifth or sixth day but this usually disappears spontaneously after a further week to ten days. Do not hesitate to ask for painkilling drugs or sleeping tablets if you need them and to tell the nurses or doctors if you feel depressed.

Getting back to the ward to be among relatively well people is a great relief to most people. When you wake up from your anaesthetic you will have no sense of time and will probably feel you have only just gone off to sleep. Many people fear that they will feel sick after an operation (especially if they have previously had an anaesthetic many years ago), but nausea and vomiting are rare today compared with even a few years ago, such have been the improvements in anaesthetic agents. If you do feel sick, tell someone and a nurse can give you an injection. Many people are thirsty when they wake up because, as was pointed out earlier, the pre-med injection dries up the mouth. Take very small sips of water or suck a piece of ice. Always check with the nurses before drinking anything immediately after an operation. If you have had an operation on the bowel or indeed if you have had any major procedure you may wake up with a tube down your nose (see page 403) and a drip in your arm (see page 396). This drip will be continued after an abdominal operation until the intestine is working properly again. A drip will replace body fluids so you will not feel as thirsty as if it were not there. Contrary to popular belief, such drips do not usually *feed* the person but simply replace fluid. If the operation has been a major one, the intravenous drip may contain blood to replace that lost at the operation. If you have a nasogastric tube, it will be sucked clear every hour or two to keep the stomach empty so as to rest the intestine. Some hospitals have an electric pump by the bedside which does the same thing, but continuously.

Pain is a very variable experience and people who have had the same operation complain of very different amounts of pain. Many people experience little or no discomfort and others need a lot of painkillers. Abdominal and chest operations seem to be the most painful afterwards. One of the commonest complaints people have about operations is that the control of their pain post-operatively was too little and too late. There is no method of measuring pain so it is up to you to tell the nurses when you are in pain so that they can do something about it. They cannot read your mind. Morphine and pethidine are still the most commonly used drugs although there are many alternatives if either of these disagrees with you. Post-operative pain is usually supervised by doctors who simply write up the medication to be given by nurses as and when the person requires it. This often means that you have to take the initiative when you feel pain. Do not worry that the nurses will think you cowardly or demanding: pain is not helpful to your recovery and anyway can be easily relieved. There is considerable evidence that pain is more easily controlled with smaller doses of drugs if it is caught before it becomes too severe. Do not wait until you are in agony before asking for pain relief: anticipate the pain on the assumption that, at night especially, it can take half an hour or more actually to receive the drug. This is because many of the drugs are so powerful that they have to be given under the supervision of a senior nurse who may be busy at the time they are needed. Ask sooner, rather than later, and you should never have to tolerate unbearable pain.

When the surgeon closes up the wound after some operations he inserts a drainage strip or tube which projects out of the wound and is covered with a thick pad of absorbent dressing. This allows blood and body fluids to escape rather than build up inside the body. Sometimes the tube type of drain is connected to a vacuum bottle beneath the bed or even clipped on top of the bed. The drain is left in place until the fluid stops flowing and is removed little by little until after three or four days it has been completely withdrawn from the wound. You can walk around with your drainage bottle (if there is one) and some people fix them on their dressing gowns when they get out of bed. Be guided by the nurses about this but do not think that just because you have a drain you will have to be in bed for days.

After three to five days most of the equipment and bulky

dressings will have to be removed and you will be as mobile as people who have had minor operations. Most people can eat soon after minor, non-abdominal operations but at the other extreme, stomach or intestinal operations will mean the bowel must be rested for several days.

On the same day as the operation you will probably see the house surgeon who will come round to see how everyone is. Ask him what was done or discovered and he will explain. The chances are very high that he was actually at the operation. He will also tell you how quickly you will recover and will put your mind at rest over any strange sensations or feelings you may have.

Most people feel pretty wretched immediately after an operation but it is amazing how quickly this feeling goes. Within a day or two after even quite major procedures most people feel remarkably good. How you feel is greatly determined by your mobility. If you can get up and go to the lavatory, wash yourself gently and sit at a table to eat, you feel a lot better sooner and this is one reason why patients are now encouraged to be out of bed very soon after an operation. One of the things that makes you feel miserable after an operation is having to use a bed pan or bottle because opening your bowels and passing water is always more difficult lying down. As soon as the nurses think you are well enough they will let you up to do as much as is wise in the circumstances.

The vast majority of people recover without a hitch and are out of hospital within a few days of their surgery. However, certain things can go wrong, the commonest of which are an infection of the wound, a chest infection, deep vein thrombosis in the legs, or an inability to pass urine. After an abdominal operation the bowel usually takes some time to get working normally again. This is called an ileus.

**WOUNDS** are normally closed with stitches in layers. The most superficial (skin) stitches only hold the skin together and the major tissues are held with thicker and stronger dissolving stitches quite independently of the skin ones. Some surgeons use metal clips to close the skin. Most skin stitches or clips will have to be removed in a few days. This is usually pain-free if done carefully. The wound is covered with a dressing which varies from a glorified Elastoplast to a thick pad of gauze and some surgeons use a spray-on plastic dressing. Which is used depends entirely on the choice of the surgeon and there is nothing significant about what your dressing is made of. Some people are sent home with their stitches in and asked to return to the ward or to the out-patients' department to have them removed at a later date. This is increasingly common as the demands on beds increase and hospital stays become shorter.

Dressings can be left in place until the stitches come out (a good idea because this reduces the chances of infection) or will be dressed several times a day if there is any sign of infection. Infection occurs because of germs introduced into the wound at the operation or because of contamination of the wound by bacteria that were freed when the intestine or bowel was opened. Operations on the bowel and gall-bladder, for example, as well as those for peritonitis, produce wound infections more commonly than do most operations. Some surgeons give a very few doses of antibiotics immediately before and after the operation to try to prevent infection in wounds that are particularly at risk.

For several weeks after the operation the area may feel tender and hard and the surrounding skin may be numb. This is normal. If the wound discharges pus or becomes red, hot and painful you should tell someone, whether you are at home or still in hospital, because these are signs that it has become infected. Careful dressing, possibly with the use of radiant heat, usually clears up such infections but sometimes the pus is helped to clear by the nurse or doctor inserting a probe into the wound.

**CHEST INFECTIONS** can occur, especially in smokers, because the anaesthetic itself produces more mucus in the lungs and many smokers find it difficult to cough this up. Post-operative pain also makes people less willing to cough and this, together with shallow breathing, means that the lungs become a breeding ground for bacteria. Physio-therapists can work wonders simply by encouraging people to breathe properly after an operation and this alone can often cure the problem. Most hospitals combine active physiotherapy with a course of antibiotics and adequate pain relief if a serious chest infection occurs. These unpleasant infections that could prolong your stay in hospital by a week can for the most part be prevented if you stop smoking for at least a week before your operation.

**DEEP VEIN THROMBOSIS** is a common condition after an operation although often it is so minor that it causes no trouble. It has been calculated that thirty-five per cent of general surgical patients over the age of forty will have a deep vein thrombosis, as judged by the most modern isotope tests, and nearly three quarters of old people with hip fractures will have one. In this potentially life-threatening condition, blood stagnates in the legs both on the operating theatre table and while the person is lying immobile in bed afterwards. This stagnation, together with the fact that an operation in itself seems to make blood more likely to clot, means that even fit, healthy people can be affected by this condition.

The stagnant blood may then clot and, in a few, causes pain in the calf which in itself is unpleasant enough but can turn into tragedy if a piece of clot breaks off and travels up to the lungs where it can cause death. Five thousand people a year die in the UK from such an embolus in the lung and many of these are people who have just had an operation. There are two and a half million operations per year, so the incidence of fatal embolism is very low. Even so, doctors are trying hard to find ways of reducing this real, if uncommon, hazard of surgery.

Because of this serious risk people are encouraged to get out of bed as early as possible to prevent stagnation of the blood in the legs. Some hospitals use gadgets that apply pressure to the legs in the operating theatre so that the blood is not static even during the operation and other hospitals give anti-clotting drugs before, during and after the operation. Not every pain in the calf is caused by a deep vein thrombosis but if you have any pain there at all, do tell a nurse or a doctor.

An **INABILITY TO PASS URINE** is not uncommon after abdominal operations, after operations of the prostate or after certain procedures on the female pelvic organs. Some patients will wake up with a urinary catheter in place (see page 372) and this will overcome the problem before it starts. If you cannot pass urine easily, tell someone. There are several tricks they can try before having to pass a catheter, which may never be necessary.

**PARALYTIC ILEUS** is a condition in which the intestine stops moving after an abdominal operation. It usually lasts for about 48 hours but affects different parts of the intestinal tract in different ways. After most abdominal procedures the stomach returns to normal activity fairly quickly (within 24 hours) and the small intestine within a very few hours. The large bowel, however, remains inactive for about 48 hours and it is this that produces the persistent swelling that is so characteristic of the post-operative abdomen. During this time (until the doctor can hear bowel sounds and until you have passed wind) you will not be allowed to eat anything and may be on an intravenous drip (see page 396).

# VISITORS

Visitors are something of a double-edged sword. On the one hand they keep you in touch with the real world and are usually welcome if they are close to you, but on the other they can be wearing if you are not feeling well and exhausting if they stay for too long or come too often.

It is natural that all your family will want to know how you are progressing, especially after your operation. Do ask one particular person (preferably your spouse) to act as co-ordinator for visitors and for telephoning in. This saves the nurses a lot of time in answering repeated calls about the one patient. If the co-ordinator always has the facts and everybody phones him or her then everyone's life is made easier.

This goes especially for visiting. There is little point in people travelling to see you only to find that you have a crowd of people with you already. You will be exhausted if you try to see them all and they will be disappointed if they do not see you. By getting someone to organize a visiting rota you need not have any visitors at all if you do not feel up to it. Many hospital patients complain that they would rather see fewer people but do not know tactfully how to keep the others away. This is not a job for you immediately post-operatively, so leave it to someone else.

Unless someone has been a surgical patient himself it is difficult for him to realize how tiring it is, especially early on, to have visitors for very long periods. Several surveys have shown that surgical patients prefer two relatively long visiting periods a day and other research shows that open visiting (except for children) is not popular with patients. As you get better you will feel more up to visitors and by the time you feel well enough to go home you will not mind how many come. Many hospitals allow up to two people per bed at a time only. This is essential on a big open ward or the whole place would be so crowded and noisy that it would cease to function as a hospital for those who are too sick to cope with this onslaught.

The day after the operation your relatives may want to make an appointment to see the houseman so that he can explain what was done or found. This is the best time because the operation will be fresh in his mind and because knowing the facts early enables both relatives and patient to come to terms with the situation before their imaginations run away with them. Always get this sort of information from a doctor, not a nurse. On occasions the doctor will tell a relative more than he will tell you, the patient, simply because he may feel that the relative will know better how to put the facts across to you – after all, your spouse knows you better than any doctor does.

People feel very strongly about their children visiting them. Most people want to see their children quite often, especially if they are maternity patients. Older people (who often make up nearly half of the ward population) tend to be less tolerant of children visiting: about one in five patients in one study were totally against the idea. Some people feel that it is too upsetting for children to see ill people and give this as their reason for not wanting children to visit but there is no evidence that children are upset in this way. On the contrary it probably does children (especially young ones) a lot of good to be able to see a hospital working in case they one day have to be admitted as patients themselves. The familiarity takes a lot of worry out of the situation, especially if the accompanying parents explain things that may cause concern. Technically, you are allowed to have your children to visit you at visiting times, and the DHSS has asked hospitals to allow children to visit their parents and other close relatives in hospital frequently and regularly if the patient so wishes! Naturally, the children should be well behaved and relatively quiet.

# YOUR LEGAL RIGHTS

Most people are happy with their stay in hospital, as several surveys have shown, but sometimes things go wrong or differently from the way you expected and it is helpful to know your rights as a patient.

There are many different levels of complaint that people have when they are in hospital. If there is a dirty washbasin, you are hardly going to complain to the Minister of Health, but there are circumstances in which you can and should do so, though today the Health Service Commissioner (the Ombudsman) handles the majority of unresolved and more serious complaints.

Generally, minor complaints about ward life should be addressed to the sister or senior nurse on duty. She will do all she can, given that there are lots of other people she has to think of too and that her hands are tied by the hospital. She cannot work miracles but will usually do everything possible to help.

If you are in any way dissatisfied with the *medical* care, you should take this up with a doctor. Start with the registrar or consultant and see if you can resolve the problem. The majority of problems arise from poor communication. Start by talking carefully with the doctors because very few complaints and problems in fact arise from poor or negligent medical care. Just in case you are involved, here is what to do.

Your most important right as a patient is to be treated with reasonable care and skill, both of which can only be defined by other members of the medical and nursing professions. A doctor who fails to provide such care and skill is said to be negligent. If you suffer as a result of negligence, you are entitled to compensation by law and you can resort to law before, after, or instead of complaining through 'the usual channels' (see below). Damages may be payable for the pain, suffering and inconvenience to which you have been put and your loss of earnings and out-of-pocket expenses can be claimed. These rights are the same whether you are a private or an NHS patient. However, legal cases against doctors are often lost and, even if the case is won, you may not get compensation.

The trouble is that if you feel you have been negligently treated you could have some difficulty in proving it. To do this you will need an expert opinion to support your case. The British Academy of Forensic Sciences will supply a patient's solicitor (but not the patient himself) with the name of a specialist who is prepared to act as an expert witness. The solicitor can also apply for a High Court order which obliges the disclosure of the relevant medical records. If you cannot get a solicitor, legal advice can be obtained from a Law Centre or through a Citizens' Advice Bureau and Legal Aid can be granted if you do not earn enough to be able to afford your own solicitor. However you seek the help of a solicitor, make sure that he is experienced in medical litigation.

Patients are also protected by law against assault. It is technically an assault on a patient or trespass to the person if a doctor does anything at all without his consent.

Most often this causes no problem because if you are conscious and you allow a doctor to do something to you it will be held that you consented, by implication at least, because you did not object. We have discussed consent forms for operations already (see page 47). The difficulties arise (and these not very often) when people feel they are being used in research trials or experiments without their permission.

If any doctor wants to use you in a research project he must explain carefully exactly what is involved and in some hospitals he will even ask you to sign a consent form. If any experiment is conducted upon you without your consent you have redress in law.

So how then do you complain? 'With difficulty' seems to be the answer because most people do not know how to complain and when they do, they find the procedure slow and complicated, according to a survey carried out by the Consumers Association. Also, a major problem with the system is that area health authorities are allowed to conduct the whole matter internally and so end up as both judge and jury, which in other spheres of life would be considered unacceptable.

The vast majority of complaints about hospitals are about simple organizational inadequacies and are nothing at all to do with the medical care. They should be made in writing to the hospital secretary (or administrator). You can also write to him in the first instance on matters of suspected medical negligence. A simple letter laying out the facts as you see them may well get results without having to take the matter further. When writing any letter of complaint, try to be balanced and rational. If you make out that everything went wrong and that all the staff were incompetent, this is unlikely to do anything but put the recipient into a bad frame of mind because he knows that this simply cannot be true. Praise the bits that went well and point out simply what went wrong in your view. The hospital secretary (or administrator) will investigate and get the staff involved to report back to him. The whole matter will then be taken to the District Administrator who is accountable to the area health authority for your area.

He will consider the complaint and write a letter of explanation or apology to you. This is usually the end of the matter in the UK where we are, as yet, not very litigation-conscious. If, however, you are not happy, you can write to the Health Services Commissioner (the Ombudsman). His office will investigate the complaint further and, if necessary, instigate an independent inquiry into the matter. If you are a private patient in an NHS hospital your complaints against NHS personnel are handled in the same way as if you were an NHS patient but any complaints against the consultant are between you and him alone, as the health authorities are not responsible for this contractual relationship.

The office of the Health Services Commissioner for England (the Ombudsman) was set up by an act of parliament to investigate complaints from members of the public that involve injustice or hardship as a result of a failure in a service supplied by a health authority; a failure of the authority to provide a service it should have done; and areas of maladministration generally. The Commissioner (Ombudsman) does not deal with matters of medical judgement or negligence.

Before the Ombudsman can investigate any complaint against a health authority, the person must have complained to the responsible authority and have given them reasonable time to investigate and reply. Complaints must reach the Commissioner within one year of the day on which the subject under complaint occurred and he cannot investigate anything that you have already taken to a tribunal or a court of law. Complaints to the Commissioner should be sent, in writing, to the Health Services Commissioner for England, Church House, Great Smith Street, London SW1P 3BW, giving your full name and address, the authority concerned, the full name and address of the place where the matters complained of occurred and, of course, a full account of the events surrounding the complaint.

When the Commissioner receives the complaint he will decide whether it is in his sphere of jurisdiction and if it is not he will send you a letter saying why. If it is in his jurisdiction he will start an investigation during which he can examine a health authority's internal papers and take written and oral evidence from anyone he thinks would be valuable. You can claim expenses and be reimbursed for your time if the Commissioner calls you for an interview, and legal expenses may be partly covered if the Commissioner thinks legal representation is necessary.

Community health councils – the 'consumer' councils of the NHS, to be found on many high streets – can do nothing about individual complaints. They can, however, tell you how to go about complaining and have a duty to do so. In some areas someone from the Community Health Council may accompany you to meetings with hospital administrators, nursing staff and doctors when complaints are being discussed. This can be very helpful because the Community Health Council may have had similar complaints from other patients before and these may add weight to your case. In Scotland the equivalent of community health councils do *not* take up individual complaints.

Now that you have seen how to complain, here are a few areas in which patients often do not know their rights. Only rarely do most of these problems ever arise but if they do it is good to know where you stand.

**THE RIGHT TO LEAVE HOSPITAL.** You can leave a hospital whenever you wish: legally the staff may not detain you against your will. If you decide to discharge yourself you will be asked to sign a form saying that you have done so and that you take full responsibility for what happens. Similarly, you have no right to stay in hospital if they want you to go. If you insist on doing so you are trespassing.

**ACCESS TO INFORMATION.** Doctors sometimes withhold information if they think it is best for you and they cannot be made to give it to you. If the matter is causing you concern, contact the Patients' Association (see page 65 for address). They will try to resolve the problem and have been successful in some such cases.

**SEEING A PARTICULAR CONSULTANT.** A patient has no right to see a particular consultant under the NHS, nor can a general practitioner insist that his patient be seen by a particular doctor. If your family doctor specifically wants you to see a particular consultant, more often than not you will end up seeing him (even if you do not see him at your first visit).

**ACCESS TO RECORDS.** Patients under the NHS have no rights to their X-rays or medical records. Even private patients have no rights to their medical records but are usually entitled to their X-rays if they have paid for them.

If you are thinking of taking legal action on this you can apply to the High Court which may issue an order for the relevant document to be made available. Take legal advice on this.

**VISITING CHILDREN IN HOSPITAL.** The DHSS has strongly recommended 'unrestricted' visiting of children on children's wards and has asked hospital authorities to do all they can to make it possible for mothers of young children to be able to stay with them. This has not been achieved in the majority of hospitals, often for reasons quite beyond the hospitals' control. Legally you can be thrown out of a hospital after visiting hours but this is almost never done unless you, the parent, are causing a nuisance. You cannot legally put down a camp bed beside your child's if there is no accommodation for mothers but you will probably be allowed to if you ask tactfully and pleasantly. For more details of children in hospital see page 74.

**CONSENT FORMS.** As we saw on page 48, a consent form is not a legal document but simply protects the surgeon from a possible allegation of assault. He or one of his staff must tell you what he intends to do and you will sign to say that he has explained everything to you. You are entitled to alter the form so that you consent only to certain things and not to others.

**REFUSING TREATMENT.** You can refuse any treatment or investigation (unless you are detained under a compulsory order) but this may lead to the hospital asking you to leave if they cannot treat you adequately or in a different way.

**EXPERIMENTS AND RESEARCH.** In teaching hospitals especially, patients are used in trials of various treatment methods. You can only be used in such a trial with your *informed* consent. Any attempt to do anything other than this is assault and actionable in law. Most people are, however, quite happy to help doctors with research if it does not hinder their recovery or jeopardize their treatment in any way. No one can give legal consent to any procedure being carried out on any other person which is not to his benefit – not even parents in the case of their own children. If a patient's valid consent cannot be obtained, the procedure or research must not be carried out.

**TEACHING HOSPITALS.** Just because you go into a teaching hospital does not mean you have to submit to examinations by or in the presence of students. Most people are perfectly happy to have students present and they often lighten one's stay in hospital but some people, especially those with personal problems, would rather be alone with a doctor. You can insist on this but the consultant may ask you to wait until the students have gone or may get one of his assistants to see you. You may not be asked if you mind being taught on, and the doctors may give the impression that you cannot refuse, but this is not so.

**DONATING YOUR BODY OR ORGANS.** Some people want to leave certain organs or their whole body to medical research. If you want to leave your body you should put this in a letter and leave it with your next-of-kin who can then tell the hospital immediately after your death. All expenses are paid by the medical school to whom you leave your body. Details of how to bequeath your body can be obtained from the Anatomy Office (01-407-5522) or from HM Inspector of Anatomy, 16–19 Grosse Street, London W1, tel: 01-636-7584.

If you want to leave your eyes, you will need an eye donor form from the Royal National Institute for the Blind, 24 Great Portland Street, London W1. Make sure you tell your next-of-kin beforehand so that the corneas can be removed without delay.

You can also leave your kidneys. Get a kidney donor form from your family doctor or the DHSS, sign it and carry it with you. This is essential because kidneys have to be removed very quickly if they are to be of value to someone else.

If you have any queries about your legal rights as a patient either in or out of hospital, contact the Patients' Association, 11 Dartmouth Street, London SW1, tel: 01-

222-4992. This Association is an advisory service and a collective voice for patients. It receives a small grant from the DHSS but is independent and is mostly financed by subscriptions from its members. Its aims are to represent and further the interests of patients; to give help and advice to individuals; to acquire and spread further information about patients' interests; and to promote goodwill between patients and the medical profession. The Association produces helpful leaflets which are available on request from the above address. It is also active in the political sphere and tries to put the patient's voice in the corridors of power, often when new health legislation is under consideration. Since its inception in 1963 it has contributed to or directly brought about the appointment of the NHS Ombudsman; a code of practice for the medical profession on using patients for teaching; improved visiting hours; improvements in drug safety; and reduced hospital waiting lists. If you would like to become a member, write to the above address.

**Some useful addresses for use when complaining or in other legal situations.**

British Academy of Forensic Sciences, c/o Dept of Forensic Medicine, London Hospital Medical College, Turner Street, London E1.

Legal Aid, New Legal Aid, PO Box 9, Nottingham NG1 6DS.

District Administrator
Area Health Authority
Board of Governors
   (Teaching Hospitals)
Regional Health Authority
} The Community Health Council will have the address; the hospital will forward letters

Community Health Council. Local address from town hall, hospital, post office or library; the Patients' Association will also advise (see below).

Health Services Commissioner, Church House, Great Smith Street, London SW1.

NHS Tribunal Clerk, N. Colley, Solicitor, Great Smith Street, London SW1.

General Medical Council, 44 Hallam Street, London W1.

General Dental Council, 37 Wimpole Street, London W1.
General Nursing Council, 23 Portland Place, London W1.
Patients' Association, 11 Dartmouth Street, London SW1,
 tel: 01-222-4992.

# GOING HOME AND CONVALESCING

As you begin to recover from your operation the registrar or
consultant will tell you when you will be able to go home. He
will usually give you a few days' notice but he may say 'today'
or 'tomorrow', especially if the sister needs a bed for a
particular patient. Such a speedy discharge can come as a
shock because it may give you very little opportunity to get
your domestic life organized. One survey found that a third
of all recently discharged patients were dissatisfied, mainly
because they were given too little notice, so be warned.

Before you are told you can go home be prepared to set the
domestic wheels in motion. Organize someone to bring your
clothes in and be sure to collect anything you have left with
the sister in the way of valuables. Collect your certificate for
being off work, collect your drugs and if possible get a friend
or relative to pick you up by car. Waiting for transport to take
you home can be a very flat and depressing experience
especially when you are keen to be home. If you cannot get
anyone at short notice to see you safely home and see that
you have food and so on, do tell the medical social worker.

Before you go, the nursing staff may ask if there is any
reason why you should not go home but often they do not, so
it is up to you to mention any problems or difficulties there
may be. There are things the hospital can do to help if you
have domestic difficulties. Do not pretend that everything is
all right at home for your return if it is not but be honest with
the staff and yourself. Over 100,000 patients are discharged
every week from hospital beds in this country and very many
of them need to get further professional help when they go
home. This help may be of a medical nature, in which case it
will be your general practitioner who will look after you; of a
nursing kind, in which case a community nurse will visit; or

of a domestic nature, when a home help could be of value. Every hospital has a medical social work department (which used to be called the Almoner's office) which can send a member of staff to discuss any problems you have before you leave. They can mobilize local authority, medical and even volunteer help. In some hospitals there is a co-ordinator for voluntary services.

When you are in hospital you are very much the centre of the stage. Doctors and nurses are there to care for you and visitors make a particular effort to be pleasant and make more of a fuss of you than they normally do in the outside world. After a few days the ward setting becomes familiar and even cosy because the problems of the outside world are held at a distance from you. Once you leave hospital, though, life changes very dramatically and even though you may not be feeling very ill by hospital standards you will soon realize how poor you feel by comparison with your normal health. Emotionally too you may feel low even when you get home, especially if you do not have a close family network to look after you. It is a good idea to let your family doctor know that you are back home because although the hospital will send him a summary of all your in-patient details he will not get these for a week or more and will be somewhat in the dark until then. He may come and see you or may ask a community nurse or health visitor to call to see you. Most often he will leave it up to you to get in touch with him if you are at all worried.

Do not expect miracles in terms of recovery speed; it takes far longer than you'd imagine to get back to normal. One survey of 257 patients found that two or three weeks after discharge from hospital 180 of the patients were not back to normal. There is also no link between the length of the hospital stay and how long it takes to get back to normal, but older people tend to take longer than young ones to feel normal again.

If you live alone you are going to need help from relatives, friends or neighbours and possibly from the Social Services Department at the town hall. The latter can arrange a home help, meals on wheels and other useful services, depending on your needs. Volunteer organizations can be very helpful, especially if you live alone. They may help with shopping, taking you out, taking you back to the hospital for out-patient appointments or may simply chat when you want company.

Before you leave the hospital you will have been given any drugs you should take and also an appointment for the out-patients' clinic, if necessary. You will probably also be given a short note to give your doctor. This summarizes in a few words what was done and the drugs you are on.

Consultants like to follow up the results of their efforts and will usually want to see you at least once after your operation to check that all is well. At this time you can check once more what you should and should not do after your particular operation and many people ask at this stage about returning to their normal sex lives. The doctor will also advise you when to return to work but if you are at all unsure, discuss the matter with your family doctor. You do not necessarily need to be off work until this hospital visit has taken place.

After a major operation many people complain of tiredness, perhaps for several months. This fatigue goes on for a long time after the wound has healed and the body is apparently back to normal. Long convalescence does not prevent it and patients often notice it after returning to work. There is very little research being done into this common experience but that which has been done shows that intellect and performance are reduced temporarily after an operation in some people, especially after serious operations. This syndrome of post-operative fatigue seems to have attracted far less attention than it should and more research needs to be done.

# PRIVATE SURGERY

Increasing numbers of people contribute to private medical insurance schemes and many companies pay the premiums for such insurance for employees as part of their terms of employment. The question of private medicine in NHS hospitals is clearly a controversial one, but I do not intend to examine the various political issues here.

Many people opt for private surgery because they feel they will get better treatment, but this is not necessarily so. It is true that by going privately you ensure that the consultant himself operates on you and if this gives you peace of mind, that is fine. However, as any of us who have worked in surgery can attest, many registrars and senior registrars are fine operators and some are even better technically than their bosses! The major advantage that most people enjoy when having an operation privately is that the surgeon takes much more time to explain things to them and this makes many people feel a lot happier right from the start.

If you want to see a surgeon privately, ask your family doctor for a letter to take to the particular person you have in mind or ask your doctor to arrange the appointment. A surgeon who has a private practice will usually see you in his private consulting room or he may have rooms in an NHS hospital. The thing to remember is that if you go privately you (or your insurance company) will have to pay for everything: each blood test, X-ray and so on. Even if you have these carried out in an NHS hospital you will still have to pay because the hospital charges you or the surgeon direct. Even if you first see a surgeon on a private basis and have all your investigations privately, when you hear the cost of the operation itself you may want to transfer to the NHS to have it done. You can do this and the surgeon will understand perfectly. He will put you on his NHS waiting list along with his other patients awaiting operation.

Conversely, you can change from being an NHS patient to being a private one and many people do this after learning that there is a long wait for their operation to be done. Some people hope that by seeing a surgeon privately first they can then become NHS patients and jump the waiting list queue. This has happened and still goes on in a few places but it is basically unfair to the others on the waiting list and gives the whole of private medicine a bad name.

Wherever you see a surgeon, he may operate on you in the hospital in which he holds his NHS appointment (assuming it has private beds), or may suggest a private hospital for you. Although private hospitals often turn out to be a little more expensive than private beds in NHS hospitals, they are often purpose-built and frequently provide a level of comfort and service that surpasses even the private wings of NHS hospitals. Also everyone there will be as you are, paying for the surgery, and this avoids any feelings of 'them and us' that can occur both among the staff and the patients of an NHS hospital.

Not only can you choose your surgeon but you can choose when to have the operation done. This can be invaluable for the self-employed or for those with considerable family responsibilities. It is the endless waiting and the possibility of being called in at a moment's notice that so upsets people waiting on NHS lists. However, just because you are going privately, does not mean that you will not have to wait at all. Sometimes there is a wait for the few private beds in a particular NHS hospital and ironically in certain hospitals you would get operated on sooner under the NHS. Your surgeon will advise you on the best course of action to take.

The costs of operations are increasing all the time and vary to some extent from surgeon to surgeon but here are some typical operations and their costs at 1981 prices. These prices include hospital room expenses, surgeon's, anaesthetist's and all other fees for an average length of stay, but remember the hospital is paid for by the day.

| Operation/treatment | From | To |
| --- | --- | --- |
| appendicectomy | £ 560 | £1060 |
| hernia operation | 560 | 1060 |
| hysterectomy | 1000 | 1900 |
| duodenal ulcer | 940 | 1550 |
| cataract | 880 | 1250 |
| tonsillectomy | 440 | 880 |
| slipped disc repair | 1500 | 2900 |
| gall bladder removal | 1060 | 1650 |
| varicose veins | 560 | 1060 |

| | | |
|---|---:|---:|
| bunion removal | 750 | 1250 |
| knee cartilage | 1000 | 1900 |
| heart operation | 3500 | 5000 |
| breast lump removal | 500 | 940 |
| hip replacement | 2100 | 3100 |
| prostate removal | 1000 | 1900 |
| nasal polyp removal | 500 | 940 |
| prolapse repair | 1000 | 1900 |
| bowel resection | 1500 | 2250 |

(Figures provided by Private Patients Plan.)

If you have private insurance cover, remember to check that the operation you are about to have is covered by the policy you have. If you pay your own premiums make sure you keep up with adequate cover for in these inflationary times you may find that just when help is needed your expenses are only half covered. The fact that you have been paying for fifteen years does not impress the insurance company. They are only interested in the amount of premium you paid for the current year. Get a claim form from the organization you are with and send it with the bills (or receipts, if you have already paid) to the organization. You do not need to get a claim form or even contact the organization until the operation is completed and you start getting the bills. The claim form must be signed by a medical practitioner: either your family doctor or the surgeon who did your operation (although your GP may charge). The insurance organizations pay very quickly: usually within a couple of days. The cheque will be made out to you and it is up to you to settle the bills. You do not have to wait for all the bills to come in before claiming anything and only one claim form is needed, not one per bill.

## NATIONAL INSURANCE BENEFITS

Before going into hospital you can claim sickness benefits if you cannot work because of your illness. You have to have been ill for three days before you can claim (unless you have recently been ill or unemployed) and you will need to take or send your medical certificate (supplied by your family doctor) to the local office of the DHSS after signing it. The address is in the telephone book or can be obtained from a local post office. If you have a dependent spouse or any other dependants you should say so on the back of the medical certificate because a separate form will be sent so that you can claim for these dependants. Do not forget to fill in your national health insurance number on the certificate. This is *not* the same as your national health service number or your hospital record number. Send in the certificate within six days of becoming ill (21 days if it is your first ever certificate) or you may lose benefits.

The first payment may take a little while but after that the payments are made weekly by Giro. For each week you receive sickness benefit you do not have to pay a national insurance stamp: this is paid for you, so you do not lose out on your contributions.

To qualify for Sickness Benefit you have to have paid at least 26 class 1 (employed) or class 2 (self-employed) contributions ever and must have paid at least 50 class 1 or 2 contributions within the relevant contribution year. Talk to your local DHSS about your 'benefit year' because this does not necessarily mean the 12 months preceding your claim.

Earnings related supplements are payable in addition to your Sickness Benefit unles you are self-employed. There are other conditions of payment of these supplements so get details from your employer or local DHSS office. An earnings related supplement is not usually payable though until you have been off work for 12 days or more and cannot be paid for more than 156 days in any period of interruption of employment. You can never receive more than 85 per cent of your average weekly earnings from all these benefits and supplements but all the money is tax free. Sickness Benefit is replaced by an Invalidity Benefit after 168 days (excluding Sundays). These 168 days do not have to be in a continuous period. (You can claim if you have been unable to work for spells of two days or more and if all these add up to more than 168 days.) Form NI.16A outlines Invalidity Benefit in more detail and is available from DHSS offices.

A good general rule is always to tell your local DHSS

office if you or a dependant is going into hospital and to let them know the discharge date as soon as possible.

Under normal circumstances, social security benefits are paid to help with your needs at home. When you are in hospital some of these are being met by the hospital (food, board and lodging etc), so your benefit may be temporarily reduced or withdrawn. If you are paying the whole cost of your stay in hospital, no reduction is made in your social security benefits. Normally though your Sickness Benefit, Invalidity Benefit, retirement pension, Widow's Benefit and other social security benefits are reduced after eight weeks in hospital. If you come out of hospital but have to be re-admitted within four weeks, the two periods are counted as one. During the first eight weeks in hospital all your social security benefits continue as normal, including Sickness Benefit. DHSS leaflet NI.9 has more details about all this.

If you have not claimed any Sickness Benefit up until the time you go into hospital the ward sister will give you the necessary certificates to claim. This claim should be made within 13 weeks of your admission date unless you are discharged before this, in which case you may claim within three weeks of being discharged. Always claim as soon as possible because you may lose benefits if you leave it too long.

When you are still in hospital the Giro cheques can be sent to you there or you can authorize a named person to cash them for you by signing on the back of the Giro order. Each Giro is only valid for three months, so if you are in hospital for a long period, do not forget to cash them in plenty of time.

# CHILDREN IN HOSPITAL

You may be surprised to learn that by the age of seven, one child in two will have been an in-patient in hospital. With three quarters of a million children being admitted to hospital each year, it is likely that one day it will be your child, so it is well worth taking the time to work out what you could do to make the experience easier for you both and how you could protect your child from the emotional damage suffered by thousands of children every year in hospitals.

Most children of school age fare perfectly well in hospital if you visit them very frequently but children under four or five will need you to spend a lot of time with them or even to stay in hospital all the time. This can be difficult to arrange if you have other children but is well worth while and will save you a lot of problems later.

Preparing a child for going into hospital cannot start too soon. Talk about the hospital as you would talk about any other part of your child's daily life. As you pass it going about your normal life, point it out and casually mention what it is for: to make people better when they are ill. If your child is old enough, encourage games of doctors and nurses and read books about children in hospital. Ask the playgroup leader to include games about hospitals in her play programme or the teacher at school to buy suitable books about hospitals for the classroom library. If you have to go to the doctor or hospital, let your child come too so that he can see that there is nothing to be afraid of, but play down any anxiety you feel because children are very sensitive to such feelings. Letting a child visit someone in hospital with you can be a good way of making a hospital seem less forbidding. Never threaten your child with the hospital or the doctor but build up an image of the hospital as a good place and doctors and nurses as kind people. In short, be positive rather than negative.

Some parents belong to the National Association for the Welfare of Children in Hospital (NAWCH), which was set up in 1961 by a group of mothers to help spread awareness of a child's emotional response to hospital and to encourage ways of giving him security in this situation. NAWCH is an active organization with 58 local groups and welcomes all parents – whether or not their children have been in hospital – as well as non-parents.

For the child in hospital, NAWCH may provide toys and day clothes where needed, furnishings and equipment for mothers' units and visitors' accommodation; transport to the hospital if there is poor public transport or if the mother has financial problems; crêche facilities for brothers and sisters; childminders for children at home; and voluntary play-workers to run playschemes in hospital wards.

Young children find it hard to understand why they have to be separated from their parents, homes and families and may not realize, especially if they are under five, that their hospital stay is only temporary. In fact studies show that many children believe thay have been deserted by their parents and left for ever in the care of strangers in hospital. Even if his mother says she is coming back, the child may feel angry at being left there against his will, a feeling which can be followed by a sense of betrayal and rejection. Unfortunately, on getting home, some children take a long time to re-establish their previous happy relationship with their mothers and a few never do. Detailed research work has shown all too clearly that this sort of emotional response is *normal* in the under-five who is left in hospital without his mother.

Luckily, *you can prevent many of the emotional problems by being with your young child in hospital as much as possible.*

If you are with your child, you can cushion him from the strange and perhaps frightening experiences he will have and help him cope with his anxiety. Most important, though, is that he will not blame you for putting him through it all, as he might if you left him alone. If a blood test or a physical examination is done, your presence will reassure him. Your absence (sometimes unfortunately at the staff's request, thinking it would be easier if you were not there) might make him think you had deserted him in his time of need. Similarly, your presence before and immediately after an operation will help your child, though you should be ready to fade into the background immediately if asked.

By being with your child, you can take a lot of work off the nurses simply by feeding, changing, bathing and playing with him and you can even help with other children. Ask the nurses what they would like you to do: you might even be able to help the ward teacher or play leader.

Ideally, you should be with your child all the time, day and night, if he is under about four or five. Some hospitals provide overnight accommodation for mothers, sometimes in the form of camp beds by their children's beds, and this means that if your child wakes at night you can be there to reassure him. However, you may be unable to stay at night for various reasons and some hospitals are resistant to the idea, unless the child is very ill. If you cannot stay, try to be there for as much of the waking day as possible and not necessarily only at visiting times. If your hospital has restricted visiting times, you may be able to persuade the ward sister to allow you in for longer periods. In 1959, the government's Platt Report recommended 'unrestricted' visiting for children in hospital (ie visiting at any time during which children could reasonably be expected to be awake). The Report also recommended the provision for the mother's admission if the child was under five. Unfortunately, hospitals are a long way off meeting these recommendations but with continued pressure from parents and from organizations such as NAWCH, arrangements for visiting and staying with children in hospital have improved a lot.

A ward where visiting is frequently neglected or discouraged is the special care baby unit. Surprisingly, mothers often think that their newborn babies do not need them. They do, and research stresses that mother-child bonding may be damaged if the mother is not with her baby as much as possible. There is mounting evidence that a baby separated from his mother does not thrive or feed well, sleeps badly and is irritable. Whenever possible, stay in hospital with your baby. This also makes breast feeding easier, though it is possible for the staff to give expressed breast milk that you have sent in from home. This can be given by tube or spoon. Bottle feeding with expressed breast milk is not generally a good idea if you plan to breast feed, as a bottle-fed baby may never subsequently take to the breast properly.

Most children are unsettled when they get back home but with patience and extra love they get over it quickly, especially if you have stayed in hospital with them. An older child may quite enjoy his stay in hospital and may even come out more confident after such an 'adult' adventure.

# Part II
# An A–Z of Operations

# ABORTION

**What is it?**

The termination of a pregnancy by removing the fetus from the womb artificially. The term abortion is also used by doctors to describe the spontaneous loss of a fetus before it is 28 weeks old. The lay term for this is a miscarriage.

The subject of abortion is a highly contentious one that raises moral as well as medical issues. There is no room in a book such as this to go into the whys and wherefores and legislation differs from country to country. Suffice it to say that for many women, both married and single, an unwanted pregnancy, be it the result of a chance sexual encounter, a miscalculated risk, or a genuine failure in contraception technique, will make them consider an abortion. Some women will seek an abortion on discovering that their fetus has an untreatable abnormality after an amniocentesis test (see page 352).

All abortion methods are basically the same in that they remove the fetus from the womb artificially before it would normally be ready to be born. The methods used are becoming increasingly sophisticated but which method is actually used depends upon the age of the fetus when the abortion is to be done.

**Why operate?**

To remove the unwanted, diseased or malformed baby.

**How?**

The dividing line for deciding which method to use is usually taken as 12 weeks after the first day of the last period. This is because up to this time the fetus is small enough (as gauged by its head size) to be removed surgically through the cervix and thus through the vagina. After this age, the uterus either has to be opened during an abdominal operation (as in a Caesarean section) or the fetus has to be 'born' forcibly. Unfortunately, because of medical and other delays, too many women have an abortion too late. It makes sense to get medical help as soon as you possibly can because the earlier an abortion is done the simpler and safer it is. Do not waste time going to a doctor you know is unsympathetic on this issue – go straight to a clinic or doctor who will help you with your decision at once.

**UP TO TWELVE WEEKS.** Until recent years the commonest way of aborting a fetus of this age was to do a D and C (dilatation and curettage see page 166). By scraping out the lining of the uterus the fetus was removed. This has now been almost entirely superseded by the vacuum method of abortion which is usually carried out under general anaesthetic because enlarging the cervical canal is painful. A local anaesthesia can be injected into the cervix but is not often used. This method is sometimes called a D and E (dilatation and evacuation) and is rising in popularity. Almost all private abortions are of this kind (if the fetus is less than 12 weeks old).

During pregnancy the uterus enlarges but in the early months the cervix or neck of the womb stays tightly shut. If the doctor wants to remove the fetus through the cervix, he has to dilate it carefully so that the delicate elastic and muscle fibres are not permanently damaged as this could possibly lead to the inability of the woman to retain any future baby in the early months of pregnancy. The doctor enlarges the tight cervical passage so as to enable a hollow metal or plastic tube to be inserted into the uterine cavity. There are several methods of vacuum extraction: one commonly carried out involves using a Karman catheter. This is made of flexible plastic with two openings at the side, is fairly fine and does not involve much stretching of the cervix to insert it. The catheter is moved around inside the uterus to break up the fetus, then the uterine contents are sucked out. After checking that no pieces are left inside, a drug is given to make the uterus contract so that the area where the fetus was attached stops bleeding. Such a vacuum extraction is much less traumatic to the cervix than a D and C, for example.

Post-operative bleeding is not uncommon and after a somewhat heavy loss early on the bleeding settles down to that of a normal or heavy period. Some women report some period-type pains but these are usually cured with simple painkillers.

**AFTER TWELVE WEEKS.** A hysterotomy is an operation rather like a miniature Caesarean section (see page 131). It is now little used as a method of abortion because it has been superseded by injection methods. Abortions after 12 weeks are surgically, emotionally and in many other ways more complex and dangerous than earlier ones.

Because the fetus is too big to come out without excessive dilatation of the cervical canal after 12 weeks and because excessive dilatation of the cervix could permanently damage it, abortions after this time have to be done in other ways. In recent years salt or urea solutions have been injected into the uterus and these have been made reliable by adding a natural hormone called a prostaglandin. Sometimes a prostaglandin is used by itself.

The skin of the abdominal wall over the uterus is disinfected and a local anaesthetic injected into the skin. Once this has taken effect, a long fine needle is passed through the pain-free area of skin into the uterine cavity. The chosen chemical is then injected. Prostaglandins are complex hormones that are especially plentiful in male semen, the uterus and placenta. They have many effects in the body but the one being harnessed here is the power to make uterine muscle contract. Thus they induce a sort of artificial labour. The ideal time to perform this sort of abortion is at 14–18 weeks. Almost no one would consider aborting a fetus over the age of 24 weeks. In most cases 20 weeks is considered the upper limit of acceptability, expect perhaps in cases of mongolism (Down's syndrome) or spina bifida.

## Post-operative progress

Up until 14 weeks it is practically safer to have an abortion than to carry on with the pregnancy but after this there are real potential hazards. The two main ones are bleeding and infection. Serious complications only occur in 2.5 per hundred thousand women having a vacuum abortion, but are more common with injection methods and rise to 250 per hundred thousand with a hysterotomy. As has been mentioned, future pregnancies may be threatened because overstretching the cervix may render it unable to hold a baby inside the uterus. If this problem occurs it can be overcome by inserting a circular stitch around the mouth of the womb early in the next pregnancy. This holds the fetus in and is removed just before delivery.

If the aborted fetus had rhesus positive blood, and the mother was rhesus negative, there used to be a danger if a rhesus positive baby was born in a later pregnancy because the aborted fetus' blood might have sensitized her. This can now be prevented by giving all rhesus negative mothers a protective injection called 'Anti-D' when they miscarry, have an abortion or give birth to their first baby.

Long-term psychological problems after abortions are very difficult to assess because (i) the studies carried out are not comparable; (ii) it is very difficult to find out women's true feelings after the event; (iii) most investigations do not look deeply into the emotional and spiritual changes in the woman but simply look for frank psychiatric disease; and (iv) results of surveys differ according to the outlook of those conducting them. There are as many opinions on this subject as there are workers researching it but the best study (over three decades) in Norway shows that of a follow-up of 897 women, 82·5 per cent were glad they had had the abortion or had no reservations at all. The remainder were classified as having 'late mental effects'. Nearly 10 per cent were satisfied but doubtful; 3·8 per cent not happy but realized it had been necessary; 3·7 per cent were repentant; and 4·3 per cent had a serious mental disturbance. In another, perhaps more telling study, Dr P. Aran followed up 100 women from Malmo, Sweden, who, after having had an abortion, went on to have a normal pregnancy. He found that 35 per cent were content; 17 per cent were content but had a bad conscience; 25 per cent had mild guilt feelings; and 23 per cent had severe guilt feelings. Commenting on the last group he said that the guilt feelings were so severe that the women had suffered for a varying length of time from nervous disorders, insomnia and decreased work capacity. Other surveys have shown that women whose moral or religious convictions are affronted by an abortion fare especially badly after having one. All women about to have an abortion need careful and sympathetic support which should be continued after the operation. This may well protect most women from the emotional after-effects.

Two distinguished workers in this field summarized the position as follows: 'the more mature and motherly the woman, the more likely such feelings (of guilt or loss) were, and the more immature, psychopathic or unmotherly, the more the patient was unaffected by a termination of pregnancy'.

Most women who have abortions are adamant that they will never have an unwanted pregnancy again but the facts tell a very different story. On average, 40 per cent of unsterilized women who have had an abortion are pregnant again within two or three years and one survey found 58 per cent pregnant again within one year. In two Swedish studies, 61 per cent of these went on to have a normal delivery. All existing evidence suggests that early abortions have little or no effect on subsequent pregnancies. Whether or not late abortions have any substantial effect is still an open question.

If you have had an abortion, do not forget to tell your obstetrician next time you are pregnant because knowing about your abortion could help him.

# ABSCESS

**What is it?**
A collection of pus in the tissues. Most of us are familiar with a boil on the back of the neck or the abscess that may follow a finger prick but abscesses can also affect deep structures of the body such as the lung and the brain.

Abscesses occur as a result of an infection with a bacterium called Staphylococcus pyogenes. Just why any one individual should suddenly get an abscess is not clear because many people can be exposed to exactly the same environmental hazards but only a few will develop an abscess. Abscesses seem to occur most readily in people who are run down physically; in those who are suffering from debilitating diseases; and in those on steroid drugs. Staph. pyogenes is very widespread indeed, living as it does in our noses. In fact, so widespread is it that it is surprising that more people do not suffer from abscesses. That they do not is partly due to the skin's natural resistance to infection and also to the presence of infection-fighting white blood cells that tend to limit bacteria and remove them by engulfing and digesting them.

Once the infection has taken hold, the surrounding tissues react by producing more tissue fluid and the blood flow to the area is increased. Because of this increased blood flow the area is red, hot and painful and the leakage of fluid makes it swell. Millions of white blood cells engulf the bacteria and then die. This mass of dead white blood cells is what makes pus. As the pus builds up it actually destroys surrounding tissue which is damaged by physical pressure and toxins and for this reason an abscess can leave a serious and permanent tissue deficit. An abscess may also produce a fever, especially if it is large.

An abscess tries to expand into areas of least resistance so that it can discharge its pus and thus release the pressure. This usually means that it 'points' towards the skin, where it can discharge. Ideally, an abscess bursts at this stage and releases its pus. The swelling then subsides and allows healing tissue to fill the cavity slowly over several weeks. This process is altered if the person takes antibiotics because these modify the body's response to the infection – often for the worse if the pus has already formed, because the treatment for an abscess is to get rid of the pus. Antibiotics may well kill the bacteria in an abscess but then leave a sterile bag of pus which becomes walled off with fibrous tissue and forms a permanent hardened lump or mass.

Deep abscesses which will not point to the skin may need surgical drainage combined with antibiotic therapy.

### Why operate?
To let out the pus so as to relieve pain and allow healing to occur.

## How?

Basically the treatment for an abscess is either to encourage it to 'point' to the exterior and discharge its pus or to incise it surgically and ensure that it drains effectively. Once the pressure is off and the pus gone, healing occurs naturally. If an abscess occurs at the seat of a hair follicle (as in a stye, the armpits and at the back of the neck) then pulling out the hair itself may be enough to start drainage. Most often though, if local heat – in the form of a poultice or covered hot-water bottle – produces no discharge of pus, a doctor will have to incise the abscess.

Small or medium-sized superficial abscesses need only a local anaesthetic before they are incised. In fact a really tense boil may be so painful that a short sharp stab with a scalpel is less painful than giving a local anaesthetic and then incising it. After the pus has been squeezed out, the wound is dressed with absorbent material to soak up any further pus produced, and bandaged or covered with an adhesive dressing. A really large abscess will have a wick or drain left in place to ensure that all the pus comes out into the dressing.

This treatment produces immediate relief to the sufferer and proves effective in the vast majority of cases.

Certain abscesses deserve special mention because their treatment is different. A gumboil or peri-apical abscess occurs at the root of a tooth and can be exquisitely painful. This can be drained either by drilling up through the tooth's root or by opening the bone immediately over the affected root. Either way, the pus is removed and normal healing takes over.

An appendix abscess is a serious condition and is discussed on page 99. Abscesses can also occur in the genital tract as a result of venereal or other infections. Most common of these are abscesses of the small Bartholin's glands in the labia of a woman's vulva. Incision may be necessary.

Amateur attempts to cure abscesses or a self-administered course of antibiotics can be very dangerous. Squeezing and poking boils can spread the infection and damage local tissue, so making it more likely that the infection will spread. If an abscess is caught very early, it may be aborted by a course of the right antibiotic but once it is painful and swollen then the chances are that pus will already have formed and that it will need to be incised.

Lastly, abscesses may spread. Should an abscess affect a tissue through which large blood vessels pass, it is possible that the inflammation will cause the blood (in a vein especially) to clot. A fragment of infected clot may then break away and lodge in an organ at a great distance from the original abscess site. This is how infection can get to the kidneys and brain from an abscess a long way away. A brain abscess can also occur as a result of direct spread from an ear infection.

Abscesses must be taken seriously and treated by a doctor as quickly as possible. Today, treatment is quick, simple and pain-free and can prevent many of the long-term problems that were seen with abscesses in the past.

# ACHALASIA OF THE CARDIA (CARDIOSPASM)

**What is it?**
A condition in which the lower end of the oesophagus (gullet) is in an abnormal state of contraction at the point where it goes into the stomach.

Typically, this condition affects young adults and may follow toxaemia of pregnancy. Difficulty in swallowing, vomiting and weight loss are the main symptoms and at night the oesophagus may fill up with saliva and flow back to spill into the lungs, causing coughing and pneumonia.

Non-surgical treatment includes dilating (stretching) the area in spasm using a bag filled with mercury (at the end of a catheter) swallowed just before a meal. Drugs can be tried but are of very limited use.

**Why operate?**
To cure the unpleasant symptoms and prevent irreversible damage to the oesophagus.

### How?

There are two operative procedures that can be used. The first involves the insertion of a special bag into the oesophagus down an endoscope (see page 387) under general anaesthesia. The area in spasm is then stretched as the bag is inflated with water. Sometimes this results in a complete cure.

By far the best results are obtained using a true operation at which the junction of the oesophagus and stomach is exposed (through the chest or abdomen) and the muscles of the oesophagus and stomach cut down to the lining membrane, which is left intact.

The slit is about twelve centimetres long and heals without any stitches. The abdomen and chest are stitched up in the normal way.

### Post-operative progress

If there are no complications, the person is out of bed within a day or so and can drink fluids soon after. Soft or puréed foods are then eaten, until by a week he is eating normally and allowed home.

The best results are achieved if the condition is caught early. If the oesophagus has already become very stretched and lax above the area of spasm, it will probably never return to normal. Many people have some heartburn after this operation but it can be cured by raising the head of the bed at night; sleeping with plenty of pillows; taking antacids; avoiding stooping and bending down; avoiding tight-fitting belts and underwear; and by keeping slim.

## ADRENAL GLAND OPERATIONS

The adrenal glands are small organs that sit one on the top of each kidney. They produce hormones which are passed directly into the blood stream. Each gland has two parts, an inner medulla and an outer cortex. The medulla produces adrenalin and the cortex many hormones, including those controlling the body's salt and water balance, those handling proteins and sugars and some sex hormones.

These valuable little endocrine glands are rarely the site of malignant tumours but benign tumours can occur. A PHAEOCHROMOCYTOMA is a benign tumour of the adrenal medulla. It causes bouts of high blood pressure, anxiety, difficulty in breathing, palpitation, headaches, trembling and sweating as excessive amounts of adrenalin produced by the tumour surge around the body. The tumour is diagnosed using special X-rays (intravenous urograms or angiography see pages 423 and 419) and by examining the urine for a special substance. The condition is cured by removing the tumour.

Tumours of the adrenal cortex produce all kinds of effects, depending on which cells are stimulated or destroyed by the tumour. CUSHING'S SYNDROME (in which the person has a rounded face, a hump at the back of the neck, and a pot belly) is caused by a tumour that produces too much of the gluco-corticoid hormones; ALDOSTERONISM (in which there is an increase in blood pressure, muscle weakness and spasms and a loss of potassium salts) comes about if there is an excess of the hormone aldosterone produced by a tumour; and the ADRENO-GENITAL SYNDROME (producing abnormal sexual development in children; masculinization of a woman, or feminization of a man) comes about when sex hormone-producing cells are affected. Such tumours are treated by removing part or all of the affected gland.

Because the adrenal glands play such a vital role in the body's hormone balance, some surgeons remove them to control hormone-dependent malignant tumours elsewhere in the body (in the breast, for example). This is not as common an operation as it used to be because other methods of treatment have been found to be as effective without depriving the person of such valuable glands.

The operation to remove the adrenal glands is carried out under general anaesthesia through an incision in the back or in the upper abdomen. The procedure is a major one but the person is up the day after surgery and home in two or three weeks. In the long term, hormone replacement will be necessary if both adrenals have been removed, and these tablets will be life-saving. If one gland is removed the body usually copes perfectly well.

If you are on steroid drugs either as a replacement therapy after removal of your adrenals or for another medical condition, be sure to carry your steroid card around with you and especially if you go into hospital for any treatment, particularly surgery. If in doubt, always tell your medical attendant that you are on steroids.

# AMPUTATION

### What is it?

The removal of a limb (or part of a limb) because it is so badly damaged that it is considered non-viable; because it is damaged by disease or affected by gangrene; or because it is cosmetically or functionally unacceptable to the owner.

Amputation is one of the most ancient of operations. Neolithic skeletons have been found with amputated bone stumps and in the fifth century BC, Hippocrates described amputation for gangrene. During the Napoleonic wars amputation became common and Napoleon was himself an amputee. Methods in those early times were crude but today amputations, whilst by no means pleasant operations, are technically more sophisticated, safer for the patient and easier to live with in the long term.

### Why operate?

With the increase in automobile accidents, injuries at work, arterial disease and diabetes, amputations are being done more in peacetime today then ever before even though surgeons go to almost any lengths to preserve a limb. This growth in numbers has also been brought about by better emergency treatment: a few decades ago a seriously injured person would have died of shock before he reached hospital and so would not have lived to have an amputation. Today, even in war (as in Vietnam recently) very seriously damaged men were 'patched up' in the field and given plasma to tide them over until they could be treated in a field hospital.

Having said this though, the majority of amputations today are done on elderly people with arterial disease.

The difficulties of deciding whether to amputate are considerable for the doctor in an emergency situation. Long-term diseases such as arteriosclerosis come on slowly and give both patient and doctor time to decide the best way to proceed but, even then, gangrenous changes can occur suddenly and will call for an instant decision. In accident cases it is often very difficult to know how things will turn out if the patient is left with a badly damaged limb which is cosmetically unacceptable and even possibly a disadvantage to him in his normal life. Luckily, this type of decision is more easily made today as plastic and reconstructive surgery advances and makes the long-term outlook more acceptable.

Even so amputation is an agonizing decision for doctor and patient alike. In several conditions, such as arterial disease, TB of the bone, leprosy and osteomyelitis, the underlying condition can now often be treated, which enables the patient to avoid an amputation altogether. Certain malignant tumours (notably some sarcomas) spread rapidly and still call for speedy amputation of the affected limb. Some congenital deformities require amputation. An extra toe or finger can be amputated simply, for example.

### How?

Methods of amputation vary according to the part involved but basically the principle is to cut away all dead, gangrenous or cancerous matter and leave only healthy tissue. Considerable psychological preparation is necessary before anyone undergoes an amputation. A good centre will explain exactly what will happen and will introduce amputees to the patient so that they can show him what life is like for them. With this encouragement, many people can more easily resign themselves to the loss of a limb.

Once the amputation site has been selected, the skin is cut away in flaps so that it can later be re-sewn over the bone stump to form a comfortable, rounded end. The surgeon then cuts through the muscles surrounding the bone. Very often a tourniquet is applied above the level of the incision so as to reduce blood loss but anyway the patient will have an intravenous drip going to ensure that blood can be given if necessary. Today's surgeon takes great pains to ensure that haemorrhage is kept to a minimum. This is important not only during the operation itself, when the patient should not lose valuable blood, but is also important post-operatively because in the event of small blood vessels leaking into the amputation stump, large collections of blood can occur which may become infected, slow wound healing, cause a painful stump, or even all three. Because even the most meticulous surgeon cannot stop all the minute bleeding, a drainage tube is usually left protruding from the skin wound so that no fluid builds up inside.

The muscles and other tissues are cut through and left sufficiently long to be able adequately to cover the sawn end of the bone. This is essential because a stump of bone covered only by skin would be painful and eventually ulcerate.

The bone itself is then cut through and the end sealed with wax if necessary. The muscles are sewn over the end and the skin sewn up to enclose it all in as neat and comfortable a way as possible. Good surgery at this stage makes all the difference to having a comfortable stump that will enable the patient to use a prosthesis (artificial limb) quickly.

A common concern expressed by potential amputees is just how much of their limb they are likely to lose. As we have seen, this is governed by the extent of the gangrene, cancer, damage or deformity and is sometimes difficult to forecast before the operation. More usually though, the surgeon will give a very accurate idea of what will be removed. If, in a leg, the frostbite or gangrene has affected only one toe and the rest of the foot is healthy, then only the affected toe is removed. If all the toes are affected (as they can be in diabetes, for example) the foot can be amputated across the middle and still leave a stump on which to walk. If a larger piece of the foot has to be removed then it is best to remove the foot and leg to just below the knee. This 'below-knee' amputation is also widely used for cases of gangrene resulting from arterial disease. Because the arterial disease results in a poor blood supply to the area, even one gangrenous toe may have to be treated by a 'below' or even an 'above' knee amputation. When a below-knee amputation is performed the good stump provided lends itself very well to a prosthesis and an intact knee joint means that very good movement is preserved.

The above-knee amputation is the next most commonly performed and enables a jointed leg prosthesis to be fitted effectively. Rarely the whole leg may have to be amputated.

In the arm, the position is somewhat different from the leg because our hands are so valuable. Even one finger and one thumb are worth saving as no prosthesis is anywhere near as good as the real thing. This means that emergency surgery is done to patch up and preserve tissue where possible and further reconstruction operations done later.

### Post-operative progress

The operation is over surprisingly quickly (almost always within one hour) and the patient is then on the way to recovery. The stump is bandaged several times a day with a supporting bandage which helps the swelling to subside. After a few days the drain is removed and after about ten days the stitches come out. Very soon after the day of the operation physiotherapists give post-operative exercises to strengthen the muscles in the affected limb because strong muscles are essential if the person is to do well with an artificial limb.

Fitting a prosthesis (an artificial limb) is not quite as easy as it sounds and involves skill and care by surgeon, prosthesis experts and all of those in the rehabilitation team. The most important member of the team is the patient himself. Unless he is keen on the new limb and willing to play his part, the whole undertaking is a waste of time.

Once the stump has healed, a temporary limb may be fitted. This gives the patient a chance to get used to an artificial limb and gives the experts a few months to assess the patient and prepare a permanent limb for him. Most people are only too grateful to the medical and other staff that something can be done to get them mobile again and so cooperate very well but co-operation can be hampered by post-operative depression or by the phantom limb syndrome.

Some people who have had a limb removed have the sensation that the limb is still present and causing pain. This occurs because the brain's pain centres are so used to receiving such stimuli that they cannot turn off once the stimuli stop coming. The pain is characteristically dull, boring and aching but it can be shooting and stabbing. It is often brought on by psychological stress or external stimulation. The body naturally re-adapts to this quite quickly and often after a few days there is no further problem. Some people continue to have the pains on and off for years, however. Two things can make phantom limb pain persist. Firstly, the person may be super-sensitive to pain and keep on reacting to the non-existent limb for months or years or, secondly, a swelling may form on the cut nerve stump – a neuroma – which is then irritated by the pressure of the prosthesis. Either way, phantom limb pain can be extremely unpleasant and is virtually untreatable. Many methods of treatment have been tried, including hypnosis, psychotherapy, the injection of local anaesthetic into the stump, cutting the sympathetic nerves (see page 273) and even leucotomy. Commonly prescribed painkilling drugs have no effect at all. It is scarcely surprising that treatment is so ineffective, given that we often have no idea of what causes the condition. It is a good thing that only about 5 per cent of amputees experience this unpleasant syndrome.

With a modern, lightweight, well-engineered prosthesis an amputee can be mobile again within days of the operation and completely independent within a few weeks of healing of the stump. Losing a limb is never pleasant but today it need not be the tragedy it used to be. Unfortunately, many amputations are done for arteriosclerosis which means that many patients also have cardiac or cerebral problems. These can slow post-operative progress.

# ANAL FISSURE

## What is it?

An anal fissure is a painful laceration (crack) in, or ulceration of, the skin at the opening of the back passage (anus). It is usually caused by passing hard stools. A fissure starts off as a small tear in the anal skin which is re-opened at each bowel movement. This tear can bleed and cause painful spasm of the anal sphincter on defecation.

## Why operate?

Treatment is necessary because of the extreme pain which produces a reluctance to open the bowels and creates a vicious circle of constipation – more tearing – constipation. An operation may also be advised if other measures have failed to cure the condition.

## How?

There are three simple ways in which an anal fissure can be treated. The first is the simplest and works in many cases, especially if the fissure is caught early. The sufferer should eat a high-fibre diet (rich in vegetables, wholemeal bread and bran-containing breakfast cereals). This, together with an adequate fluid intake, so softens the stools that the tear heals spontaneously.

The other two methods are operations and involve a stay in hospital.

The simpler of the two involves a stretching of the anal canal by the surgeon's fingers under general anaesthetic. This frees constricting bands of tissue that form over the months of constipation and, together with a high-fibre diet post-operatively, gives good success rates.

The third method involves cutting part of the anal sphincter muscle under local anaesthetic.

## Post-operative progress

Neither of the two operative methods involves more than a couple of days in hospital and both are likely to be successful if the person continues with a high-fibre diet post-operatively. Some people suffer from faecal incontinence (leaking) but many of them are better within two to three weeks. When someone has had this stretching procedure, he will return to the ward with a sponge in his back passage to help stop bleeding. This is removed one hour after the operation.

If you ever have bleeding from the back passage, do not simply change your diet to one containing more fibre and assume that the cause of the bleeding is an anal fissure. It may well be, because fissures are common, but any bleeding from the back passage should be reported to your doctor as it may be caused by a malignant growth in the rectum (a growth which needs urgent medical attention) or by haemorrhoids (piles).

# APPENDICECTOMY

**What is it?**
The surgical removal of the appendix.

The appendix is a small tube, the width of a pencil, that hangs down from the right side of the colon. One end is closed and the other opens into the caecum whose contents are fluid and flow in and out of the appendix. If a hardened mass of food (a faecalith) becomes lodged in the appendix, the muscular wall of the appendix cannot force the faecalith beyond the obstruction, so it swells, becomes red and starts to cause symptoms and signs. Pain is at first felt around the navel and then settles beneath a point at the junction of the middle and outer thirds of a line joining the navel with the easily felt bone at the front of the pelvis. Appendix pain can, however, be very different from this and the condition is often notoriously difficult to diagnose.

As time goes by, the obstructed appendix fills with pus and eventually bursts, spilling its infected contents into the abdominal cavity and producing a potentially lethal condition known as peritonitis. It is to prevent such a calamity that operations on the appendix are carried out. Sometimes a

surgeon will remove a perfectly sound appendix even when
there are no symptoms because it can cause problems should
it become obstructed. For this reason gynaecologists often
remove the appendix at Caesarean section and people in jobs
that take them far away from access to surgery, such as
astronauts, mountineers and long-distance sailors may
choose to have their normal appendices removed so that they
cannot be caught out and die unnecessarily.

Why appendicitis occurs in certain populations of the
world and hardly at all in others has never been adequately
explained but it looks increasingly as if it is something to do
with food. Countries in which highly refined foods are eaten
have very much higher levels of appendicitis than do those in
which plenty of roughage is eaten. There have also been
'epidemics' of appendicitis when a country or even areas
within a country have changed over to eating refined
'modern' foods.

Appendicectomy is the most frequently performed
emergency operation in the western world. Unfortunately,
the diagnosis is often difficult to make because the signs and
symptoms are not always typical and can mimic many other
conditions, especially in children and old people. This is
particularly dangerous because children and old people fare
especially badly if they are not operated on early for
appendicitis. For this reason surgeons have tended to operate
if in any doubt at all. This is now changing with the
realization that many of the appendices removed are normal.
In the US especially this has led to far greater care being
taken lest the patient sue for having had an unnecessary
operation!

### Why operate?
To remove an appendix which has, or might, burst so as to
prevent peritonitis or the formation of an appendix abscess.

### How?
Under general anaesthetic the surgeon makes an incision
about eight centimetres long in the skin of the lower right
abdomen over the appendix area. Once the abdominal cavity

is opened he assesses the situation. Sometimes, in severe cases, pus flows out of the abdomen and this has to be removed by suckers and swabs. Once he has assured himself that appendicitis is indeed the condition, he proceeds to remove it. He frees the appendix from its tethering tissue and then, after clamping and tying the base and inserting a circular stitch close to it, he cuts the appendix off with a knife and puts it in a bottle for pathological analysis. The circular 'purse string' stitch at the base is then pulled tight as the appendix stump is pushed back into the bowel and the appendicectomy is complete. The whole procedure up to this stage can easily be completed within ten minutes in some patients. However, the appendix may sometimes be situated abnormally and be difficult to find. In other cases the appendix may have formed so much pus that it has stuck to surrounding organs and formed an abscess. If this has occurred, the operation takes much longer. In these cases especially (but sometimes routinely) a plastic drainage tube is inserted into the appendix area so that the pus formed will drain to the outside once the wound is closed. On occasions the appendix looks completely normal so a surgeon will make a thorough search for an explanation of the signs and symptoms that made the operation necessary at all. This is highly skilful and even a very experienced surgeon may find nothing obviously wrong. He will remove the appendix anyway as a preventive measure and then close up the wound.

The appendix itself goes off to the laboratory for examination and unless a diagnosis is very obvious at operation the pathologist will have to search for other explanations. In children threadworms can cause trouble and a course of anti-worm treatment is necessary post-operatively. Rarely, a benign tumour is found. This requires no further action as it has by definition been removed along with the appendix. Most often though the appendix is simply inflamed and a small obstructing faecalith may be found.

**Post-operative progress**
The operation is over quickly in most cases and the patient

can get up the following day. Apart from feeling sore there should be no side-effects if the inflammation was caught early enough. These patients can expect to go home within a few days.

The patient whose appendix bursts and produces peritonitis is not so lucky. Because the intestines are often paralysed by the toxic waste and pus, a person with peritonitis cannot eat anything by mouth and has to be given food and fluids intravenously until the intestines start to work normally again. A tube is swallowed into the stomach (see page 403) and the fluid sucked back up at intervals. This lets the bowel rest and recover its activity slowly. The tube also allows gas to escape and so reduces the pressure inside the intestine. With these measures and the careful use of antibiotics when indicated, even severely ill people with peritonitis can be saved. Until fairly recently, peritonitis was looked upon with dread because it so often ended fatally. Today this is not the case and with careful management mortality is very low. Even so, it can take several days for the bowel to start functioning normally again and because there may be an abdominal drain in place, the wound does not heal so quickly. The person with peritonitis will probably be in hospital for two weeks and some have to stay in much longer. There can be problems in the long term as well after peritonitis. In some people, tight fibrous bands called adhesions are formed which stick the contents of the abdomen together and can themselves cause problems later. On occasions the bowel can become twisted or obstructed by these bands and another operation may be necessary to free it.

Appendicitis is a serious condition and far greater effort should be put into preventing it. It was always thought that the appendix had no role in man and that it could easily be dispensed with in the event of disease. Recent research is questioning this and it now appears that lymphatic tissue clustered in and around the appendix may play a vital role in certain of the body's immune systems. Perhaps a change to a high-fibre diet (which would enable many people to keep their appendices) could be justified for this reason alone. After all, the symptoms of diverticular disease (see page 173) can be abolished by eating dietary fibre, so why not try to prevent appendicitis? The evidence looks encouraging and the remedy is always at hand.

# ARTERY OPERATIONS

Although the commonest reason for operating on arteries is to redress the ravages of degenerative diseases such as atheroma and arteriosclerosis, which are often caused by smoking, surgeons also operate on congenital arterial abnormalities and on damaged arteries.

When the coronary arteries (that supply the heart) become narrowed, they produce the well-known symptom of angina. This narrowing can and does occur in other arteries of the body too and can produce angina-like pains elsewhere, especially in the legs on walking. When it occurs in the legs it is called intermittent claudication. Arterial surgery has come a long way in the last decade and can now be performed on very small arteries if necessary, using stitches as fine as a human hair. Synthetic materials can be used to bypass trouble spots and patches sewn on to larger arteries where they are weak or have burst.

An **ENDARTERECTOMY** is a procedure during which the surgeon removes or cores out the inner lining of a narrowed artery. This is rather like de-scaling a furred-up water pipe. The artery to be cleared is exposed and the centre cored out. New arterial lining regrows within several weeks. The incision in the artery is closed with many fine sutures so that it cannot leak. Results from this kind of operation are dramatic, provided that the rest of the artery is not so diseased as to prevent good blood flow after a local operation. Even if the chances of success are not very high, many surgeons will operate as thoroughly as possible, simply because the alternative is often amputation. The surgeon is helped in his decision by careful pre-operative X-ray studies called arteriograms (see page 419). Endarterectomy operations may take many hours because of the delicate nature of the surgery.

**BYPASS OPERATIONS** are now often performed when an endarterectomy cannot be done for some reason. The diseased area can be bypassed, so taking blood from one good artery to another. Synthetic, flexible, inert tubing materials are now used routinely to achieve this. Some surgeons use a long vein from the leg as the bypass channel. This is stripped out carefully from the leg, turned upside down (so as to render the vein's valves ineffective) and carefully stitched into place just as a synthetic tube would be. These vein grafts work very well and are commonly used in the heart.

Both endarterectomies and bypass procedures are commonly used in the legs to overcome the angina-like pains (intermittent claudication) that occur there in some people with generalized arterial disease. These pains can be cured in selected people by one or both of these procedures, so enabling the person to walk long distances, perhaps for the first time in years. The upper end of the graft starts above the obstruction where the blood supply is still good and the lower end is inserted beyond the obstruction in the lower part of the thigh. It is worth remembering that 70 per cent of those with claudication get some spontaneous remission with *no* treatment and many can live with mild claudication. Those with serious trouble are investigated and some of these will be suitable for operation.

A **SYMPATHECTOMY** is a procedure in which the sympathetic nerves that automatically control the width of arteries are destroyed. It is thought that some people have too much activity in their sympathetic control system and that because of this the leg arteries, for example, are in a constricted state for much of the time, resulting in a poor blood flow. Trials can be done with local anaesthetic to deaden the sympathetic nerves that supply the legs to see if doing so improves the person's condition. If it does, then a permanent deadening can be achieved by operating on the nerves themselves. Sometimes this is done with a further special injection which produces a permanent effect. The nerve trunks lie in the back on either side of the spine, and are reached through an incision which starts just outside the navel and runs horizontally around towards the back. Other types of sympathectomy can be performed if other areas of the body are affected.

A sympathectomy may also be carried out for reasons other than arterial blood starvation. It is sometimes done for excessive sweating; strange types of pain; and even rarely for severe period pains.

After major arterial surgery many patients will go to an intensive care unit for a few days (see page 51).

Another type of arterial operation sometimes performed is called an **EMBOLECTOMY**. In this a clot that is blocking off an artery is removed at an open operation. Such clots can occur in the femoral (main leg) artery, in the arteries behind the knee, in the armpit or in the artery that supplies the lungs. Their removal results in immediate restoration of blood flow to the area.

For coronary artery surgery see page 156.

# ARTHRITIS

**What is it?**
A family of conditions which produce pain in a joint or many joints. There are millions of people in the western world suffering from arthritis at any one time but by far the commonest of all the reasons for pain in the joints are rheumatoid arthritis and osteoarthritis.

**RHEUMATOID ARTHRITIS** is a generalized, whole body disease which happens to manifest itself most dramatically as painful, swollen joints. It is a disease that affects women more than men and often begins in early adult life. It may be of sudden onset or come on slowly over several years with non-specific signs. Generalized body symptoms often precede joint pain and swelling. Most typically there is pain in several small joints of the hands and feet. It is often symmetrical. Some people start off with one painful swelling of a single large joint, for example, the knee, while others begin with a soft tissue problem such as the carpal tunnel syndrome (see page 135) or an inflammation of the tendons.

Typically, the affected joints are painful, stiff and swollen. Large joints may accumulate fluid and the skin overlying an affected joint can become red and moist. Morning stiffness is a classical symptom of the condition and one which disappears as the day wears on.

Eventually, there is a loss of muscle power and bulk and resulting deformity of the affected area, especially in the hands and feet. Sometimes these deformities are so severe that the person cannot lead a normal life and may have to stop working, eventually even becoming crippled. In addition to these 'arthritis' signs there may be generalized body signs which include fever, weight-loss, tiredness, excessive sweating, swollen lymph glands, an enlarged spleen and eye troubles.

The management of the condition is almost entirely non-surgical. Mild, early cases respond to bed rest, splinting of the affected areas to rest them (especially at night) and drug therapy. Physiotherapy, special appliances, injections of steroids and powerful anti-inflammatory drugs are then tried. If all fails, surgical treatment of the affected joints may become necessary to reduce pain and cure deformities.

**Why operate?**
To reduce pain, increase joint function and return the person to as normal and independent a life as possible.

**How?**
Surgery for rheumatoid arthritis is very varied and what is done depends on what the problems are. Some of the things a surgeon can offer are: a repair of ruptured tendons; the transfer of tendons to replace damaged ones; the freeing of nerves (in the carpal tunnel for example, see page 135); the release of constricting bands of connective tissue; the fusion of painful joints so that they become rigid and pain-free; total joint replacement; and the removal of the synovial linings of joints (especially of the knees).

After operation, intensive physiotherapy is carried out and the person is taught how to use gadgets and aids to daily living, if necessary. Occupational therapy is often helpful to get the person used to new ways of coping with her disability.

**OSTEOARTHRITIS** (more correctly, osteoarthro*sis*, because often there is no actual inflammation which is what *-itis* means) is a degenerative, longstanding, wear-and-tear condition, affecting mainly the large joints. Both sexes are affected but as there are more older women about, it appears to be more common in women.

The joints involved are mainly the weight-bearing ones, including the joints of the spine. The end joints of the fingers are affected too, sometimes with knobs, known as Heberden's nodes. The affected joints are stiff and painful but only occasionally swollen. The problems are caused by joint wear; episodes of inflammation of the synovial lining of the joint; and degeneration and inflammation of the ligaments around the joint.

Pain is worst on weight-bearing and the stiffness is made worse by rest. People with this type of arthritis complain of a difficulty in getting going but unlike the stiffness of rheumatoid arthritis, it is not especially marked on waking. There may be a limitation of movement of the joint and eventually the muscles acting on the involved joints become weak and wasted. X-rays help confirm the diagnosis but blood tests are of no use (whereas they are useful in rheumatoid arthritis).

Rest is a key to successful treatment as are special exercises for the muscles acting on the affected joints. Physiotherapy at a hospital will relieve pain, build up muscles and increase the range of movement in the affected joints, and various combinations of wax treatment, electrical muscle stimulation, hydrotherapy and traction prove helpful in many cases. Drugs help relieve the pain in the joints and splints can be used to restrict the movement of painful joints during acute flare-ups or to correct deformities.

**Why operate?**

Surgery may be necessary if the pain cannot be relieved by any other methods or if there is considerable deformity or instability of the joint.

As severe deformity and loss of use are rare in osteoarthritis, people rarely have to change their jobs or way of life, unlike those with severe rheumatoid arthritis.

Surgery does not cure either of these types of arthritis but can restore use, relieve pain, improve the appearance of the affected area and enable the person to get back to productive work. Early surgery can also save neighbouring joints from being irreparably damaged by preventing the person from putting unnatural stresses and strains on them.

**How?**

Apart from the special operations that can be done for rheumatoid arthritis (see page 104) the following are commonly used in the surgical management of arthritis in general.

An **OSTEOTOMY** is a procedure in which a bone is cut across and re-fixed in a different alignment. An arthritic hip, for example, may be realigned to cure a limp.

A **SYNOVECTOMY** is an operation to remove diseased synovial membrane from a joint. This is a commonly performed operation suitable for many joints. Under normal circumstances the synovium produces lubricating fluid for the joint but in rheumatoid arthritis it becomes inflamed and swollen. This swelling stretches the ligaments that hold the joint in place and the joint can become unstable and disorganized, especially in the fingers. Removal of the affected synovial membrane reduces pain and can give the person normal use of the joint again.

An **ARTHRODESIS** is a procedure in which a diseased, often painful, joint is fused solid to prevent it from moving. There are several methods of joining the bones together, but they usually involve removal of the cartilage on each surface which allows new bone to link the two surfaces (as when a fracture heals). Steel pins or screws then hold the bones closely together.

Once a joint is arthrodesed, there is no real joint and, in time, the two original bones fuse into one. While all this is taking place (which can take up to six months) the area will have to be held immobile in a plaster cast if screws or pins have not been used, so as to give the area immediate immobility. An arthrodesis certainly relieves otherwise incurable pain in many people with severe arthritis but has its drawbacks, especially when it comes to the big joints. A fixed knee or hip is awkward to live with and it is often these people who end up having artificial joints to replace their diseased ones.

An **ARTHOPLASTY** is an operation to rebuild or replace a joint. A diseased hip, for example, is re-shaped by an extensive operation which may or may not include the replacement of part of the joint with artificial materials. Sometimes a joint is rebuilt using the person's own bone as a graft. Most often today arthroplasty takes the form of a whole or partial joint replacement. For more details of arthroplasties see Joint Replacement on page 236.

# BLADDER TUMOURS

### What are they?
Although benign growths can affect the bladder, most are malignant and affect men twice as often as women. There is a link between certain bladder tumours and carcinogens in urine. These are especially often found in men who work with benzidine and naphthylamine. Those working in the rubber industry are screened for bladder cancer regularly.

The first signs of a growth are blood or pus in the urine which is painful to pass. A cystoscopy (see page 163) confirms the diagnosis and a biopsy specimen is taken to be sure of the pathological changes before the final operation is performed.

### Why operate?
To remove the tumour and prevent its spread.

**How?**
Many bladder tumours are rather like warts on the inside of
the bladder lining. These can easily be removed using
electrical cutting equipment down an operating cystoscope.
The majority of bladder tumours can be removed like this
without an open abdominal operation. Cure rates for such
tumours (called papillomas) are very high because they have
not invaded the bladder wall and certainly have not spread to
the rest of the body. Even if such a growth recurs, it can be
removed in a similar way once again.

If a growth penetrates the bladder wall, the tumour or
even the part of the bladder containing it will have to be
removed. Rarely, the whole bladder will have to be excised. A
piece of small bowel (ileum) can be used to make a new
bladder which is then made to open on to the abdominal wall
and to empty into a detachable plastic bag.

Radiation therapy can be used for certain tumours,
especially inoperable ones. Occasionally, smaller tumours
can be treated by implanting radioactive gold grains, radium
or tantalum wire but external beam therapy is necessary for
most tumours.

As bladder tumours tend to recur, your surgeon may ask
you to return at regular intervals for a check cystoscopy.


# BOILS AND CARBUNCLES

**What are they?**
Collections of pus in the skin with local inflammation. Boils
occur most commonly on the back of the neck, in the
armpits, on the buttocks and on the face. They are painful as
they become tense and are especially so when they occur in a
tight area of the skin that has little 'give' as the swelling
grows.

A carbuncle is a boil that is deeper seated in the skin and
underlying tissues. It usually has several openings, may make
the person feel unwell and may cause a fever.

Heat in the form of a poultice or a covered hot-water bottle can be used to bring a boil to a head. The top eventually comes off and releases the pus. Pain is relieved at once and a dry, clean dressing is all that is required for a few days while the area heals itself.

If you have repeated or multiple boils you should see your doctor. He will test your urine for sugar because untreated diabetics tend to have more boils than do other people. You may also get more boils if you are severely run down, so again it is worth seeing your doctor.

## Why operate?

A boil may need surgical intervention if it does not heal itself or come to a head and burst. Some doctors prescribe antibiotics for boils, especially if there are many of them, but incising a boil is the best treatment.

## How?

Often, no local anaesthetic is used as the needle used to administer it causes more pain than the lancing of the boil. In addition to simply letting the pus out, the doctor may incise it and leave a wick coming from inside so that the cavity drains into a dressing placed over the boil.

Boils drained in this way, even if very large, heal quickly and often all that is needed is a painkilling tablet or two while the worst of the pain subsides.

See also Abscesses, page 85.

# BONE CANCER

Bone can give rise to both benign and malignant tumours. A malignant tumour of the bone marrow is called a *myeloma*. Bones are also commonly the site of secondary tumours from cancers elsewhere. The first sign of non-marrow tumours is often a bony lump or pain but in these the diagnosis cannot be made with certainty until a biopsy (sample) is taken and examined under a microscope.

Bone can be the site of primary cancers (though these are

very uncommon) but is very much more likely to be involved as a result of the spread of cancers from elsewhere in the body. An orthopaedic surgeon will see only one or two patients a year with a primary bone tumour but will see many with secondary deposits in bone. Many tumours, most notoriously breast cancer, spread in the blood to the bones where they may cause pain and fractures. Other tumours that commonly spread to bone are those of the lung, kidney, thyroid and prostate.

The presence of these secondary deposits can be confirmed with ordinary X-rays or by a special bone scanning procedure, neither of which is unpleasant to have done. When the secondary deposits depend on hormones for their survival, treatment with hormones can be very successful. Others may be helped a lot by radiotherapy. Usually, the underlying primary cancer will have to be treated but ironically it is often these bony secondaries that cause more problems to the cancer sufferer. Many distinguished research units all over the world are looking for ways of treating bone secondaries, so hopefully an answer will be discovered in the future.

MALIGNANT TUMOURS of bone are of many kinds but the commonest is called an *osteogenic sarcoma*. Sadly, it is often seen in young people and children and initial radiation therapy or drug therapy gives the best chance of a cure. The tumour spreads via the bloodstream to the lungs very early, so chest X-rays may be taken to look for this. If the lungs remain clear of the cancer for three months after the radiation therapy, then the limb can be amputated with a good chance of a cure. About a third of such people then live for at least five years. This is a far higher survival rate than used to be experienced when amputation alone was used.

BENIGN TUMOURS of bone can often be left untreated. If they are troublesome they can be cut away easily. Any pain there may have been is cured by removing the lump and these benign tumours do not recur.

# BOWEL CANCER

**What is it?**

Cancers occur both in the large and small bowel but very much more commonly in the former. Cancers of the small intestine are rare yet cancer of the colon is the second biggest cancer killer in the western world. Non-malignant tumours of the colon are also extremely common.

Rectal or colon cancer may show itself as a change of bowel habit; the presence of blood in the stools; weight loss; a loss of appetite; or even as general weakness. Anyone who has any of these troubles should consult his doctor.

The diagnosis can almost always be confirmed by a barium enema X-ray examination (see page 422) and a sigmoidoscopy (see page 407) will enable most of the tumours to be seen and biopsied. A stool sample may be taken to check for blood which may not be apparent as the red fluid most of us expect to see. In those people in whom the diagnosis is difficult, colonoscopy has revolutionized the accuracy of diagnosis and enables the surgeon to perform biopsies and even to operate on small cancers. For more details of this procedure, see page 386.

No one knows why cancer of the colon occurs, let alone why it is so common in the West. There are several theories but too much fat in the diet and too little dietary fibre (roughage) are two favourites.

Another problem in the large bowel is the benign growth on a stalk called a polyp. Very small ones occur in about one in ten of the adult population but they rarely cause symptoms. Larger polyps which cause symptoms occur and these need removal, as some become malignant if left.

**Why operate?**

Surgery is essential to remove the growth as it will eventually obstruct the bowel and threaten the person's life.

**How?**

Under general anaesthesia an incision is made over the

tumour for a length of about 20 cm. The tumour is located and the section of colon containing it cut away and removed. The two healthy ends of the colon are then rejoined at the same operation or possibly at a later one, perhaps leaving the person with a temporary opening of the bowel on to the surface of the abdomen (a colostomy, see page 147) in the meantime. This is especially often done if the growth had been causing bowel obstruction. By allowing the faeces to come to the surface of the abdomen, where they are collected in a bag, the obstructed area is rested and the person enabled to recover enough for the major operation to remove the tumour. Some people will have to have a permanent colostomy if the tumour occurs so low down near the rectum that the colon cannot be joined to the remaining rectal tissue. Many polyps and small tumours can be removed using a colonoscope (see page 386).

The length of the operation depends on how major a procedure is being undertaken at the one operation. A colostomy to relieve obstruction can be performed in half an hour and this may well be the longest that the surgeon would want to operate on a frail old person. The removal of the tumour itself takes between one and two hours and the most major of all these colon cancer operations takes about four hours.

A special word about bowel preparation is important here because today's good results at operation depend greatly on the state of the bowel at the time. Some surgeons will put the person on a low-residue diet and laxatives for a week so as to clean the bowel but others feel a shorter regime of total bowel washout is better for the patient because it is completed in 48 hours and produces a much cleaner bowel on which to operate. In this method the person has up to 12 litres of fluid passed down a nasogastric tube over a few hours. This runs through the bowel from end to end and completely clears it out. Many surgeons also use antibiotics pre-operatively to sterilize the contents of the bowel so as to reduce wound infections, which are common after bowel operations.

After the operation the bowel is rested completely by sucking all the stomach's juices straight out up a nasogastric tube. Fluid balance is maintained with an intravenous drip while bowel function returns to normal. This usually takes about five days after which light fluids and meals can be taken. This caution is very important because the stitching in the bowel could be torn apart if craggy lumps of faeces were allowed to force their way past the repaired area.

Recent advances with automatic stapling devices are making the joins more safe but most of the above precautions are still necessary.

## Post-operative progress

This varies according to the severity of the operative procedure carried out. The simple removal of a polyp via a sigmoidoscope can be done as an out-patient procedure but anything more serious entails more invasive surgery and so greater and more prolonged aftercare. As we saw above, you will have a drip for intravenous fluids and a nasogastric tube to keep the bowel empty, both of which will stay in place until the bowel's function returns to normal. This often takes about five days but can be longer. You will be able to sit up out of bed within a day or two of the operation and should be completely mobile again in about a week. If all goes well, most people are home again within two weeks or so of the operation unless it has to be performed in stages, in which case the stay could last for a month or two, depending on the person's state of health.

Success rates with operations for cancer of the colon are fairly good. Benign tumours and polyps are, of course, 100 per cent cured by an operation. Taking people with all stages of colon cancer (the very severe and the very early), about half are still alive at three years, and 40 per cent at ten years. If the growth has not spread outside the colon, more than 70 per cent survive for ten years. The most recent surveys suggest that people with cancers found even before they produce symptoms (as chance findings on X-rays, for example) have even higher survival rates than this.

The long-term problems after such surgery are few. Even if you have a permanent colostomy, you can still lead an active life and do exactly the same as everybody else (see page

148). It is amazing how people get used to caring for their colostomy and contrary to their expectations can often control it just as they did their bowel motions before the operation.

When a large section of colon and back passage are to be removed, people often wonder if it will affect their sex lives. The answer is a definite 'no' in women as they can achieve orgasm, suffer no loss of sexual drive and have babies normally. However, in men there may be a problem. Many of the nerves to the penis and its surrounding structures are removed with the tumour, especially if it is very low down and affects the rectum. If the rectum is removed for ulcerative colitis, the surrounding tissues are not removed, so sexual function is left unchanged. Many cancer patients, however, who have had the rectum removed complain that they have lost their sex drive or the ability to have an erection. This can be very unsettling and needs medical help but may cure itself over the first year or so.

Today's outlook for patients with this – the second commonest of all cancers – is brighter than ever and things are improving all the time as surgical techniques become more sophisticated.

# BRAIN TUMOURS

**What are they?**
The brain is the control centre for the whole of our nervous system and is contained in the rigid, bony skull for protection. It is an organ weighing nearly one and a half kilogrammes, consisting of nerve cells (on the outside mainly) which form the brain's grey matter and nerve cell connecting systems (on the inside) which make up the white matter. It is divided into several distinct parts which control specific body functions such as speech, mood, movements, eyesight and so on. Having said this though, we do not know for certain what most of the mass of the brain does.

Brain tumours can be diagnosed in several different ways. The person's story and a careful clinical examination are most valuable but specialized tests are used too. An EEG (electroencephalogram, see page 382) tells doctors what is happening to the brain in electrical terms and in the past several unpleasant investigative procedures involving the introduction of air into the cavities of the brain were used when brain tumours were suspected. These have now been almost entirely superseded by more accurate and totally painless procedures of which the best known is computerized tomography (see page 424). This invention has revolutionized the diagnosis of conditions inside the skull. It means that fewer exploratory operations are now performed and that once a surgeon decides to operate, he does so with a very good idea of what he will find.

Brain surgery is a very emotive subject because quite naturally we feel uneasy about a surgeon interfering with such a vital organ. However, even though surgeons obviously have to be extremely skilled to do brain surgery, most of the brain withstands surgery very well. A wrong move at an operation on certain parts of the brain can render the person paralysed or destroy an essential body function, so the surgeon is especially careful when operating in these particular areas.

Some simple brain surgery can be carried out by removing a small, one to two centimetre diameter plug of skull bone. Such a 'burr hole', as it is called, can give a surgeon enough room to evacuate a blood clot, for example. More extensive conditions will need a *craniotomy*. At this procedure several small holes are drilled in the skull and are then joined up with an air drill so as to make a flap of skull bone like opening a window on the brain. This gives the surgeon a much bigger opening than a burr hole through which to inspect the brain. Once the brain is exposed it has to be kept moist (as it is naturally used to being bathed in a fluid) and any bleeding is stopped as soon as it appears. Operating on the brain is a delicate job but there is no special magic about brain surgery.

Brain tumours are the most emotive conditions affecting the brain that need surgery but contrary to popular fear, the combination of tumour and brain is not necessarily a fatal one. Over a third of all brain tumours are benign and a further third are very slow growing and do not spread much.

Almost any of the specialized tissues in the brain can be affected by growths but about a fifth are growths of the outer covering of the brain – the meninges. These **MENINGIOMAS** are relatively easily removed and a complete cure is always the outcome. The same goes for **NEUROFIBROMAS**, tumours on nerves inside the skull.

**PITUITARY TUMOURS** account for 10 per cent of all brain growths and these can be operated on up the nose (the gland lies at the base of the nose in the skull) or via a craniotomy. Sometimes cures are effected with radiation therapy and no surgery is required. An **ACOUSTIC NEUROMA** is a benign tumour on the hearing nerve deep in the head. The tumour itself is not malignant but as it grows it presses on neighbouring brain tissue and can permanently damage it. Removal is often difficult but produces very high cure rates of the troubles caused by the tumour. Total deafness on the operated side is the rule.

The largest single group of brain tumours are the **GLIOMAS** and arise from connective tissue in the brain. The severity of the operation needed to remove a glioma depends entirely on where it is sited. Deep ones are difficult if not impossible to remove without damaging an unacceptably large amount of normal brain tissue and radiation therapy may be all that can be offered.

Brain surgery takes a long time, depending on the procedure, and operations lasting four hours or more are not uncommon. There is very little post-operative pain and the person is usually home in two to three weeks. Unfortunately it is necessary to shave all the hair off the person's head before the operation. This means that he will be bald until it regrows and this ironically can be more distressing than the operation itself. A wig usually makes all the difference.


# BREAST SURGERY

The breasts can become diseased like any other body organs. However, anything wrong with the breasts has especially unpleasant overtones for many women because breasts have become inextricably linked with sexual attractiveness in our society and, as a result, women quite naturally fear breast diseases more than many others.

By far the most important disease of the breast is breast cancer, which is the biggest cancer killer in women in the western world and accounts for about a quarter of all malignant tumours in women. Because one in 20 of all women dies of breast cancer today, it causes great concern and any lump in the breast is often immediately feared to be a cancer by a worried woman and her relatives.

If you think you have discovered a lump you must see your doctor who may send you to a surgeon. Often he can reassure you but even if he agrees there is a lump there is still a four to one chance that it will be innocent (not malignant).

Pain in the breast usually signifies an inflammation of some kind and most malignant lumps are not painful. A discharge from the nipple is always worth telling your doctor about because it can be an early sign of an underlying cancer. Having said this though, a discharge from the nipple is much more common in women with benign breast disease than in those with a carcinoma. A blood-stained discharge is a more reliable sign of an underlying cancer and should never be ignored.

Fortunately, the breast is an accessible organ and can easily be felt by the examining doctor. Experienced doctors get the diagnosis right more than eight times out of ten on clinical examination alone but mammography (soft-tissue X-rays of the breast) and biopsies of lumps play a vital role in confirming the diagnosis, sorting out confusing diagnoses and telling the surgeon the type of pathology involved. Mammography is particularly valuable in older women who do not have as much active glandular tissue in their breasts. In younger women this tissue can cause problems with interpreting the X-rays. A mammogram is done as an outpatient and so is a needle biopsy (see page 362).

The surgeon may then advise either an excision biopsy just to remove the lump or a biopsy for frozen section examination (see page 363) with a view to proceeding to mastectomy at the same operation if necessary. The sample of the lump is removed and then examined by a pathologist while the woman is still under the anaesthetic and on the operating table. His result comes back in minutes. If there is a cancer the surgeon removes the breast or part of it, whichever is appropriate for that particular woman. Because this procedure is carried out while the woman is under the anaesthetic, she will have had to have given consent to removal of her breast *before* the biopsy operation, thus giving the surgeon the permission he needs to go ahead if necessary. Of course, the breast is only removed if the biopsy shows the lump to be malignant or pre-malignant.

## Benign (non-cancerous) tumours of the breast

A FIBROADENOMA is a common non-cancerous tumour of the breast. It is a painless, firm lump and occurs mainly in young women aged 15–30. In young women such lumps are hard, very mobile and difficult to grasp. Because of this they have been called 'breast mice'. In older women these tumours grow larger and are softer. Such tumours are composed of fibrous and secretory tissue and do not become cancerous.

The treatment involves removing the lump just in case it turns out to be cancer.

A DUCT PAPILLOMA is a benign tumour (wart) that causes bleeding from the nipple. Such bleeding is not uncommon in young women and is usually caused by a benign condition. Nipple bleeding in an older woman (around the time of the menopause) is more likely to be caused by a cancer. Papillomas are easily removed through a small incision.

CYSTS are common because the breast is made up of glands which produce milk after the birth of a baby. Chronic mastitis is a poor term often used to describe the formation of many cysts in the breast, especially of middle-aged women, in whom it is common. There may or may not be pain but usually the first sign of trouble is the feeling of a lump. The breasts are firm and nodular and there may be pain or tension just before a period. The lumps may enlarge slowly or quickly.

A cyst can be 'needled' to remove its fluid and this is all that is required in many cases. If this does not cure the condition, it is probably best to have the lump removed to be safe, although the fluid the doctor takes off at the needling will often be carefully examined for cancer cells.

Removing a cyst is a simple procedure involving only a day or two in hospital.

Chronic mastitis can also rarely occur in men and can be induced by giving them oestrogens (as in the treatment of prostatic cancer, for example).

Surgery is not always necessary for this condition in women – many need nothing more than reassurance that cancer is not the cause of the lump and will be relieved of their pain by wearing a well-fitting brassière. The treatment of pre-menstrual tension with hormones helps too and usually this is all that is needed.

It has never been proven that chronic mastitis is a direct cause of cancer and as both diseases are common they can exist at the same time in the same woman. Perhaps the same underlying hormonal mechanism produces both diseases. This is a possible explanation as women who have had chronic mastitis are more likely to develop breast cancer.

## Breast Abscesses

Nearly ten per cent of all breast-feeding mothers with a blocked duct or mastitis will go on to develop a breast abscess in the weeks after the birth of their babies. However, these abscesses are almost entirely preventable and arise only because we in the West feed our babies in such a strange way. Because we breast feed by the clock (if indeed we breast feed at all), the breasts usually become engorged (swollen) and the pressure within them can block a milk duct. The blocked duct shows as a red, hot, tender lump in the breast and this often makes the woman shivery or feel 'flu-like.

First-aid measures for a blocked duct include feeding the baby more frequently (to empty the breast); massaging the lump gently but firmly towards the nipple; ensuring that the bra does not press on any particular area of the breast; varying the position in which the baby feeds at each feed and even within a feed; and using hot or cold compresses (whichever gives best relief). Antibiotics are only necessary to prevent infection if all these methods have not dispersed the lump within 24 hours.

If a blocked duct is caught early it will not go on to become infected and form a proper abscess (a walled-off, pus-filled structure within the breast) – indeed most blocked ducts do not become abscesses if treated as above. Once an abscess does form, though, it will (like abscesses elsewhere) need to be incised by a doctor to allow the pus to escape. If you have a breast abscess you should not feed the baby from that breast but you can continue to feed from the other one. Once the abscess has cleared up you can feed again from that breast. In the meantime, express milk from the affected breast and discard it.

### Cancer

As we have seen, this is now the commonest cancer among women in the West. It occurs in men too but does so 100 times less commonly than in women. It affects young women more frequently than any other cancer but the peak age of occurrence is at seventy.

The search for a cause for this killing disease has occupied many of the best academic and surgical units around the world for years. There is still no definite promise of a cure, even after all this research, and much effort is being expended on looking for causes with the hope of being able to prevent the disease.

There are, however, certain features in common in the backgrounds of women who have a breast cancer. Women who breast feed for long periods on an unrestricted basis and who have children young seem to be less susceptible to breast cancer but a lot more research needs to be done to see just how important this is. Unfortunately, so few women breast feed exclusively and for long periods (one year or more) in the West that it will be a long and difficult job to gather statistically significant groups to compare. Women with a close relative who has had breast cancer (a sister or mother) are twice as likely to suffer from this cancer as are the general population. Infertile women are at greater risk but child-bearing for the first time before the age of 30 seems to reduce the risk. It is commoner in unmarried women who have never had children and frequent pregnancies seem to protect against the disease. Dietary factors may be important and there seems to be an increased risk among women who eat a lot of fat and cow's milk.

The natural development of breast cancers is that some grow rapidly and others slowly. Some have already spread to bones around the body by the time they are first discovered and some remain contained in the breast for a long time. Survival rates for *untreated* breast cancer are depressing. About a fifth of women live for five years, although some live much longer. With the best treatment of the earliest cancers, more than three quarters of affected women are alive five years later and about a half ten years after the diagnosis is made.

### What can be done about breast cancer?
As with so many conditions in which there is no single cure-all technique, the field of breast cancer is a battle ground for the exponents of the many, varied treatments. There are no hard and fast rules and if one were to listen to twenty top breast cancer specialists discussing how they would want their wives' cancers managed, they would all have an individual viewpoint. Basically, the way that breast cancer is managed depends to some degree on what stage it has reached by the time the diagnosis is made.

In essence the idea is to control the local growth of the disease but some larger centres will perform several screening tests to see if and how far the growth has spread to bones and other organs. Many of these tests are done so that the doctors can learn more about this common and unpleasant cancer. In most hospitals not involved in research the average woman will not have lots of tests.

In order to see exactly where the tumour has spread the

doctor will examine the breast thoroughly. He will then take a biopsy specimen to ensure that it definitely *is* cancer. In some centres he will order a mammogram (soft-tissue X-ray of the breast), a chest X-ray and a series of X-rays of the skeleton to look for secondary deposits in bones. This latter may well be done in parallel with a radioactive bone scan or liver scan to look for secondary deposits in these areas. The team involved then decides upon the course of treatment to follow, taking each woman as an individual case.

Very simply, a cancer confined to the breast has a 90 per cent chance of complete cure but one that has spread to the lymph glands has only a 50 per cent chance of a cure. One that has spread to involve the bones and other organs is not cured by surgery alone but radiotherapy and other treatments will help.

**EARLY BREAST CANCER** is treatable with surgery alone or surgery in combination with radiotherapy and/or anti-cancer drugs. For many years now experts have disagreed about the extent of surgery necessary for cancer of the breast. It is now being discovered that radical (ie major) operations on the breast involving the removal of the whole breast together with muscle and lymph nodes under the armpit disfigure the woman badly yet produce no improvement in survival rate.

Because of this, today's surgeon does not usually recommend them. This change of practice is having a positive side-effect on women who, previously scared about being disfigured, now come to their doctors earlier and can be treated more easily. A recent survey in Cardiff showed that 20 per cent of women with breast lumps delayed getting medical advice for fear of being told they had cancer.

However, a crucial part of the treatment is still to get good local control of the disease. Because breast cancer can cause unpleasant ulcers if left untreated, it is most important to treat the primary lump adequately. For this reason many surgeons feel the best operation is to remove all the breast tissue by mastectomy together with some lymph nodes from the armpit for assessment by the pathologist.

A new operation is coming on the scene and has obvious attractions. In this operation, called a subcutaneous mastectomy, all the breast tissue is removed with the cancer inside yet leaves the skin of the breast intact. A silicone bag is implanted at the same operation and the woman comes round after the operation with a normal-looking breast. Some surgeons remove the lump and its surrounding tissues or excise the breast leaving plenty of skin and then insert an implant at a later date when the area has settled down. Other methods of achieving this same end are radiotherapy alone; simply removing the lump without radiotherapy; and removal of the lump with radiotherapy. Although a cure is more important than worrying too much about one's figure it is encouraging to know that more surgeons today are trying to reduce the psychological insult involved in losing a breast to the woman with breast cancer. Unfortunately, the successful treatment of most cancers involves removing the breast.

Even if the breast cannot be preserved, simply removing it and possibly taking out any affected glands under the armpit are all that is required for early cancer. Subsequent treatment depends greatly on the centre you are at. Some give radiotherapy and others reserve it until and if further trouble occurs. If radiotherapy is advised, it is not urgent but is usually started within a few weeks.

Most experts now agree that the term 'early breast cancer' is a misnomer because the latest research shows that even when the growth appears to be confined to the breast, it has often already spread throughout the body. Because of this one must sincerely question the value of women feeling their breasts each month for lumps as has always been suggested by health educators. If, as is now known to be the case, breast cancer has often already spread by the time a lump is felt, the way we currently manage breast cancer will have to be re-assessed. True, it is better to have a small lump removed than a big one but that is probably all that can be safely said. After that the disease, if it has spread, will have to be treated as for late cancer. Having said this though, it has been shown that women with small tumours live longer than those with large tumours, so perhaps there *is* a reason for continuing to feel for lumps and detecting them early. This is just one of many dilemmas and confusions surrounding the management of breast cancer.

**LATE BREAST CANCER.** Once a breast cancer has spread to involve the rest of the body, the management of the whole condition is carried out in this light. The lump in the breast may simply be removed to prevent it ulcerating through the skin and this may be combined with radiotherapy. Often, the simplest of operations is done for the most severe form of disease as the surgeon does not want to subject the woman to unnecessarily major surgery. Radiotherapy may also be used to treat secondary cancer deposits in bones so as to reduce the bone pain, which it does very effectively.

As breast cancers seem to be influenced by a woman's hormones, various kinds of hormonal manipulations have been tried as forms of therapy. Women who are pre-menopausal or within five years of the menopause can have both ovaries removed. About one third will have breast cancers that respond to this measure within three months of the operation. At the first sign of a recurrence these women can have their adrenal glands removed, which again seems to buy more time. As a last resort, the pituitary gland can be removed, thus removing the last hormone-producing gland that could affect the growth and spread of a hormone-dependent tumour. The last two operations are less common now as anti-cancer drugs are improving.

In those women who do not respond to the original ovary removal, male hormones can be tried and women who are too ill to have their adrenal glands removed at an operation can have them suppressed by a drug called dexamethasone.

Anti-cancer drugs have a place in the treatment of breast cancer but they are often reserved as a last resort after other things have failed. Several drugs are used together and the treatment may last for months. In pre-menopausal women but not in post-menopausal ones, anti-cancer drugs have been shown to lengthen the disease-free interval after mastectomy in some trials but not in others.

**Results**

The survival of women with breast cancer has hardly changed over the last ten years. Many trials have been carried out yet there have been no improvements worth talking about. There is, however, better control of the disease on the chest wall and of the secondary spread. There are many newer ways of treating problems, so the disease and the treatment cause much less trouble to patients than in the past. Newer treatments have fewer side-effects than the older ones so the quality of life is better even if the expected survival has not improved.

Women who have smaller cancers have been shown to have a significantly higher survival rate and a reduced probability of dying of cancer than those with large tumours but, having said this, eight out of ten women with breast cancer will die of the disease eventually although they may have no trouble at all for 20 years or more.

The trouble with any studies of treatments for breast cancer is that one has to know how many women would have died each year in the normal (non-cancer) population. Using these figures from life expectancy tables, a recent 20-year follow-up study of 982 women treated for localized, early breast cancer found that the number of deaths was twenty times that expected in the normal population.

This raises the question of screening the female population for breast cancer. Efforts to do this, using clinical methods and mammography (now thought to be the best screening method), have proved too expensive as they yield so few positive results, even among high-risk groups. Whether or not women should be encouraged to feel their breasts repeatedly for lumps is also a matter for debate, as we have seen. Undoubtedly, some early cancers that have not yet spread will be picked up and treated successfully, yet others will already have spread by the time they are found.

Women almost always wonder how successful treatment will be but it is very difficult to give guidance in any particular woman. We now know that breast cancers are such variable and varied tumours and behave so unpredictably that it is often quite wrong for a doctor to tell a woman she will have an X per cent chance of surviving five years. Each woman is unique in response to her tumour and it is impossible to draw hard rules. Medical knowledge is still so poor in this field that even the best expert cannot tell you with any certainty what your outlook will be.

Women's reactions to the diagnosis of breast cancer vary considerably, as would be expected. According to some recent research, those who cope well with the diagnostic label 'cancer' do better than those who do not. One recent study in a London teaching hospital looked at the psychological response of 69 women to their breast cancers and followed them for five years after their operations.

There was a statistically significant difference in the outcome of the disease five years later, which correlated well with the woman's psychological response to her cancer. Women who denied (to themselves) that they had a cancer and those who had a 'fighting spirit' survived cancer-free for longer than the others in the groups whose response was stoic acceptance or a feeling of hopelessness. No one knows why this should be but there are known links between the brain and the hormone-producing organs which may well be activated in the 'fighter' and 'denial' groups. A lot more research needs to be done on the links between mind and body in cancer before any final answers can be given on this subject.

### Post-operative progress
This depends very much on what was done. The simplest operation to remove the lump (often called a *lumpectomy*) causes very little pain, a small scar a few centimetres long and the woman can be home in a few days. Even the scar of a major operation is not unpleasant and fades quickly, being scarcely visible by one year.

More serious operations can produce considerable discomfort (ask for a painkiller) and possibly some swelling of the arm on the affected side. The swelling is caused by an accumulation of body fluid because the drainage system in the armpit has been tampered with. Movement helps reduce the swelling and physiotherapists will help with this. Most women are up and about the day after the operation and home within a week or two, even after the most major procedures. You will almost certainly have suction drains in the wound for a few days after the operation to remove any blood and tissue fluid that accumulates after any major operation such as this. These prevent infection, reduce bruising and help healing and are removed after a few days by the ward staff. The stitches come out at about ten days.

Some women complain of pins and needles or darting sensations across their chest after the operation, but these pass quickly.

If the surgeon has *not* inserted an implant at the time of the operation (which is most often the case), you will be given advice on a prosthetic device (a false breast). In the early weeks you can use a simple, inexpensive, light-weight, foam rubber pad to fill out your bra on the operated side and this makes most women feel a lot better about having to have their breast removed. It is also more comfortable to sleep with a light-weight prosthesis like this in a light sleeping bra. About six or eight weeks after the operation you can have a more realistic breast prosthesis fitted. This can be supplied free on the NHS or can be bought from a specialist firm or mastectomy centre. The best ones are made of liquid silicone gel in a silicone bag, are skin-coloured and feel (through a bra) just like a real breast. They come in various sizes, take up the body's own temperature and can be washed easily. Most women who have these are extremely pleased with them and people who do not know about their mastectomy are never able to tell that the breast is a false one. You do not necessarily have to have a special bra, although your hospital will fit a pocket inside your own bra (free of charge) so that your prosthesis can fit into it. You can buy special swimwear to take a prosthesis but most women find a normal swimsuit is just as good.

But looking normal to outsiders is only part of coming to terms with a mastectomy. As with so many medical conditions, people who have been down the same path before can be very helpful and mastectomy is no exception. The Mastectomy Association, 1 Colworth Road, Croydon,

Surrey, was started by a mastectomy patient and helps doctors and patients who want to know more about living after a mastectomy. Their sensitive and practical advice helps many of the thousands of women who lose a breast every year and this help often extends to their families and medical advisers too. That such an organization is needed can be seen from a recent study which found that one year after surgery for breast cancer a quarter of all the women needed treatment for anxiety and depression (compared with 5 per cent of a control group of women with non-cancerous breast lumps). One third had moderate or severe sexual difficulties (8 per cent in the normal group). Sympathetic help from people who have been through the same experience undoubtedly reduces the negative feelings and insecurity experienced by most women at some time after a mastectomy and many find that helping others in a similar situation helps them to come to terms with their problems. A woman's sex life continues exactly as before after her mastectomy – indeed the mutual understanding between a woman and her husband is often deepened by the experience. Many women have married after a mastectomy. If you are having periods, you may find you will get the same sort of discomfort on your mastectomy side that you would normally have had in the breast at this time of the month.

Remember that talking about it with your husband, family and friends is bound to help. Slowly they will all come to terms with your new condition.

# BROKEN NOSE

Broken noses are common and need treatment if there is displacement of bone and good cosmetic results are to be obtained. Sometimes there is simply a crack visible on the X-rays with little or no displacement of the bone. These cases are best left alone. Because the nose is so important a landmark on our faces, most men and all women are extremely keen to have deformities of their noses treated promptly and effectively. The diagnosis is made easily if the nose is very obviously broken but otherwise needs X-rays to confirm the break and to ensure that no skull fractures were caused by the same trauma.

A broken nose will almost always be re-set under general anaesthesia although in a few cases the bones can be pushed back gently after the application of a local anaesthetic in an out-patient clinic. Instruments are inserted into the nose and this, together with pressure from the outside, straightens out the pieces, which then unite.

The nose may be packed inside and a plaster of paris splint may be placed over the outside if the bone fragments are unstable. This stays on for a few days. There may well be extensive bruising and you could have black eyes for a week or so. Swelling is common and can take up to a month to go.

# BRONCHIECTASIS

## What is it?

A longstanding disease of the lungs in which widening of the bronchial tree (airways) is followed by infection. It can be congenital (present from birth) but is more often caused by measles or whooping cough in childhood. All chest infections in childhood should be properly treated and because they usually are, bronchiectasis is a relatively uncommon condition today. Bronchiectasis occurs in adults too in association with cancer of the lung, tuberculosis or after the inhalation of a foreign body.

A cough is the most common sign and this comes and goes. Lots of foul sputum is produced. There is often a fever, the person feels unwell and, if a child is affected, his growth rate is poor. Rarely, an abscess forms on the brain or the person coughs up blood.

X-rays help confirm the diagnosis so that non-surgical treatment can be started. This consists of very active physiotherapy to drain the affected segments of the lungs. Breathing exercises and lessons in coughing up the pus help enormously. Antibiotics may be used too.

**Why operate?**
If the disease is confined to one segment of the lung, the removal of that segment produces excellent results.

**How?**
Under general anaesthesia an incision is made in the chest over the affected area. A segment of lung or a whole lobe is then removed after getting the person as fit as possible before the operation. Surgery is uncommon for bronchiectasis today because the condition is now so rare and because antibiotics and physiotherapy control those cases that do occur.

# BUNION

**What is it?**
An acquired deformity of the big toe caused by wearing too tight or narrow a shoe. The shoe rubs on the first joint of the big toe and produces a painful, swollen lump. It is much more commonly seen in women than men.

**Why operate?**
To remove the painful, swollen lump and to improve the appearance and use of the foot.

**How?**
Under a general anaesthetic an incision is made over the affected area and either the bunion is trimmed off or a more extensive operation performed in which the bone and joint from which the bunion arises is cut off. The simple operation takes twenty minutes.

**Post-operative progress**
After the operation the person must not wear shoes that press on the scar and will need exercises, with or without electrical stimulation to the muscles of the foot. Normal walking can be resumed without pain after several weeks.

# CAESAREAN SECTION

**What is it?**
An abdominal operation to deliver a child from the uterus in a woman in whom a vaginal delivery is impossible, or dangerous to either the mother or the baby.

A Caesarean section is an operation that has become more widely used over the last fifty years than ever before. Although it was first performed (as we understand the procedure) in the sixteenth century and undoubtedly caused a sensation in earlier days, it is now commonplace and unremarkable – thanks mainly to great improvements in anaesthesia and operative technique. Many people believe, erroneously, that Caesarean sections get their name from the emperor Caesar, who was supposed to have been delivered in this way. This is thought not to be true but that the word Caesarean comes either from the Latin *caedere*, to cut, or arose as a result of a Roman law during the time of the Caesars that required that a pregnant woman who died before the birth of her child be delivered surgically immediately following her death. Caesar could not have been delivered in this way because his mother was alive during his life. Today, Caesarean sections are performed to save the baby's life and we tend to take the mother's survival for granted.

Early Caesareans involved making a vertical incision in the uterus' thick upper part that is well supplied with big blood vessels that bleed very profusely once the baby is removed. This problem has been overcome in two ways. First, the incision used today is made at the lower, thinner part of the womb and is transverse as opposed to vertical. By using such an incision not only is the baby more easily pulled out but the major blood vessels of the uterus are not cut. The uterus also heals much more strongly using this 'lower segment' operation and so presents less of a problem in future pregnancies.

The second great advance is the use of a drug which, when injected intravenously, causes the uterine muscle to contract, so compressing those blood vessels that are cut and closing them off.

With these two advances and the safety and availability of blood transfusions, if necessary, a previously somewhat heroic and potentially lethal operation is now performed safely millions of times a year all over the world.

## Why operate?

There are many reasons why Caesarean sections are carried out and they have undoubtedly saved many children, but no responsible obstetrician will undertake a Caesarean section lightly as it is a major operation and has its problems, as we shall see. Women with very small pelvic bones may have to have a 'Caesar' simply because the baby has insufficient room to come down the birth canal. In some women the uterus does not contract properly and thus endangers the baby by holding it too long 'in transit' in the pelvis. These babies have to be delivered quickly by Caesarean section to avoid possible brain damage caused by the shortage of oxygen that a prolonged delivery causes. Certain badly positioned babies have to be delivered abdominally or they would not come down the vagina at all. Maternal conditions such as an abnormally positioned placenta that would be in the way of the baby (*placenta praevia*); a placenta that separates too early (*abruptio placentae*); diabetes; severe, high blood pressure; certain cases of heart disease; fetal distress; a poorly-functioning placenta; previous Caesarean sections (especially in the United States); and genital herpes infections are all possible reasons for having to have a Caesarean section.

## How?

Under general anaesthetic or epidural analgesia (see page 391) the surgeon makes an incision twelve centimetres long in the midline below the navel or horizontally just below the bikini line. Once the abdominal cavity is opened the uterus is easily visible as a lilac/purple coloured mass, crossed by a lattice of arteries and veins. The surgeon quickly cuts horizontally through the thin lower part of the uterus, taking care not to damage the baby that lies directly underneath. He then inserts his fingers into the uterine incision and extends the hole. This displays the glistening sac of amniotic fluid which usually breaks spontaneously but may have to be cut. The fluid is sucked away by electric suckers.

The next step is for the surgeon to put his hand into the uterus and rotate the infant's head so that it appears in the cut in the uterus. Then, using either his hand or a special pair of obstetric forceps (see page 185) he delivers the head whilst an assistant applies pressure on the top of the uterus to help the baby out. About this time, an injection of ergometrine (a drug that makes the uterus contract and stops bleeding) is given and the rest of the baby delivered. The placenta is delivered and the uterine and abdominal walls sewn up in layers as in any other abdominal operation. The whole procedure up to the birth of the baby can be as quick as two or three minutes but once the baby is born the rush is over and time can be taken to close up the abdomen carefully. Because so many people suffer from appendicitis, some surgeons feel it wise to remove the appendix while they are doing a Caesarean section.

### Post-operative progress
A Caesarean section is painful post-operatively and effective doses of painkilling drugs are necessary for most women during the first day or so. After twenty-four hours in bed, many women feel like getting up gently and can start eating a light diet. Most women are up and about after forty-eight hours, but still experience some soreness, as would be expected after any abdominal operation. For this reason and because she may well still be suffering the after-effects of the anaesthetic, the woman may not relate well to her baby as quickly as she would after a normal delivery. A good hospital will encourage her to hold and feed her baby as soon as possible and this can be achieved more easily if the woman has her Caesarean section carried out under epidural analgesia. This enables her to take more part in the birth, to handle the baby as soon as it has been delivered and even put it to the breast while the operation is still under way.

Mothers allowed to do these things suffer less post-operative pain.

Although some women think a Caesarean section might be a 'chic' or easy way out of having a baby, nothing could be further from the truth, especially for a normal mother and baby. Any operation can be followed by post-operative troubles, from constipation to life-threatening pulmonary embolism (see page 36) and so should not be undertaken lightly. It probably takes as long as six weeks for the Caesarean-delivered woman to become as fit as her normally-delivered sisters and in the meantime the mother/baby relationship may suffer because she feels 'low' or is in pain. Most women who have a Caesarean section are in hospital for seven to ten days.

Some doctors nowadays feel that a Caesarean section is a contra-indication to breast feeding as it is an 'added strain' to the mother. It is true that a doped, post-operative mother may not feel as willing or able to feed as a normal mother but if a woman really wants to feed her baby there is no reason why she should not after a Caesar. The only problem is finding a comfortable position in which to lie so that both mother and baby are happy. This can be tricky in the early days especially as the milk takes longer to come in after a Caesar.

One of the greatest worries women who have had a Caesar have is whether they will be able to have a baby normally again. Opinions vary on this. In the United States the principle, 'once a Caesarean, always a Caesarean', is widely adhered to but in the Commonwealth, many patients previously delivered by Caesarean section are allowed, under proper hospital conditions, to try for a normal delivery. Studies show that only 0·25 per cent of lower section uterine scars rupture in late pregnancy or labour if a normal delivery is embarked upon. Also there are very real dangers to repeated abdominal operations. Although post-operative mortality is less than 0·1 per cent, all post-operative patients have pain, many require blood transfusions, most develop some bowel distension, fevers are not uncommon and wound infection occurs in 1·5 per cent of women. Add to this the hazards of any operation (see page 54) and you can see that a normal birth is best, if at all possible. Some women though have to have repeated Caesarean sections and the procedure can probably be safely repeated at least three times before considering sterilization.

After a Caesarean section a woman's figure is just as firm or flabby as it would have been after a normal delivery and, provided she follows post-natal exercises as instructed by the doctor, she should have no muscle weakness. The scar usually heals well and if made low enough can be completely covered by pubic hair as it regrows after the operation. It takes about a year for the scar tissue to look like normal skin and eventually it can only be seen with difficulty as a very thin white line. If a repeat Caesarean section is necessary, the old scar is re-opened.

Women who have had Caesarean sections can return to sex as early as (or even earlier than) their normally-delivered sisters. Fertility is not altered because although the uterus is scarred this is not in the area in which the egg usually implants, so all is well.

Most women are going about their daily life as usual by four to six weeks after the operation but it is advisable not to do anything but the lightest housework for the first month.

# CARPAL TUNNEL SYNDROME

**What is it?**
A condition in which there is pressure at the wrist on a nerve to the hand as it goes through the 'tunnel' formed by the bones of the wrist behind and a tough band of fibrous tissue in front.

There are many causes of this condition, which is more often seen in women than men. A fracture of the wrist; arthritis of the wrist; inflammation of the tendons in the wrist; generalized water-logging of the body (oedema); an underactive thyroid gland; and pregnancy are all possible causes.

Typically, the woman complains of pain early in the

morning which may waken her. She gets relief by swinging her arms as she paces round the room. The pains radiate up the arms and doctors may mistakenly think that arthritis of the neck is the underlying trouble. The diagnosis can be difficult to make but several tests can be done to help. A blood pressure cuff put around the upper arm and inflated often reproduces the symptoms of the condition; nerve conduction tests are sometimes abnormal (because of the pressure on the nerve in the tunnel); and there may be a loss of sensation in part of the hand.

### Why operate?
To relieve symptoms and prevent further damage of the nerve to the hand.

The method of treatment used depends to some extent on the underlying cause of the condition. A pregnant woman who is getting trouble because of a build-up of water in the tissues in the carpal tunnel will not want or need an operation because when she has given birth she will be free from her symptoms. A woman with an underactive thyroid gland needs treatment for that and effective treatment of arthritis affecting the wrist may also mean that an operation will not be necessary.

Most women, though, do not fall into these groups and will need an operation if other conservative measures fail. Local injections of hydrocortisone into the carpal tunnel work in a percentage of sufferers, as do night splints made of plaster or plastic and some doctors get good results using small doses of diuretic (water) drugs which encourage the kidney to put out more urine. If all these fail, an operation may be necessary.

### How?
The operation is simple and takes about half an hour. It is done under a general anaesthetic. An incision is made in the band of fibrous tissue at the front of the wrist. This relieves the pressure in the tunnel. The skin incision is very small and is unnoticeable after a few months. This operation cures the condition in many cases but the result is not always

perfect. Various studies show that from one per cent to 25 per cent of sufferers have residual symptoms after the operation. New work in the US is beginning to suggest that the condition may not require an operation at all and that it might be caused by a deficiency of zinc in the body. More research is under way on this.

# CATARACTS

### What are they?
Opaque areas in the lens of an eye that can cause impaired vision. There are many different types. Some are present at birth; some occur after injury to the eye; others are a reaction to toxic substances; but by far the most common are senile cataracts.

With a cataract the lens of the eye becomes less transparent, either all over or in spots or stripes. Most cataracts are invisible from the outside without special instruments until the lens becomes milky-coloured and nearly opaque. At this stage it looks as though the person has a milky white or grey pupil. The person who has a cataract notices that his vision is gradually worsening, becoming more 'frosted' over the years.

Opacity of the lens in the eye is probably a sign of normal ageing but most very old people can still see perfectly adequately even with some 'frosting' of the lens. The condition progresses very slowly in old people but more actively in young ones. Some diabetics get cataracts which progress very rapidly. There is no drug cure for cataracts.

### Why operate?
Early on, glasses can correct the visual problems but surgery is the only permanent answer for severe cataracts. Unfortunately, many of those seen by an ophthalmologist for cataract removal are already very old and have poor retinae (the light-sensitive linings to the backs of the eyes). Surgery in these people often provides very little improvement.

## How?

No longer are people prepared to accept the poor vision caused by cataracts: they get treatment earlier and are completely cured in the majority of cases. New instruments, fine sutures (stitches) and enzyme treatments have all revolutionized the surgery of cataracts in the last decade. Nearly everyone can have his lens taken out safely, whatever its state, under local or general anaesthesia.

When cataracts are present in both eyes both can be done at once though most often one will be done before the other and the worse eye is operated on first. If both eyes are done at the same operation this will totally confuse the sufferer because he will see things so differently afterwards.

Using a low temperature cryoprobe to hold the lens and an enzyme (alpha-chymotrypsin) to dissolve the structures that hold it, the lens can be removed whole, making cataract surgery safe, quick and with the minimum of side-effects. In one operative method the incision in the eye is only three millimetres long and the lens is broken up with ultrasound and sucked out. All the methods enable the person to be up and about quickly and to watch television the day after the operation. After the removal of the lens, the eye is sewn up with extremely fine sutures. Such delicate operations on the lens (and indeed on the eye generally) are made easier (and even possible in some cases) by the everyday use of operating microscopes.

## Post-operative progress

One of the great advances in the management of cataracts has been the improvement in post-operative care. In order to be able to see after a cataract removal the person has to have a substitute lens. Ideally, the replacement should be in the same position as the original lens but intra-ocular lens implants are still fraught with difficulties so spectacles or contact lenses are the only answers. Because these lenses are further away from the retina than Nature's lens, they have to be less powerful to get things in focus.

If the person has only one lens removed his other eye will

produce a normal-sized picture of the world. This bombards the brain with two images, one bigger (produced by the eye without a lens) than the other and this can be very disturbing. If only one eye is affected, the eye with the better vision is left in case the better eye suddenly fails because of another condition. Should it do so, the other eye and its spectacle lens can take over and prevent the person being 'blind' until the cataract is removed. Even with spectacle lenses the going may not be easy because it is only at the centre of a powerful lens that objects are viewed in perfect focus. At the edges of such a lens there is unpleasant distortion. Contact lenses are the ideal answer but some old people who do not have good manual dexterity do badly with them and even young people still need glasses for near work such as reading. This is because the eye loses its ability to focus on near and far objects without a lens. Bifocals can overcome this problem if contact lenses are not suitable for some reason.

All cataract sufferers do very well after an operation and may be home within a week. Double cataracts fare slightly less well and some surgeons use intra-ocular implants to return them to normal. Implants are useful in the elderly, in people who have a cataract on one side only and in those who would not manage well with contact lenses. When intra-ocular implants work they are very successful indeed.

# CEREBRAL ANEURYSM

### What is it?
A 'blow out' in the wall of an artery in the brain. The causes are uncertain but there can be a weakness from birth in an artery in the brain. The aneurysm usually produces no symptoms, until it bursts. When it does so it causes a stroke.

### How?
Surgery is required to seal off the aneurism. More rarely today the carotid artery in the neck that supplies that side of

the brain can be tied off. Surgery to clip or tie off the actual 'blow out' area is left for a few days until the person is fitter.

# CERVIX OPERATIONS

## Biopsy
If a Pap smear (see page 374) suggests malignant changes in the cells of the cervix, a surgeon may recommend that he takes a biopsy (sample) of the tissues so as to get a larger piece to examine under a microscope. The operation is simple and is performed in a few minutes under general anaesthesia. A woman with the pre-cancerous condition known as *carcinoma-in-situ* will be cured simply by removing completely the tiny amount of tissue required for this microscopic examination. Follow-up smears will confirm that this has occurred. In some specialized units a low-powered microscope called a colposcope can be used to look at the cervix without the woman having to be admitted to hospital at all. Colposcopy, with special staining of the cervix, may enable a specialist to identify abnormal cells and so ensure their removal at biopsy.

## Cauterization
Vaginal discharge can be caused by many conditions but an inflammation of the cervical canal (*endocervicitis*) is one easily treatable cause. Chemical or, more usually, electrical burning (cauterization) of the superficial tissues of the cervix, often done without an anaesthetic, cures the condition. New methods using cryosurgery (very low temperatures) are now widely used too. There may be a slight brown discharge for a few weeks and bleeding may occur for a few days after the procedure but otherwise there are no side-effects.

## Cancer
Cancer of the cervix is the second most common cancer in women and is the most frequent type seen in the genital

system. It is becoming less common, perhaps because more women are being caught early as a result of cervical smears (see page 374) being done widely. Once a Pap smear has proved positive, a biopsy will be done to confirm the diagnosis. Treatment depends on the stage of the disease but radiation and surgery may be used singly or in combination.

Radiation techniques are improving and as the procedure is less troublesome than surgery, it is increasingly used for this cancer. In certain cases, surgery will be essential to remove the cervix, upper vagina, uterus, fallopian tubes and even the ovaries.

The results of treatment are excellent if it is started early. Sixty per cent of all women with cervical cancer (including the very severe cases) are still alive five years later and for women who have localized cancer, the figure is nearer 80 per cent.

It is not entirely proven that cervical smears reduce the incidence of this disease or even that *carcinoma-in-situ* progresses to become true carcinoma. Obviously the smear programme has been helpful in picking up some cases and is probably worth continuing. However, there is evidence that the group of women most at risk are not the ones having Pap smears done (see page 374).

# CIRCUMCISION

**What is it?**
The removal of the foreskin of the penis in males. Female circumcision, in which part of the external genitals is removed and/or sewn up, is not practised in the West and will not be described here.

Circumcision is not often carried out today but may still be done for religious or, more rarely, medical reasons. Whereas the operation used to be favoured by doctors and parents alike, doctors are now loath to do it unless there is a good reason. The days of routine circumcision have gone. This change has come about because it has been realized that circumcision can lead to infection, bleeding and scar tissue formation and that there are always some dangers involved in general anaesthesia, however small.

Some doctors still carry out circumcisions at birth without an anaesthetic but many think this unreasonable because it is obviously very painful and is usually unnecessary. Jewish boys are circumcised on the eighth day after birth and Muslim boys between their third and fifteenth year.

A newborn boy's foreskin is united to the tip of the penis and only becomes separated later. This separation usually occurs by the third or fourth year but can be later than this, so do not worry about consulting your doctor if your son's foreskin cannot be pulled back before he is five. The first school medical examination is the time to mention any problems.

The best way to look after your baby son's foreskin is to leave it alone. However, once it becomes easily retractile, pull it back gently to wash behind it at bath time. This enables you to clean away any white matter (smegma). If you force the skin back you could tear the tissue and make subsequent circumcision inevitable.

### Why operate?

There are very few reasons for doing a circumcision today. Religious reasons are now the major ones but there are a few medical ones too. Repeated infection of the tip of the penis (*balanitis*) or a foreskin that looks like being permanently non-retractile at the age of five are two such indications. A tight foreskin (*phimosis*) that balloons out as the child passes water can be a real nuisance and may need to be treated by circumcision. In adults a circumcision may be done if there is difficulty or pain on intercourse, if the foreskin is tight, or for repeated infection of the penis tip.

### How?

Whilst traditional Jewish methods involve the use of no anaesthetic and a few doctors still perform this procedure in infancy without anaesthetic, this is now unusual.

Circumcision is a simple procedure. The foreskin is pulled back by the surgeon and freed so that it retracts easily. He then cuts it around its base, removes the excess skin and stitches up the cut edges around the rim at the base of the head of the penis.

## Post-operative progress

Most babies can be out of hospital either the same day or the next and there are usually no complications. The stitches will dissolve on their own within a few days as the area heals. The operation performed in adults may leave the man a little sore for a few days but is usually as uncomplicated as that in children. Intercourse can be resumed when healing is complete, in about two to three weeks. Many men feel conscious that their penis tip is very sensitive as it rubs against their underpants. This is because the skin of the penis has been protected for so long and now needs some time to become desensitized to constant stimulation. This sensitivity usually disappears in a few weeks.

Many men are concerned about whether a circumcision will affect their sex lives. In short, it should have no effect at all. Women like penises whether they are uncircumcised or not and surveys show that both types appeal equally. In the early days when the penis tip is very sensitive a man may find he ejaculates sooner than he would like to but the effect soon wears off as the penis skin sensitivity returns to normal.

# CLEFT PALATE AND LIP

## What are they?

Defects, present from birth, in the roof of the mouth and the upper lip. The conditions come about as a result of imperfect development before birth in the ninth week of fetal life but no one knows why this should happen. Genetic and environmental factors have been blamed.

The child may have either a cleft lip (hare lip) or cleft palate or both together and the degree of tissue and bone loss can vary considerably. Cleft lip occurs in about one in a

1000 babies and cleft palate in one in 2500. Twelve per cent of these children have a relative with a cleft palate.

A cleft palate or lip is usually first noticed at birth but some cleft palates only come to light when the baby does not feed properly. Breast feeding may be difficult but breast milk can be expressed (by hand expression or using an electric pump) and the milk given using a special teat or with a spoon. A special plate appliance can be fitted by an orthodontic surgeon to help the baby suck properly. A cleft lip on its own rarely causes a feeding problem.

Cleft lips are usually repaired surgically by the age of three months but another operation may be needed at about four or five years to improve the cosmetic appearance of the area. The timing of a cleft palate repair depends on each individual case.

The treatment of a cleft palate and lip begins soon after birth and can take years to complete. If the infant has clefts affecting both sides, the bones of the upper jaw may need realigning. This is usually achieved using a prosthesis supplied by an orthodontist. After each feed the prosthesis has to be removed and washed before being replaced.

**Why operate?**
To improve the child's appearance; to enable him to eat, speak and drink normally; and to ensure the proper development of the upper jaw and its future teeth.

**How?**
The baby is admitted two days before the operation to check that he is not anaemic and that his nose and throat are free from infection. If there is infection the operation is postponed while antibiotic therapy eradicates it. Cleft lips can be relatively easily repaired but a cleft palate may need several operations to get a perfect result.

**Post-operative progress**
Immediately after the operation the baby is watched very carefully and his mouth and pharynx sucked out to keep the

breathing passages open. The baby's arms are splinted so that he does not pull at the lips or the stitches while they are healing. This takes about ten days.

Feeds are restarted about four hours post-operatively. The baby is fed with a cup and spoon which he will already have been used to pre-operatively. If there is a lot of saliva that he cannot swallow, apply a barrier cream to prevent soreness of his face. Ensure that after each feed his mouth area and around the stitches is cleaned with saline and gently dried. The stitches come out on the seventh day but a device may be used to take tension off the stitches up to as long as the tenth day.

Although the first operation makes the child look substantially normal, further operations may be necessary as he grows. A very good result can now be obtained in all but the most severe cases.

A cleft palate is usually operated on much later than a cleft lip – at about 15 months. These children tend to get more upper respiratory infections than other children and such infections need careful and immediate treatment if they are not to spread up the eustachian tubes to cause middle ear infection.

Although 80 per cent of children with a cleft palate repair end up speaking normally, some have problems later with certain sounds, especially 'k', 'p', 't', 'g', 'b' and 'd' and need long-term speech therapy. There may also be long-term dental problems and hearing loss.

Teamwork between the surgeon, dentist, orthodontist, speech therapist and parents is essential if the child is to end up substantially unaffected by his cleft. This is usually available but requires considerable strength and perseverance on the part of the parents over several years and may be worrying and wearing for them. Most agree that the effort is well worthwhile.

# CLUB FOOT

**What is it?**
A deformity of one or both feet, present from birth, in which one or both point unnaturally upwards or downwards or are twisted so that the sole faces inwards or outwards.

Many babies are born with feet that are positioned strangely, often as a result of the way they were lying in the womb. If the bad position can be easily corrected (as is usually the case) the condition rights itself; perhaps with the aid of simple exercises. If only one foot is affected, or if correction is difficult or impossible, medical treatment will be needed.

Although most children with a club foot have the deformity as a result of their position in the uterus, others may inherit it and yet others have it in conjunction with spina bifida. More unusually, club foot can be acquired in later life, for example with cerebral palsy or poliomyelitis.

**Why operate?**
The condition will need treating if the child cannot put his foot down flat to walk. He may then develop irreversible deformities of the bones of the feet and so be unable to walk properly. As most babies with club feet are otherwise completely normal, it is essential to get treatment early.

**How?**
Treatment can be started soon after birth. A physiotherapist straps the feet and ankles three times a week and shows the mother how to do it at home herself. Special splints and casts can be used to hold the feet in a more normal position until they stay there of their own accord, but more serious cases will need surgery. Tendons can be lengthened or shortened as necessary and fibrous tissue stripped away from the bones. A plaster cast is then applied to retain the normal position while healing occurs. Older children may need to have certain foot bones joined rigidly together in order to correct the condition.

## Post-operative progress

The plaster stays on for four weeks, after which it is removed and physiotherapy exercises for the foot and ankle are resumed.

# COLOSTOMY

## What is it?

An opening on the abdominal wall through which a piece of colon (large bowel) discharges food residue to the exterior. It is performed when the colon and rectum have had to be removed, usually for cancer or inflammation. It may be temporary (as with diverticular disease, see page 173) or permanent.

Colon tumours that are high up in the organ (far away from the back passage) can be removed and the colon joined up again. However, if the trouble is in the rectum it is more difficult to make the join safe so a temporary colostomy may be necessary to allow time for the area to heal. If the tumour is low in the rectum it may be necessary to remove the back passage as well, thus leaving a permanent colostomy. Surgeons are developing new ways of avoiding this situation for some, but in a really low growth it is still best to have it removed fully and to accept a colostomy.

A colostomy is different from an ileostomy (see page 224) in that the opening is flush with the skin (an ileostomy protrudes beyond the surface); the faeces are formed and discharge intermittently (an ileostomy produces fluid faeces which are discharged continuously); and there is no irritation of the surrounding skin (an ileostomy is easily irritated and the surrounding skin made sore by the fluid contacting the skin). A colostomy can, however, be smelly whilst an ileostomy is usually odourless.

The action of a colostomy in some cases can be controlled in the same way as normal bowel movements and with some practice many colostomists live perfectly normal lives while some do not wear a bag at all – they know when their bowel actions will be.

Colostomies have got a bad reputation because they are often used to relieve obstruction caused by an underlying cancer. This leads many people to think that because their friend or relative died within a relatively short time of having a colostomy, they will too. This is, of course, not true. Many people have colostomies for other reasons and a colostomy itself does nothing whatsoever to shorten life.

Many of the general remarks about ileostomies apply to colostomies so the reader should turn to page 224 for more information. More detailed information is available from your doctor or specialist. There is a self-help group for colostomists just as there is for ileostomists (see page 429). This has branches all over the country and currently helps 7,000 colostomy patients each year. It has useful literature and trained voluntary visitors who can help both before and after the operation. Some hospitals have their own nursing sister to help with these problems. She is called a stoma therapist.

# CONGENITAL HEART DISEASE

**What is it?**
Heart disease present at birth, usually taking the form of a malfunction or maldevelopment of a part of the heart. The heart is a complex organ and abnormalities are relatively common. Also the circulation of a fetus is different from that of a newborn baby and faults can occur during the changeover from one system to the other. The last decade has seen great strides in the treatment of children with congenital heart defects and today most can be treated satisfactorily.

No one knows what causes these diseases. Drugs taken early in pregnancy when the heart is developing have been examined but there are no definite clues yet. German measles suffered by a pregnant woman certainly is a cause of some of the defects but apart from this we are none the wiser.

Doctors divide congenital heart diseases into those that

make the baby blue (*cyanotic*) and those that do not (*acyanotic*).

A careful examination of the heart forms part of the doctor's routine examination of every newborn baby. Similarly, during early childhood, it is well worth having your child's heart listened to routinely by your clinic or family doctor, as a heart condition may otherwise go unrecognized. Though some congenital heart conditions improve spontaneously, others get worse as the child grows older and may sometimes prove fatal without medical or surgical help.

Many newborn babies have heart murmurs but the vast majority of these murmurs are innocent – they do not represent an abnormality and often disappear in a short time. There are many sorts of murmurs, some of which point to an underlying congenital heart abnormality which will usually need investigation and perhaps even treatment. Some congenital abnormalities of the heart are apparent at birth but others are not diagnosed until the child is older.

The abnormalities which may be present in the heart at birth include narrowing of the heart valves; a hole between the upper or lower chambers of the heart; the persistence of fetal blood vessels which normally close around the time of birth; and more complicated conditions such as Fallot's tetralogy, the classical blue baby condition, in which there are several defects. Some children are born with a normal heart in the right side of the chest instead of the left.

A blue baby is one with a heart abnormality which causes a mixing of the blood from the two sides of the heart, so that the arteries of the body are supplied with blood which is poor in oxygen. This should not be confused with the blueness affecting some newborn babies after a difficult labour. A severe heart abnormality may lead to signs of heart failure, including poor colour, very quick breathing and swelling of the limbs and face.

An older child with a congenital heart disease will need an antibiotic if he is to have any operation (even a tooth extracted). This prevents dislodged bacteria from the tooth socket reaching the abnormal heart tissue via the blood stream and setting up an infection in the heart.

Children with serious congenital heart conditions can often do a surprising amount. Most can be trusted to rest when they are tired and they sometimes get into a squatting position to help the blood circulation. The child grows up to be more independent if he is not constantly told to stop and rest. However, tiredness should always be taken seriously and treated by rest.

Congenital heart disease is now no longer the killer it was and in many cases there is no need for urgent surgery at all. Some children do very well even with quite severe anatomical abnormalities and unless the child is failing to grow or shows signs of heart failure, he will be watched carefully by a paediatrician or heart specialist to see whether an operation will ever be necessary.

The main danger with all but the most serious of congenital heart defects is that the parents will tend to treat the child like an invalid. Children adapt very well to their condition and usually only do what they feel able to do, whatever their parents do or say. As with so many distressing (to adults) conditions in childhood the parents react much more strongly to the situation than does the child and this can be counterproductive to the child's normal development.

Unless there is an urgent reason for operating, most surgeons would rather wait until the child is at least five years old, if only because certain conditions repair themselves and others are found not to need an operation. Also, the child is better able to cope with a stay in hospital if he is older and the operative results are better in older children.

Really severe, life-threatening conditions will, of course, be operated on immediately after birth, if necessary.

Any of us who are parents would naturally be concerned about heart surgery on a child of our own but today's operations run at about a 95 per cent success rate, so statistically the odds are vastly in favour of success. Operations for the most straightforward congenital heart troubles are even safer than this.

For details of children in hospital and their preparation for an operation, see page 74.

Children are not kept long in hospital for heart surgery and most are home in about three weeks. This obviously depends on the nature of the condition, its severity, and the age and health of the child. The vast majority of operations for congenital heart defects provide permanent cures.

Let us now look at some of the commoner congenital heart conditions.

**PATENT DUCTUS ARTERIOSUS.** In the fetus the lungs are not filled with air because there is no air in the uterus. There is a short blood vessel (ductus) that bypasses the lungs until they function at the first breath. Once the lungs start working, the ductus closes off and the right and left sides of the heart circulate their blood independently and without connections.

If this channel remains open (patent) it gives rise to the commonest of all congenital heart defects, one in which blood from the aorta is shunted into the lungs instead of around the body, where it should go. In the most severe cases, half of the output of the heart will go needlessly to the lungs. This puts extra stress on the heart as it tries to step up its output so that the rest of the body gets supplied with the correct amount of blood. Such a child may have no symptoms at all. He is not blue. There is a characteristic heart murmur that doctors can hear with a stethoscope and this helps make the diagnosis. As the child gets older he may fail to grow, suffer from more chest infections than other children, be breathless and perhaps have palpitation. Eventually, the heart begins to fail as it cannot pump out enough oxygen-rich blood to supply the body.

The operation to tie off the open connecting channel can be done at any age but is usually delayed until the child is about five years old. The operation is simple and because the duct lies outside the heart, the heart is not opened. The chest is opened and the ductus tied off and cut. The child thrives after the operation and often grows more rapidly than before. After the operation he is entirely like a normal child.

**COARCTATION OF THE AORTA.** In this condition there is a narrowing of the aorta (the main outflow artery from the heart) just beyond where the arteries come off to supply the head and neck. Beyond the narrowing, the aorta balloons out widely.

It is rare for a coarctation to produce any symptoms before adolescence and even then the diagnosis is often made accidentally when a doctor finds he cannot feel a pulse going to either leg or that there is a rise in blood pressure in the top half of the body. Occasionally, the sufferer complains of headaches, nose bleeds or visual disturbances caused by the high blood pressure in the upper half of the body.

The diagnosis is made by finding a characteristic murmur and large differences between the blood pressure in the arms and the legs. Certain X-rays of the chest show typical changes. An angiocardiogram (see page 419) may be done to demonstrate to the surgeon the extent of the narrowed area of aorta.

If the condition is left untreated, the person will die at about the age of thirty-five. This usually comes about because the aorta ruptures, the person has a stroke or his heart fails.

The surgical correction of the condition involves cutting away the narrowed segment of the aorta and joining the two ends together again. It may be necessary to use a synthetic (Teflon) graft if the narrowed segment is very long and the two aortic ends will not join up. Surgery produces a complete cure.

**PULMONARY STENOSIS.** In this condition the pulmonary valve, through which blood passes from the heart to the lungs, is narrowed. This throws a strain on to the heart as it tries to pump enough blood through and the right side of the heart enlarges and eventually pumps very inefficiently. This condition can occur alone or as a part of a multiple heart defect such as Fallot's tetralogy (see below).

A child with pulmonary stenosis will be blue because insufficient blood is getting to the lungs to be oxygenated and the ends of his fingers may also be swollen. These children often squat as they find this is the most comfortable position for reducing breathlessness. They do not grow well. They get more chest infections than other children and die young if not treated. Cardiac angiography (see page 419) confirms the diagnosis before the operation.

With the aid of modern cardiac bypass machines (heart-lung machines), the pulmonary artery can be cut and expanded so allowing more blood through. Results are good and although the operation can take several hours, most children recover well.

ATRIAL SEPTAL DEFECT. This is a condition in which there is an abnormal opening between the two upper pumping chambers of the heart – the atria. The right atrium collects blood from the venous circulation and pumps it into the right ventricle. From here blood goes to be oxygenated in the lungs from which it is returned to the left atrium. This passes it to the left ventricle which pumps it out at high pressure to the body. Clearly, a hole between the venous and arterial collecting chambers will mean that their blood will mix. Blood in the left atrium has just come from the lungs but it goes through the hole in the heart's dividing wall into the right atrium which pumps it straight back to the lungs. This extra effort enlarges the right side of the heart and produces changes in the lungs which in turn cause chest infections and shortness of breath. The diagnosis can be made clinically but is confirmed by cardiac angiography (see page 419).

The child is usually operated on between the ages of six and twelve years when, using a heart-lung (cardiac bypass) machine, the surgeon opens the heart and stitches up the hole. A really large hole may have to be patched up with a synthetic material.

VENTRICULAR SEPTAL DEFECT. This is a condition in which there is an abnormal opening between the two ventricles (lower pumping chambers) of the heart. Some such defects close spontaneously but others are so large that they need operating on in order that the child can grow normally. Because the pressures generated by the left ventricle normally pass blood around the body's circulation, high pressure blood shoots into the right ventricle and this raised pressure is transmitted to the lungs via the blood that leaves the heart to supply them. The child may have difficulty in breathing and becomes tired very easily. Such children get more chest infections than do others and may be breathless at rest if the defect is severe.

The diagnosis is made both clinically and from special X-rays of the heart and open heart surgery is the answer to the problem. If the hole is small, it can be stitched up but if large will require a synthetic patch. Unless the defect is very severe, most surgeons postpone operating until the child is three years old.

**TETRALOGY OF FALLOT (BLUE BABY).** This is the best known of the congenital heart conditions that produce cyanosis (a blue colouring of the lips, tongue and extremities caused by too little oxygen in the blood). This condition consists of four abnormalities – pulmonary stenosis, a ventricular septal defect, an abnormal aorta and an overgrown right ventricle (pumping chamber).

The diagnosis is made clinically by listening for the characteristic heart murmurs and from the appearance of the child but angiocardiography finally clarifies exactly what is wrong. Provided the infant does not go into heart failure, no treatment is necessary in infancy. These babies grow remarkably well but eventually need to be operated on using a cardiac bypass machine. Almost every child can be cured by modern surgery, often performed in early childhood.

While awaiting an operation the child may need tablets to keep the heart's strength up and blood may have to be removed to reduce the body's increased number of red blood cells produced in response to the poor oxygen-carrying power of the blood in this condition.

Should the child be too ill to wait several years for a full corrective operation, a temporary procedure can be performed. This involves taking an artery (often the subclavian artery in the neck) and using it to bypass the pulmonary valve obstruction, so taking more blood to the lungs. In this way more blood is oxygenated and the body gets more oxygen-rich blood without an open heart operation.

# CORNEAL GRAFT

**What is it?**
The cornea is the transparent part of the front of the eye through which light enters the eye. Behind it is the iris (the coloured part), the opening in which is known as the pupil.

This 'window on the eye' can be damaged by trauma or infection which scars it, makes it opaque and causes partial or complete blindness as if a thick net curtain had been drawn across the window. Having said this though, corneal scarring only causes a tiny fraction of all blindness.

Corneal grafting is a very old operation – in fact it is the oldest of all human transplant procedures. There is very little emotion on the part of most people when it comes to donating their corneas, if it will save someone's sight. This has meant that, unlike in the fields of liver, kidney and heart transplantation, people and their relatives on their behalf have been all too willing to part with corneas for so worthy a cause. The success rate of the operation is extremely high and this too makes people think that giving their corneas is a worthwhile gesture. Today, human corneas can be stored in a bank for up to 24 hours ready for use. Because they cannot be stored for long, there is a constant need for donors to replenish corneal banks.

**Why operate?**
To restore previous vision.

**How?**
If both eyes are affected, the eye with the worse problems is operated on so that if the procedure fails the better eye will be left functioning. The operation is done under a general anaesthetic using an operating microscope. The diseased cornea is cut away as a single piece and replaced with an exactly similar-sized piece of donor cornea. This is stitched to the recipient eye's cornea. It is not always necessary to replace the whole thickness of the cornea – sometimes a partial thickness graft will be done.

## Post-operative progress

The eye is left uncovered (as after most eye operations) and the person is allowed up within a few days and home within ten days. There will be careful post-operative follow up, which may be very frequent in the early weeks. Eyesight returns to normal over several months but can take a year.

Success rates, as we have seen, are very high. This has come about as a result of better operating techniques and the improved selection of donor corneas. If the procedure fails to improve matters, the person is rarely worse off, and can be operated upon again.

# CORONARY ARTERY SURGERY

Narrowing of the arteries that supply the heart itself with blood (the coronary arteries) causes angina – a pain in the chest, arm, or neck resulting from too little blood going to the heart muscle. Atheroma, a fatty substance which builds up in the arteries over the years, is probably responsible for the reduced blood supply but little or nothing can be done to clean this off the affected coronary artery lining once it is there. Small areas of coronary artery lining can be cleared of obstructing atheroma but that is all.

Prevention is, of course, the way to tackle this killing epidemic which now claims the lives of one in three middle-aged men in the West. Just how this can be achieved is not known and a book about operations is no place to examine all the theories. Suffice it to say that exclusive breast feeding as an infant; the maintenance of a slim body; a diet high in dietary fibre and low in animal fats; and no smoking all seem to be important protective factors. Ignore any of these and you increase your chances of coronary heart disease.

Many people with coronary artery occlusion or narrowing suffer pain which is worst on exertion. This comes about because the heart cannot get enough oxygenated blood for its needs and because waste products of metabolism build up in the heart muscle. The extreme end of this is the complete occlusion of an artery by a blood clot which causes death of the tissue normally supplied by the obstructed artery. This is a classical heart attack or myocardial infarction. If the area of heart affected is large, the heart may fail as a pump and the person will die then and there. Most heart attacks are not as severe as this though, and the person recovers although about half end up living with angina or other signs of heart disease.

Angina can easily be mistaken for pain which in fact comes from elsewhere. Heartburn, hiatus hernia, neuralgia, peptic ulcer or even gall-bladder disease can all cause heart-type pains and a good doctor will rule out such conditions before telling his patient he has heart disease. The trouble is that coronary artery disease is so common that the person may well have this *and* another condition too.

Medication is the first line of attack for angina. Nitroglycerine tablets under the tongue soon dissolve to exert their effects throughout the body. This drug acts by enlarging arteries. It widens the coronary arteries and thus improves the blood supply to the heart and relieves the unpleasant symptoms. However, other arteries are widened too and this gives the person a pounding headache and hot flushes which are unpleasant. These are, however, a small price to pay for pain relief. Newer drugs have been developed and there are many that are available for doctors to prescribe but, for the acute attack of angina, few beat nitroglycerine tablets. Some drugs can to some extent prevent angina coming on but many sufferers are unhappy about the possible effects of very long-term drug taking and would rather find an alternative. Surgery can be that alternative for those with severe angina which cannot be controlled with drugs. Before surgery is undertaken though, the surgeon will probably want you to try to reduce your weight, cut out cigarettes, reduce your fat intake and take up some form of exercise. Graded exercise combined with these other life-style changes can reduce angina and even cure it in very large numbers of people.

However, if all of these methods fail, there are two surgical approaches to the problem. One involves opening the blocked artery and coring out the blocking material and the other involves a bypass operation to carry blood around the obstructed area. Both of these procedures assume that the surgeon knows where the blockage or narrowing is. This entails the use of special X-rays – angiocardiography (see page 419).

In the more major (bypass) procedure the chest is opened under general anaesthesia and the whole procedure can take four or five hours. One method involves taking the cut end of the mammary (breast) artery which normally supplies the chest wall and inserting it into the diseased artery beyond the blockage. The more usually performed operation involves taking a length of saphenous vein from the leg. This can easily be spared by the person (it is the one removed to cure varicose veins). It is used to make a bypass around a blockage or narrowing so as to provide an alternative route for the blood. This can be repeated for many blocked sites at the one operation. All of this is done with the aid of a heart-lung machine so that the surgeon can operate on a still, blood-free heart.

After such major surgery the person spends several days in an intensive care unit where his heart and certain other body functions are closely monitored. The hospital stay is usually of the order of two or three weeks and the person can be back at work in six weeks or so.

Success rates are very high with this bypass operation, especially when the patients are carefully selected as a result of pre-operative X-ray studies and other tests. Fewer than ten per cent of those operated on die as a result of the operation. The beneficial results are immediately obvious and most people (about 70 per cent) live normal, active lives after the operation though only really long-term trials will prove whether such surgery should be used routinely. Some people are able to work for the first time in years. It has been claimed that having a bypass operation reduces the chances of dying of a heart attack within the first five years after surgery, but evidence on this is still scanty, and some surveys show that medical treatment produces an exactly similar clinical outcome as surgery when assessed three years after starting.

It is as yet too early to be sure that surgery offers any substantial advantage over medical therapy in coronary artery disease – more research is needed.

# COSMETIC SURGERY

### What is it?
A branch of plastic surgery. Plastic surgery is that section of surgery that specializes in the repair and reconstruction of the body. Plastic surgeons do not spend most of their time doing 'cosmetic' operations (which are by definition medically unnecessary in the majority of cases) but rather reconstruct severely burned, damaged or deformed people. With increasing wealth, though, more and more women especially are turning to cosmetic surgery to improve their looks and to patch up their self-esteem.

### Why operate?
Some women come to cosmetic surgery because they really do have deformities but most are simply displeased with their bodies in one way or another. Certain deformities are really distressing and many a woman's whole outlook on life has been changed for the better by nose or breast surgery, for example. To be fair though, many of the candidates for these operations are either bored or sexually dissatisfied and need to sort out their personal lives rather than spend fortunes on face lifts or a host of other available operations. Some cosmetic surgeons, realizing this, get the help of a psychiatrist before undertaking cosmetic work because they know from experience that surgery done for the wrong reason can backfire on them in the future. Cosmetic surgery is not something to be undertaken lightly. After all, there are real and measurable risks to having an operation of any kind, so to expose oneself to these unnecessarily or because your husband has gone off you is somewhat foolish. Also, it is important to remember that the result may not be exactly what you had in mind and this might not be the surgeon's

fault. He may come across things he could not have foreseen and you could end up more bothered by the scars than by the original condition. Having said all this, millions of women have had cosmetic surgery and are perfectly happy with the results.

## Nose operations

A nose operation can improve both its shape and size. Lumps can be removed, nostrils narrowed, the whole nose straightened and even made smaller overall. Unfortunately, nose reductions can be tricky and the woman can be left with a smaller but still crooked nose. Sometimes nose surgery reduces the nostrils' width and thereby alters the voice and even affects the sense of smell on occasions.

Almost all nose cosmetic surgery is done from inside the nostrils so there are no scars. Such operations are done under a general anaesthetic and often involve physically breaking the nose first before it can be reshaped.

The nose is put in its new shape and style and held there by a plaster of Paris visor-shaped splint which remains in position for ten days. When the woman wakes up from the anaesthetic she is usually amazed at the enormous black eyes produced by the internal bleeding that accompanies the bone breaking. This bruising is usually only slightly painful and the woman can go home in three or four days.

By ten days the swelling has gone down but you will find you are housebound for at least three weeks because the bruising looks so bad that you will look as if you have been in a fight. Wearing dark glasses is a way round this. It can be as long as a year before all traces of the operation have disappeared but most women go about their normal lives with the use of make-up after the first four weeks. In the long term, a changed nose can sag at the bridge, but this is uncommon.

## Face-lifts

These aim at removing flabby and excess skin around the ageing face. At the most simple level an eyelift can be carried out. This involves taking away some of the excess skin of the eyelid. After three days in hospital you can return home and have the stitches out seven days later. The bruising takes about ten days to disappear. The next step is to have the bags under the eyes removed too. This takes much the same sort of time to heal but of course will cost more. In both cases, a large pair of sunglasses will cover up the evidence until you feel confident enough to face the world.

A full face lift involves incisions around the ears and in the scalp. The excess skin of the face is pulled taut and removed. After a few days in hospital the stitches come out at the end of a further week and the scars heal without much trace. Many women feel happier growing their hair long so as to conceal the scars around the ears. This is an operation that is very effective in making a woman look younger but is costly and probably only lasts for about ten years before it will need repeating. Few surgeons will do a face-lift on a woman under 45.

## Breasts

There are few subjects that arouse more dissatisfaction among women than their breasts. In a breast-orientated society many women feel insecure about their breast size. Women with large, pendulous breasts may indeed have serious problems not only in finding bras to fit but in living with a real handicap. The other extreme is more commonplace though and far more women want their breasts enlarged than reduced.

Breast enlargement has been through many fads and fashions but the injection of liquid silicone under the breast (long thought to be the best way of enlarging breasts) has now been abandoned as unreliable and dangerous. Today, the breast is enlarged by the insertion of a sealed silicone bag full of silicone gel under the breast itself and on top of the chest wall. These bags do not, of course, actually enlarge the breast tissue but simply push what there is further forward. The operation is safe and quick and involves only small incisions (about eight centimetres long) through which the bags are placed behind the breasts. The scars are almost invisible as they are in the folds of skin under the breasts.

Nearly half of the bags of silicone become enclosed in fibrous tissue (a substance formed as the body naturally walls off a foreign substance) and this makes the breast harder and rounder than normal. Nipple sensation may be so heightened that the nipples are uncomfortable and this state can last for several months. About one in a hundred women rejects the implants entirely.

In general this is an operation best done in women who are unlikely to have more children, because their breast shape may alter with subsequent children. Breast feeding is not necessarily impaired.

After three to four days in hospital most women are performing their household activities within six weeks and feel normal very much sooner.

Breast reduction is a very good cosmetic operation but is only done in women whose breasts are so large that they cause real suffering. This is because the scars can be considerable and the woman may not be able to breast feed if substantial amounts of tissue are removed. Also nipple sensation is lost in half of all women having this operation and this can be an enormous problem to the woman who likes her breasts to play an important role in love-making. The operation is simple and involves removing breast fat and tissue together with a piece of overlying skin and then sewing up the edges again. This not only reduces the actual size of the breast but elevates the nipple to a more acceptable position. The scars are large and can remain red for up to a year after the operation. Breasts can also be lifted without actually removing any breast tissue but this is unsatisfactory as they tend to drop again over the years.

### Bottoms
Too droopy a bottom can be tightened by removing part of the fat from the bottom completely and then reshaping the skin. It is not often performed and leaves fairly obvious permanent scars. The patient has to remain in hospital for about ten days and will convalesce for six weeks.

## Abdomen

Two types of cosmetic operation can be done on the abdomen. The first removes flabby skin and stretch marks after pregnancy. This operation involves the removal of skin and its supporting tissue over quite a wide area and then the stitching of the skin edges together along a line across the bottom of the tummy just above the pubic hair line. Ideally the scar should not show above a bikini but it is not always easy to engineer this exactly.

This sort of operation should only be done after a muscle-strengthening programme to improve the tone of the abdominal muscles which often become weakened after having several babies. In many women weight loss and good tummy exercises can render such an operation unnecessary. Tummy muscles *can* be tightened though, if necessary, surgically. After four or five days in bed the woman is in hospital for ten days and recovering for six weeks. It is about a year before the scar has faded enough to display it.

The second tummy operation is much rarer and is called an 'apronectomy'. This is only carried out in very obese people and involves removing their 'apron' of fat. It results in a flat tummy 'overnight' but does not make the otherwise obese person thin – nor does it answer the basic question of why she was obese in the first place.

# CYSTOSCOPY

## What is it?

A procedure usually, but not necessarily, carried out under general anaesthesia in which a tubular instrument with a light at the end (a cystoscope) is passed into the bladder via the urethra (the tube leading from the outside of the body to the bladder).

There are many different types of cystoscope but they are all basically similar. They are about 30 centimetres long, have a bent end with a light at the tip, an outer jacket through which water can be circulated in and out of the bladder and a telescope eyepiece for the doctor to look down. Most modern instruments are illuminated by fibre optics (see page 385), so producing a very good light in which to diagnose and operate.

## Why operate?

The bladder has to be visualized for many different reasons. Commonly, a cystoscopy is of great diagnostic help when there are signs of bladder obstruction that suggest that the prostate gland is enlarged (see page 289). A special operating cystoscope enables the surgeon not only to see what is happening but to cut away the prostate gland in tiny bites, so preventing the need for a major abdominal operation to remove the gland. This instrument is called a resectoscope. Bladder stones and tumours are also easily visible down a cystoscope and small stones can be crushed and washed away very easily. Some kidney stones get stuck in the fine ureter as they are squeezed down towards the bladder. If this occurs, a surgeon can use a cystoscope to remove the stone if it is lodged in the lower part of the ureter. In this procedure a loop is passed up the ureter from its opening into the bladder and is hooked over the stone. In this way the stone may be moved down into the bladder from where it can easily be removed. Stones that are too big to respond to this procedure will have to be removed at an operation (see page 335). Some non-cancerous tumours of the bladder can be burned off its lining with an electrode passed down a cystoscope – again saving the patient an abdominal operation.

Certain kidney conditions cannot adequately be diagnosed using intravenous fluids that are concentrated in the kidneys and then X-rayed. In such cases fine plastic catheters are passed up the ureters that lead from the bladder to each kidney so that the radio-opaque substance can be injected backwards into the kidneys. These fine catheters are passed up the ureters using a cystoscope with its tip in the bladder near the opening of the ureters. When the cystoscope is withdrawn, two fine catheters are seen emerging from the urethra. Down these a radio-opaque substance is later injected when the patient is in the X-ray department. Once satisfactory X-rays of the kidneys and ureters have been obtained, the catheters are simply pulled out gently. Similarly, a radio-opaque substance can be injected into the bladder via a cystoscope so as to outline conditions affecting the organ.

### How?
Cystoscopy can be adequately performed under local anaesthesia, though many surgeons feel it should ideally be done under general anaesthesia. The penis is clamped for ten minutes after the insertion of local anaesthetic jelly and this ensures that there is no painful or unpleasant sensation at all. Many urologists prefer to have the patient under a general anaesthetic because it is more pleasant for the patient, gives the surgeon more flexibility and relieves him of concern about hurting the patient.

Once the person is anaesthetized his legs are put up in stirrups and he is cleaned and towelled up. The cystoscope is checked before being passed into the urethra. The irrigation system is connected and after first emptying the bladder the surgeon washes water in and out several times down the cystoscope until he gets a clear view into the bladder when looking down the telescope eyepiece. He then carries out his inspection or operation as outlined above. He can take biopsies (samples) of anything he sees and as with so many of these modern instruments can actually photograph anything interesting. Once the procedure is complete the bladder is emptied and the cystoscope withdrawn. The patient is returned to the ward or is free to go home if he is an out-patient.

### Post-operative progress
There are almost no post-operative problems with cystoscopy. Some people, especially men, complain of some soreness when they pass urine for the first time or two but that is all. If operative procedures have been carried out you may pass some blood or dark-coloured urine. This should be reported to the medical or nursing staff but is quite normal and should cause no concern. It is helpful to drink plenty of fluid after the examination to flush the bladder through.

# D AND C

**What is it?**

A D and C (short for dilatation and curettage) is a simple gynaecological procedure in which the uterus (womb) is scraped out under general anaesthesia. It is colloquially known as a 'scrape' because the surgeon uses a long-handled scraper (curette) with a spoon-shaped end to clean out the lining of the uterus.

The uterus is a hollow organ made of muscle the size and shape of a small pear. Hormones in a woman's body cause the lining of the uterus to build up and to be shed in cycles. The monthly shedding of the surface cells together with the attendant bleeding is known as menstruation (a period). It is these superficial cells that are scraped away or curetted at a D and C.

**Why operate?**

A D and C is used to treat or diagnose irregular, frequent or heavy periods; infertility; painful periods; bleeding around the time of and after the menopause; and to remove any placenta retained in the uterus after the birth of a baby. A polyp in the uterus can be the cause of excessive bleeding at period times but this is just one of many conditions that can be diagnosed at a D and C. Sometimes the cells of the uterine lining show specific changes that indicate a hormone imbalance but often the tissue shows nothing, yet the D and C cures the patient in some, as yet unknown, way.

In some cases of infertility, evidence from a D and C can help decide whether the woman is ovulating or not. A D and C for this purpose is usually carried out in the last ten days of the menstrual cycle but is being replaced in some centres by a suction catheter technique.

Most women cease to menstruate around the age of 48 years but the age varies considerably. Sometimes periods may have stopped and then the woman bleeds again. Because this might be a sign of cancer of the uterus, a D and C is often done to obtain some cells to exclude this diagnosis.

Sometimes hormone treatment (with oestrogens) after the menopause causes bleeding. Some gynaecologists think it safe therefore to carry out a D and C before starting this treatment and then to carry out an annual Vabra curettage (see below) as an out-patient.

A D and C can also be performed to remove the remains of a miscarriage from the uterus and is carried out with especially great care as the soft, pregnant uterus is especially liable to be punctured by the instruments. This procedure involves no actual dilation of the cervix because it is already soft and more open than usual in pregnancy. The opposite extreme to this is another modification of a D and C in which the cervix is stretched (or dilated) by increasingly large instruments in the treatment of painful periods. Some women have pain because clots of blood get stuck in the cervix. Because this sort of painful period is rarely seen after a woman has had a baby, doctors feel it sensible to dilate the cervix (as the baby does) so as to mimic birth from the cervix's point of view. Results of this procedure are very mixed and many doctors no longer recommend it as it can cause cervical incompetence – a condition in which the cervix is too weak to hold a fetus in the early months of pregnancy. This is a cause of early miscarriage and is to some extent preventable.

### How?

Because stretching the cervix is painful, a general anaesthetic is usually given. Local anaesthetics can be injected into the cervix but a general anaesthetic is usually preferred by most gynaecologists. The cervix is a tiny canal that in a woman who has never had a baby will only take an instrument the size of a knitting needle. In women who have had babies the canal is wider but will still not be wide enough to accept a curette. Because it is so narrow the cervix has first to be dilated or enlarged. This is done by inserting increasingly large dilators until it will accept the curette. Before this widening is carried out the direction and depth of the uterine cavity is determined by inserting a fine instrument called a uterine sound. This ensures that the surgeon does not push the dilators too deeply into the cavity of the uterus as he can estimate the depth from his measuring sound. After step by step dilatation, the cervix is wide enough (about one quarter of an inch or five millimetres across) to receive the spoon-shaped curette. This can take several minutes to achieve in young girls or old women. The curette is then inserted and dragged over the inner surface of the womb to remove the surface in strips. The material obtained is sent to a pathologist for study.

If only a very small piece of tissue is required for diagnostic purposes, a fine suction curette can be inserted through the undilated cervix. This is called a Vabra curette and because it is so small means that there is no need for an anaesthetic. Such an instrument avoids hospital admission altogether but a normal D and C may entail one night in hospital.

## Post-operative progress

Some post-operative bleeding occurs rather as if the woman had had a period (which is exactly what a D and C is like in mechanical terms). The woman's next period is not as heavy as usual because the lining that would have formed it has been removed. Ordinary bathing is perfectly safe but vaginal douching should probably not be performed until bleeding has stopped. Most women are back to a completely normal life within a week after the operation. Intercourse can be resumed after three days but contraception is essential because although it is unlikely an egg will implant in a recently curetted uterus, it could just happen. A D and C does not interfere with conception and pregnancies after are exactly the same as in a woman who hasn't had one. Some doctors feel that a D and C should not be undertaken lightly, though, because the stretching of the cervix to accept the scraper may leave the woman with a weakened area which could result in a miscarriage later. Because of this real disadvantage the Vabra catheter is being increasingly used in place of D and Cs where possible.

# DENTAL OPERATIONS

Most dental procedures are carried out by dentists working in general practice but if conditions occur that your dentist cannot deal with, he will suggest you go to a consultant dental surgeon at a general or specialist dental hospital.

By far the commonest dental operation carried out as an in-patient is the **REMOVAL OF AN IMPACTED TOOTH** – usually a wisdom tooth. A tooth is called 'impacted' if it is prevented from coming through into the mouth. The wisdom teeth (third molars) are the most commonly affected and cause pain which is not only local but can spread to other parts of the face and head. Localized infection around the tooth is also a problem. Because wisdom teeth can be in very awkward positions they are often difficult to remove in a dental surgery under local anaesthetic. This is why hospital admission is usually advised.

The operation is much like any other insofar as the person is prepared as for any general anaesthetic. After the operation there is a lot of pain and swelling and the jaw may be stiff. Ice packs and painkilling medicines help considerably. After the first 24 hours you will be asked to use a mouthwash regularly every four hours: a teaspoonful of salt in a tumbler of warm water is suitable, or something recommended by your dentist. Most people feel like taking things easy for a few days after the operation and the stitches are removed a few days later in the dental out-patient department at the hospital. Most people are back to normal in ten days.

A **CYST** or an area of infection in the jaw bone can often be removed under general anaesthesia as a day case.

Some people have many bad teeth that need to be removed and some dentists feel it is better to have these teeth removed in hospital under general anaesthesia. Dentures are fitted immediately – in fact you wake up with them in place after the operation. These may or may not be replaced at a later date with more permanent dentures once the gums are back to normal.

Occasionally, a dentist will suggest that someone with a serious medical condition who needs to have teeth removed should have them out in hospital just to be safe.

# DETACHED RETINA

**What is it?**
A condition, seen mostly in older people, in which the light-sensitive lining at the back of the eye (the retina) becomes detached, producing strange visual disturbances.

The eye is a near-perfect sphere contained within a tough outer coat of fibrous tissue which comes round to the front as the white part of the eye (the sclera). Inside this outer coat are other layers that nourish the nerve cells of the eye. At the back of the eye light is focused via the lens, which lies towards the front of the interior of the eye, on to a light-sensitive layer called the retina. It is here that light images are turned into nervous impulses which are in turn interpreted by the brain.

Should a piece of retina become detached, fluid which is normally present inside the eye leaks behind the tear and separates the retina from the coat behind.

The main thing people complain of when a retina detaches is a sensation that a 'curtain' is falling or moving across the eye. The most severe detachments produce a curtain that reduces the vision in the affected eye to almost nothing. A detachment that is left untreated will progress to complete blindness.

Diagnosing a detachment is not easy but when a doctor looks into the eye with an ophthalmoscope he may clearly see an obvious tear or even the folds of retina that the person describes as 'curtains', if they are present. There are, however, lots of less obvious changes that occur before this and they may not be easy to see. Drugs may have to be put into the eye to make it possible to see these changes.

Retinal detachments occur after trauma; in the elongating short-sighted eye and with certain diseases affecting the retina, such as diabetes. Many of the conditions causing a retinal detachment cannot be treated, so the detachment itself has to be treated. However, recent advances in certain diseases (for example diabetes) mean that more can be done than ever before to tackle the underlying problem. The doctor may suggest you stay in bed while awaiting the operation so that mild trauma or even physical effort such as stooping will not cause the detachment to extend.

## Why operate?
To seal the retina to the underlying eye coats so as to prevent blindness. Often, the procedure is done as an emergency to save the person's sight.

## How?
Under general anaesthesia, an incision is made in the white of the eye. Fluid can then be removed from behind the retinal detachment, so allowing the intra-ocular pressure to press the retina back into place. The retina can then be fixed in place by cryotherapy (a freezing technique); a beam of laser light (photocoagulation); or an electric needle. A plastic implant is often stitched to the eyeball's outside surface over the detached retinal area. This pushes the outer walls of the eye's covering into the eye to bring them close to the retina for fixing by one of the above methods.

## Post-operative progress
Although many people feel especially sensitive about operations on their eyes, such procedures are rarely painful and most eye operations have success rates that are the envy of other types of surgeon. Surgery for a detached retina is no exception. About 80–90 per cent of people are successfully treated by the operation.

The operated eye may have to be bandaged for a day or so but some surgeons do not even keep the operated eye covered for this long. Most surgeons feel that complete physical rest helps minimize the chances of a tiny bleed occurring in the eye and it certainly makes sense not to do anything rough that might dislodge the delicate tethering that was achieved at the operation. Because of this it is essential to stay off work until the surgeon is entirely happy with the results. By about two months the surgeon will be able to tell if the result looks like being permanent.

Unfortunately, recurrences are fairly frequent, mainly because the retina in many of the conditions causing detachment is very poor and thin. Re-operation is perfectly feasible though and can tide the person over for a few more months or years.

# DISLOCATIONS

A dislocation occurs when, because of exceptional pressure, a bone becomes displaced from its joint. The commonest joints to be dislocated are the shoulders, fingers and elbows.

Sometimes it is difficult to be sure of the diagnosis and even a doctor may have to take X-rays to be sure there is no fracture. The main signs are pain, swelling and an unwillingness to move the joint.

The treatment is to replace the joint as soon as possible. The vast majority of dislocations do not need open surgery as they can be pushed back by the surgeon performing the right manoeuvre with the affected part. In general this entails pulling on the part and manipulating it back into place. Once back in place, the joint immediately feels normal but there may still be some pain.

**SHOULDERS** dislocate easily because the socket into which the 'ball' on the top of the upper arm bone fits is so shallow. Under pain-relieving drug cover, most of these go back quickly and easily but a repeatedly dislocating shoulder may need an open operation to tether the arm bone so as to prevent further dislocation.

**ELBOWS** dislocate in children quite often but recurrent dislocation is uncommon.

**FINGER JOINTS** usually go back into place with a firm pull by the surgeon and no further treatment is required.

# DIVERTICULAR DISEASE

**What is it?**
A condition of the large bowel in which little balloon-like pouches appear on the outside of the organ. There may only be a few of these diverticula or there may be many hundreds. The condition is very common indeed, affecting as it does about half of all sixty-year-olds.

Just why this disease should be so common is not known but it is thought that our highly refined, low-roughage diet plays a part. A very large percentage of people with proven (by barium enema X-rays, see page 422) diverticular disease can have all the symptoms alleviated simply by changing their diet to one containing more vegetables, wholemeal-flour products and bran-enriched breakfast cereals. As recently as a decade ago doctors were prescribing low-roughage diets for diverticular disease but today it has been proved that these actually cause the condition as the low residue, hard masses are squeezed through the colon, producing the 'blow-outs' or diverticula.

Diverticula of the colon can become inflamed but the actual number of people being operated on for such inflammation has fallen dramatically in recent years as more sufferers get relief from their symptoms and prevent complications by changing to a high-fibre diet. This is a very good example of preventive medicine really working.

However, although the colon looks strange, these small blow-outs do not seem to produce trouble in the vast majority of people. If the neck of the blow-out becomes blocked off for some reason, this results in inflammation with severe, sudden onset of left-sided abdominal pain rather like left-sided appendicitis. This is called diverticulitis and is characterized by pain with chills, nausea and vomiting. Between attacks there may be diarrhoea and constipation.

Many people with an attack of diverticulitis do not need an operation. Bed rest and antibiotics together with pain-killers often allow the inflammation to settle. Anti-spasmodic drugs may be used to reduce the colon's activity and all these measures help save the person from an operation in mild cases.

## Why operate?
An operation will be necessary for those people who develop repeated severe attacks and for those with complications such as perforation. An operation may also be done to distinguish between a cancer of the colon and diverticular disease.

## How?
There are several stages of severity of the condition and what the surgeon does will be dictated by how severe the problems are.

Occasionally the operation is done for repeated attacks of diverticulitis and can be carried out as a planned procedure. In this case the procedure follows a time of cleaning out of the bowel and being given an antibiotic.

More commonly though, the operation is done as an emergency procedure to deal with an abscess beside the colon, peritonitis or one of several other complications.

Under general anaesthesia the surgeon makes a long incision in the midline or to the left of the midline of the abdomen and assesses the nature of the problem. If, as is often the case, the inflammation has caused an obstruction of the colon at the site of the diverticulum, major surgery is required. The whole manoeuvre can either be performed at the one operation or the same work can be done at two or three separate operations. The choice depends greatly on the surgeon's own individual level of experience and the clinical conditions at the time.

Either way, it is necessary to construct an opening (see page 147). In this a loop of normal large bowel is opened and brought through a hole in the surface of the skin of the abdomen. This diverts food residues away from the inflamed area and allows the trouble to subside. This procedure is called a colostomy and whilst not at all pleasant is not too difficult to put up with for a while as the doctors wait for you to get well enough to undergo the second stage of the operation.

At this, the diseased area of the colon is removed and the healthy ends joined together. This then heals well because the colostomy still bypasses the area. The third stage removes the colostomy and re-routes the stools as normal.

The creation of a colostomy takes about an hour but if the whole procedure is carried out at once it can take two to three hours.

## Post-operative progress

Emergency colonic surgery is very major surgery and as many of those undergoing surgery for diverticulitis are old and frail anyway the mortality rate is high. Younger, fitter people fare much better and of those who survive the operation about 90 per cent are cured. It is usual to have a nasogastric tube (see page 403) and an intravenous drip (see page 396).

After such a major operation, you should not expect to be up before four days and you may be in hospital for several weeks. If you are to have the operation in stages you will have to wait at least three weeks between each stage so even though you might well be at home in between operations, the whole thing takes a long time.

Many surgeons use a drain to ensure that pus and blood do not collect in the abdominal cavity. The drainage site may go on discharging for some weeks. You probably will not get back to normal for many weeks and it could easily be three months before you feel completely well.

Once the operation has been completed and you are back on to ordinary food again, be sure to change your diet to one rich in dietary fibre (roughage) so as to ensure the long-term success of the operation. Never let your stools become hard. As soon as you have any difficulty passing stools or pass hard ones, increase the amount of fibre in your diet so that your stools are always soft and easily passed, then stabilize your diet at this level of fibre intake. You cannot give yourself a new colon but you can certainly reduce the chances of ever having trouble again.

# DUPUYTREN'S CONTRACTURE

### What is it?
A condition of the hand in which the fourth and fifth fingers become fixed in a bent position and can only be straightened surgically.

No one knows why it occurs but it may be linked with a previous injury. It affects older people and occasionally there is an hereditary factor. Some people seem to get it if they grip tools repeatedly.

### Why operate?
To straighten the fingers and give the person a normally functioning hand again.

### How?
Treatment is often difficult. If caught early on, the bands of fibrous tissue that pull on the affected fingers can be cut under general anaesthesia. More severe cases will need a more extensive operation to remove contracted tissue in the hand. This may have to be followed by skin grafting. Rarely, the affected fingers may have to be amputated.

### Post-operative progress
There is not much pain after the operation but the temporary loss of the use of a hand is unpleasant, especially if it is the dominant hand. Physiotherapy and splinting of the hand may be used after the operation. Results are good, except in most severe cases in which many fingers are involved and even in these cases great improvement can be expected.

# EPILEPSY

## What is it?
A condition in which the brain fires off bursts of electrical activity for no known reason. These discharges cause convulsions of brief duration which come on suddenly.

In the classical **GRAND MAL** fit (which is what most people think of when they think of epilepsy), the person may have strange sensations (an aura) of some kind before the attack but usually the first sign is a loss of consciousness as he falls to the ground. He then makes a series of convulsive movements and may bite his tongue, foam at the mouth and wet himself. After this he goes into a coma or may simply sleep for several hours. On recovering, he has a headache.

**PETIT MAL** is a much less dramatic affair. The person (usually a child) does not lose consciousness but simply has brief, momentary lapses of consciousness. These can be noticed as brief breaks in speaking, an upward rolling of the eyes or similar signs. These short-lived attacks halt the person for a split second only.

**FOCAL EPILEPSY** is the term for an epileptic attack that originates from a particular part of the brain. The attack may be very minor and pass unnoticed or severe enough to lead to a generalized convulsion. Temporal lobe epilepsy is a common form of focal epilepsy in which the focus of the epileptic discharge seems to be the front part of the temporal lobe of the brain. The person may experience intense pleasure, or have hallucinations of taste and smell with sweating, weakness, pallor and fear. There may be convulsive movements of the limbs and smacking of the lips.

Drugs are the mainstay of all epilepsy treatment but a book such as this is no place to describe these. The vast majority of people with epilepsy today are well controlled on drugs and many can be maintained on one drug for most of their lives.

## Why operate?
Of all the epilepsies, surgery is really only applicable to focal

epilepsy and to temporal lobe epilepsy in particular. There are several criteria that must be fulfilled before any surgeon will consider operating for temporal lobe epilepsy. First, there must have been a failure of drug therapy; second, there must be good evidence (from an EEG, see page 382) that the problem arises from one side of the brain predominantly; and third, there must be some degree of certainty that a spontaneous cure is unlikely. Lastly, the person must have an IQ of more than 60.

If these criteria are fulfilled, about half of the people operated on are free from seizures after the operation. In about a fifth the fits are reduced to less than a quarter of their previous frequency.

### How?
The operation involves removing the temporal lobes and some deeper parts of the brain under general anaesthesia.

One of the encouraging findings has been that half of all those who have psychiatric abnormalities before the operation are normal mentally afterwards. All in all then, if the subjects are chosen correctly, two thirds of all those operated on for temporal lobe epilepsy are helped significantly.

# EPISIOTOMY

### What is it?
A cut made in the outer part of the vagina and in the perineum to enable a baby to be born more readily or to allow the application of obstetric forceps to the baby's emerging head.

### Why operate?
As a baby comes down the mother's birth canal, its head stretches all the mother's tissues on its way to the outside world. The walls of the vagina are very elastic and, although they seem to be grossly overstretched, do in fact return to normal surprisingly quickly after delivery. Sometimes, and

especially if the baby gets into difficulty or if the uterus stops contracting under the influence of an epidural analgesic, forceps may have to be applied to the baby's head. This enables the obstetrician to pull or guide the baby out firmly but in a controlled way. In order to produce enough room to insert the forceps, an episiotomy may have to be performed. An episiotomy may also be necessary for the safe delivery of twins or babies born 'upside down' (breech babies). In both these situations most doctors would agree that a surgical incision was necessary.

Some, but not many, obstetric units perform episiotomies routinely on the grounds that the larger the vaginal opening, the easier the birth of the baby and the better the chance of producing a normal, healthy child. It is also argued though without medical proof that women who do not have episiotomies are more likely to suffer from prolapse of the womb in later life. Between 20 and 25 per cent of women suffer spontaneous tears in the perineum without episiotomies so this is yet another reason given for doing them routinely.

There is much debate as to whether episiotomies should be done as frequently as they are but doctors who have seen a lot of women with prolapses and incontinence, or who have seen a baby's head so stretch the vaginal opening that it tears into the back passage, feel strongly that this is good preventive surgery. Episiotomies are easier to stitch up than spontaneous tears and this is one reason why many obstetricians feel they should control the situation. However, they do not necessarily heal faster or better. On the other hand though, many women feel that there is too much intervention in childbirth and that they would rather not suffer the after-effects of an episiotomy (see below). The decision is a matter of weighing the undoubted immediate unpleasant effects against the prevention of possible suffering in years to come and this is difficult for both doctor and patient to do, as neither can foresee the future. There is no reason to assume that having had one episiotomy a woman will necessarily need another. Good midwifery can mean that a woman need have neither a tear nor an episiotomy.

## How?

Towards the very end of the labour, at the height of a contraction and when the baby's head is stretching the vaginal opening into a thin rim, the obstetrician or midwife puts local anaesthetic into the skin and muscles and then makes a cut with scissors from the vaginal opening downwards and outwards for about four centimetres. The baby's head comes out soon after and once the baby and the placenta are delivered, the episiotomy can be sewn up. Further local anaesthetic may be injected but the stitching is often completely free from pain because the tissues are so stretched.

Local anaesthetic will not, of course, be necessary if the woman has had an epidural analgesic (which is very often the case, as episiotomies are needed very frequently in women who have this type of pain relief). The sewing is done with soluble catgut which means the stitches don't have to be removed.

## Post-operative progress

Once the epidural or local anaesthetic has worn off, the episiotomy area is painful. Many women say that the after-effects of their episiotomy was the most painful thing about having a baby and that this is a reason why they would rather not have had an episiotomy. Ice packs and local anaesthetic creams help the pain and it is worth taking painkillers if the pain is severe. Plenty of hot salt baths help enormously and a foam or pneumatic ring helps some mothers to sit by taking the pressure off the affected area. The worst effects of an episiotomy are over within a few days and the wound is usually completely healed within ten days. The deeper tissues take longer to heal and for many weeks the inside of the vagina may feel 'knobbly' where the stitches were.

In most cases, an episiotomy does not affect a couple's sex life for long and if intercourse is attempted in the first six weeks, the doctor should be told of any pain and discomfort when the woman goes for her post-natal visit. Some discomfort is to be expected for a few weeks but most women do not find that this puts them off sex. Should the muscles between the lower end of the vagina and the anus be weakened, damaged or badly repaired, air may be sucked into the vagina as the woman moves or has intercourse and this can embarrass her and upset her partner. This should be discussed with the doctor at the post-natal visit and he may suggest muscle exercises to strengthen the pelvic floor. Some women are unnecessarily fearful of intercourse after an episiotomy because they do not understand what has been done and worry that the area may be 'weak' and might burst on intercourse. This cannot occur.

Intercourse may be painful after birth even without an episiotomy because vaginal lubrication is not as efficient as normal during this time. According to one psychosexual expert who has studied the subject, episiotomies are sometimes used as an excuse (consciously or unconsciously) to avoid sex and it is these women who are most troublesome to both doctor and husband. Sometimes the woman fears another pregnancy but often, according to this expert, the episiotomy acts as a focal point for any sexual discontent that was present before the birth.

## EYE REMOVAL (ENUCLEATION)

There are several conditions that call for the complete removal of an eye and in all of them the eye is no longer of use and may even have become troublesome. A malignant tumour of the eye is an indication for its immediate removal which often cures the condition completely. If one eye is severely damaged or completely blind (while the other is normal) most surgeons will remove it.

When an eye is to be removed this is done under a general anaesthetic. The good eye is protected during the operation and the diseased eye removed. The socket heals remarkably quickly and an artificial eye which matches the remaining eye can be chosen with such care that no one will ever notice it is false. The tear glands are left in place so crying and washing of the surface of the false eye occur just as normal. Surgeons today can even link an implant that carries the false eye to the old eye's muscles so that the new eye moves in harmony with the remaining one. The false eyeball itself is not fixed to the eye's muscles and all false eyes can be removed for cleaning by the person himself.

We need two eyes to see things in depth. This is known as stereoscopic vision. People with one eye soon adapt to the new messages their brains receive and can drive and perform most other tasks of daily living perfectly well. Some people have never had stereoscopic vision and so do not suffer any loss when an eye is removed. If the person had good stereoscopic vision before the operation it may take months for the perception of depth and distance to return to normal.

Obviously, having to have an eye removed is an unpleasant thing to come to terms with but if it can prevent disease from spreading to the rest of the body, prevent deterioration in the remaining good eye and be cosmetically advantageous, it is usually acceptable to most people.

# FIBROIDS

**What are they?**
Fibroids are non-cancerous tumours of the uterus that cause heavy periods by enlarging the bleeding area of the lining of the uterus or by increasing the number of blood vessels in the uterine wall, or both. They are made of fibrous and muscle tissue and no one knows why they arise.

The uterus has two layers. The inner layer (endometrium) changes during each cycle and is shed every month as the menstrual flow (a period). The outer layer of the uterus is made of muscle. This contracts repeatedly and forcibly during labour to expel the baby from the uterus. Sometimes this muscle layer contracts at times other than during labour – the pains some women experience during a period and the physical sensations during an orgasm are both caused by the uterus contracting. It is within this outer layer of muscle (that forms the bulk of the uterus) that fibroids develop. Most women who have fibroids have several, even though one in particular may produce most of the symptoms and signs.

There are three main types of fibroids and they are all treated differently.

**SUBSEROUS** fibroids grow on the outside of the uterus. These often grow large and may first show as a lump in the abdomen. Because such fibroids are attached to the uterus by a stalk they can become twisted on themselves and produce symptoms which make an emergency abdominal operation necessary.

**INTRAMURAL** fibroids grow in the muscle wall of the uterus and cause it to become larger than normal. This type can show as a lump in the abdomen or may produce pressure on neighbouring organs. Frequency of urination (as a result of pressure on the bladder) is not uncommon with this kind of fibroid.

**SUBMUCOUS** fibroids grow in the cavity of the uterus and cause heavy periods.

Most fibroids cause no symptoms or problems and are only found on pelvic examination.

An internal examination usually enables the doctor to make the diagnosis with certainty but he may also do a Pap test (see page 374), X-ray the inside of the uterus using hysterosalpingography (see page 394) or do a D and C (see page 166).

Fibroids occur most commonly in women in their 30s and 40s and tend to shrink in size after the menopause when oestrogen secretion falls. Because of this some surgeons may delay surgery if the fibroids are not too large until the menopause intervenes, so tiding the patient over until nature helps solve the problem. This can save an unnecessary operation.

### How?
Fibroids are treated differently according to their type. A dilatation and curettage (D and C) will reveal a submucous fibroid in the cavity of the uterus and a thorough vaginal examination will often enable the others to be found.

Occasionally a D and C will correct the menstrual abnormalities caused by fibroids and this can sometimes delay or completely avoid an operation at all. Many fibroids do need operating on though because they are causing abdominal enlargement, pressure on the bladder or bowel, menstrual irregularity or uncontrolled bleeding, varicose veins or even severe anaemia.

**MYOMECTOMY** is the name of the operation which involves the removal of the fibroid itself yet leaves the uterus intact. Clearly this is essential for women who want more children. Because there are times when the surgeon finds the uterus to be grossly distorted and unlikely to be able to function normally in a future pregnancy, he usually gets the woman's permission to remove her uterus before the myomectomy operation but this is a safeguard which is rarely needed. Because myomectomy is accompanied by a ten per cent recurrence rate, many women who have had their children choose to have the uterus out altogether, so curing the fibroids and ensuring the ultimate in contraception. This is a less serious operation than a myomectomy and cures the condition once and for all. Hysterectomy, though, has its problems (see page 219) and should not be undertaken lightly even if the ovaries and fallopian tubes are left intact (as they usually are).

Myomectomy is an abdominal operation carried out through a horizontal incision over the uterus. It usually means a stay in hospital for two weeks because convalescence can be slower than with other gynaecological operations.


# FISTULA-IN-ANO

## What is it?
A tunnel (sometimes more than one) which leads from the anal canal to the skin outside. It results from an infection starting in the wall of the rectum or anus. The infection breaks through to the skin like any other boil but in this case leaves a track which will continue discharging pus.

**Why operate?**
An operation is necessary because these fistulae never heal spontaneously and the long-term skin irritation and abscess formation are unpleasant for the sufferer.

**How?**
Treatment consists of taking the top off the fistula and removing all of the track under general anaesthesia. If there are multiple tracks the operation can be complex and it may be necessary to cut part of the anal sphincter to lay them open. This is not usually a problem though. The time taken to do the operation varies according to the severity of the condition but a single-track fistula can be operated on in 20 minutes. It may be necessary to examine the area under general anaesthesia several times after the operation at weekly intervals so as to be sure that it is healing and to trim the edges back if necessary.

**Post-operative progress**
There will be some pain for several days after the operation and the time you spend in hospital will depend on the complexity of the operation and how many times an examination under anaesthesia is necessary. It is important to keep the stools very soft by eating plenty of high-fibre foods (see page 173) and you will find daily hot baths very soothing.

After you leave the hospital the surgeon will want to see you very regularly to check the wound so as to ensure that no bridging over of tissue closes off the track as this will encourage pus to build up again. The time for complete healing varies a lot but six weeks is not uncommon.

# FORCEPS DELIVERY

**What is it?**
The use of a twin-bladed instrument, specially designed for the purpose, to help remove a baby from the uterus in the final stages of labour.

Obstetric forceps were first used 100 years ago but have been developed a lot since then. The original instruments were flat and straight but over the years curves have been added, the handles angled and double-slotted locks built into each blade so that the blades of the instrument can be locked together. Basically, a forceps consists of two, separate blades, each consisting of an oval 'head' end and a strong handle at the other end. The head end is curved in such a way as to allow the blade to fit snugly round the baby's head. Of over 600 different types of obstetric forceps only three are widely used today. These are the Simpson type, the Wrigley type and the Kielland type.

Forceps deliveries used to be last-ditch affairs with the obstetrician making heroic last-minute efforts to 'get the baby out'. Today this is no longer the case. Forceps are used much more carefully and are in no sense a last-ditch effort. Forceps are used in a planned way in over a quarter of births.

## Why operate?

There are lots of medical indications for forceps but they fall into three main categories. The first group includes all the conditions that might do the mother or baby harm if she were to keep pushing down hard for long periods. If a mother has high blood pressure, straining can raise it still further, possibly to a dangerous level, and women with heart or lung disease might well suffer unnecessarily from prolonged pushing. Lastly, there are some women who, especially in prolonged labours, become so exhausted that the baby needs to be helped out.

The second group of indications is centred around the baby. In many big hospitals the fetus is monitored so that its wellbeing can be watched closely. By attaching a small electrode to the baby's scalp while it is still in the uterus, doctors can watch its progress and especially keep an eye on its heartbeat as it is displayed on a TV-type screen or on paper at the mother's bedside. Should anything go wrong the baby will have to be delivered quickly if it is to be born unharmed and it is in such cases that forceps can be especially useful. But as well as helping out babies with this 'fetal distress', as it is called, forceps are also valuable in protecting the soft skull of a premature baby as its immature head passes between the muscles, ligaments and bones of the birth canal.

The last group of babies that is helped by forceps are those that are held up in the birth canal because the uterine contractions are too weak; because they are lying in a poor position; or because they are too big to come out easily. Forceps can prevent many such mothers from having to have a Caesarean section. Women who have an epidural (see page 391) are also much more likely to have to have forceps.

### How?

Forceps are large, powerful instruments and can only be fitted around the baby's head when the cervix is fully open and ready for the baby to come out. If the baby has to be delivered before this, then a Caesarean section will be necessary. As well as the cervix being ready for the birth, the baby's head must be low enough down the birth canal to enable the doctor to fit the forceps and the waters must already be broken. If the head is too high, then a Caesarean section may have to be performed. A suction extractor called a Ventouse apparatus is sometimes used instead of forceps in Britain and on the continent of Europe. It is almost never used in the United States. It works by producing a strong vacuum under a cap which is placed on the baby's head. The suction gives the obstetrician a good strong grip on the baby and enables him to pull it out rather as if he were using forceps.

Once the decision to use forceps has been made, the obstetrician will usually do an episiotomy (see page 178). He then takes one of the blades of the forceps and with his left hand inside the vagina alongside the baby's head he inserts the blade with his right hand in such a way that the hollow of the instrument fits around the baby's head in just the right position in front of the ears. He then repeats the procedure for the other blade and locks the two together to form a handle which remains outside the vagina. At the next contraction the woman is asked to push down as usual while the doctor pulls on the baby's head to guide it out. In all but the very deepest of heads, this is achieved within a minute or two of applying the forceps. Once the head is delivered, the forceps are removed and the baby's body is delivered as usual.

## Post-operative progress

From the mother's point of view a forceps delivery today need present no problems compared with a normal birth. The old tales of doctors struggling to pull babies out are, thankfully, a thing of the past now that we have recourse to safe Caesarean sections as an alternative in the really difficult cases. Forceps births are potentially more painful than normal ones but, with adequate pain relief, should be no more unpleasant. Special nerve blocks are often used but as so many women are having epidurals today (see page 391), forceps are less of a problem because they feel no pain anyway. General anaesthesia is rarely used for a forceps delivery but a really difficult situation may call for it.

From the baby's point of view a forceps delivery presents few problems. When the blades are applied to the head they do not squeeze it like a wrench because the blades are hollowed out to accept the head. However, as they sit snugly around the sides of the head the forceps blades may well leave impressions in the skin for a couple of days. These are usually completely harmless but rarely a nerve in the face can be squeezed and so result in a facial weakness for a few days. When you see your new baby you may feel that the forceps have squeezed his head flatter than you think it ought to be. Don't worry though because a baby's skull bones are very soft and soon come back to normal shape. The reason the head is like this is not because the forceps have squashed it but that the condition for which the forceps were applied was probably one in which the baby's head was being squashed by the birth canal anyway. Even some quite normal, non-forceps babies have squashed-looking heads immediately after delivery.

Just because you have had forceps once does not mean you will always have to have them. Only one in five women who has forceps for their first birth needs them next time.

## FRACTURES

The body's tissues and organs all hang from and are supported by a bony skeleton made up of more than 200 bones. Bones are rigid, strong structures but nevertheless have some natural flexibility. In children, the bones are much more flexible than in adults and a special type of fracture (a greenstick fracture) occurs in children in which the bone bends but does not break right across. These fractures usually heal very well if left alone or if splinted in a plaster cast.

A fracture is a break in a bone and in theory almost any of the body's bones can be fractured. In practice, very few of the body's bones are subject to fractures, except in the most serious of car crashes, for example. Fractures can occur as the result of a direct blow to the body or indirectly by transmission of pressure from one part of the body to another. An example of the latter is the collarbone which can be broken by falling on an outstretched hand. Sometimes fractures occur spontaneously when a bone is weakened by generalized bone disease or by the presence of a secondary cancer deposit.

Fractures can be 'open' or 'closed'. In an open fracture. bone pokes through the skin but in a closed one, the fracture is diagnosed by other signs.

There are three types of closed fracture.

A **GREENSTICK** fracture is only seen in children. The bone is not broken all the way across and there is usually no displacement. It heals quickly with minimal medical intervention.

A **SIMPLE CLOSED FRACTURE** is one in which the bone is broken into two fragments only with displacement of the ends but in which the skin is still intact.

A **COMPLICATED FRACTURE** is one in which the broken ends of the bone have damaged nerves or blood vessels locally. In one in three of such fractures the bone fragments.

Open fractures are generally more serious and bone can be seen poking through the skin.

It is often very difficult to tell whether a bone is fractured or not and it may take X-rays to be sure of the diagnosis. As a general rule though, fractures are usually painful over the fractured area; there is often swelling or bruising; the bone may poke through the skin; the person is reluctant to use the affected part; and there may be a deformity of the part.

The commonest bones to fracture are (in order of frequency but depending to some extent on age) wrist, ankle, collarbone, elbow, hip, nose, ribs, upper arm, forearm, thigh, pelvis, shin, skull, fingers and back.

This is not a first aid book so the reader is asked to refer to such a text for advice on what to do in an emergency. Here, we will look at what doctors can do for fractures.

## General action
After first aid measures have been carried out to save life, control pain and seek medical help, a doctor will have to be involved. Bone is not the dead 'scaffolding' that many people think it is. It is a living tissue that can regrow and heal like any other and doctors make use of this when treating fractures. The first thing that the doctor has to do is to 'set ' the bone in its proper position again so that it *can* heal. This means that he will need several X-rays to tell him the position of the broken ends so that he knows how to manoeuvre them back into position.

If the X-rays show that the bones are still in line, no manoeuvring is necessary. Once the doctor knows what has to be done, he will render the person pain-free (with local or general anaesthesia) and then 'reduce' the fracture.

Because the intrinsic stability of the rigid, strong bones has been lost and because powerful muscles surround many bones, the whole area will then have to be immobilized in a plaster cast (to include the bone and nearby joints) or with other devices so that the broken ends are held close together, thus allowing them to heal. This type of fracture repair is the most common and is known as closed reduction because at no time has the surgeon opened up the area to do anything.

Under certain circumstances (very splintered bones, very difficult angles of bone fragments, or the close proximity of structures that could be damaged by closed reduction), open reduction is carried out. In this procedure (an open operation), the bone pieces are re-aligned and fixed with metal plates, nails, screws, pins, wires or other equipment made of special metal that does not corrode in the body's tissues. Sometimes stout pins are inserted through the skin and then deeply through the bone to obtain instant fixation yet spare the person an open operation.

Fracture healing times vary according to the cause of the fracture, the age and health of the person and the bone fractured. In children fractures often heal within three or four weeks but up to six months may be needed for complete healing in a weight-bearing bone in an adult. Most non-weight-bearing bones take at least six to eight weeks to heal.

Rarely, fractures fail to heal and an open operation may be necessary to drain any pus there may be, to re-align the bone fragments or to graft bone to aid union.

**ARM FRACTURES** are not too troublesome once fixed because the person can walk around with his affected arm in a plaster cast in a sling.

**LEG FRACTURES** are more troublesome because even though a walking heel is built into the 'foot' of the plaster cast, leg plasters are cumbersome and present problems with trousers (which may have to be split on that side), bathing, and of course walking. The leg must not be allowed to take the weight of the body; crutches or other walking aids are needed but these are easily mastered, except by the elderly.

**PELVIC FRACTURES** may or may not prove troublesome because small ones allow the person to walk within a few weeks but severe ones can mean weeks of bed rest. Unfortunately, a blow severe enough to produce a fractured pelvis may cause damage inside the abdomen and this can prove more troublesome than the fracture itself.

**SPINE FRACTURES** are of several different kinds, some of which are trivial and others of which involve months in body braces or plaster casts which at least enable the person to remain mobile. Very severe spine fractures may require long periods of complete rest but these people will often have had a bone fusion to help brace the fractures internally.

**RIB FRACTURES** almost never need operating on and heal spontaneously. The only treatment necessary is pain relief and possibly a splint of some kind (often a firm binding) around the chest to reduce the movements of the broken ends as the chest moves with breathing.

**HIP FRACTURES** are very common in the elderly and probably take up more medical time than any other fractures because they cannot effectively be treated without an operation. In a hip fracture it is in fact the upper end of the thigh bone that is broken and not the hip itself.

To obtain the best results the old person should be operated on very soon after the fracture has occurred. Under general anaesthesia the fracture is reduced and fixed with nails, screws or plates. Because this produces rigid fixation of the fracture the old person can be up and about within a day or two of the operation. This is good because elderly people immobilized for long periods fare very badly.

If the fracture is very near the head of the thigh bone, the ball-shaped head may die and will then have to be replaced by a metal hip joint prosthesis (see page 237). This may be followed by a total hip joint replacement if the results are not good after replacing the thighbone part. The results of operations for hip fractures are now extremely good but as the majority of such fractures occur in fragile, old people, they may be repaired yet the person die from the complications of surgery and old age.

# GALL-STONES

**What are they?**
Gall-stones are stones made by the body that lodge in the gall-bladder and its ducts. In order to understand the operation to remove the gall-bladder let us look at the gall-bladder itself.

The gall-bladder is a small pouch a few centimetres long that lies in the top part of the right side of the abdomen under the liver. It is pear-shaped and holds an ounce or two of bile (gall). Bile is produced by the liver on a continuous basis and passed to the gall-bladder for concentration and storage. It is discharged after meals into the first part of the intestine via a wide, thin-walled duct called the common bile duct. Bile helps the digestion of fatty foods but intermittent discharge is not essential – people whose gall-bladders have been removed seem to fare perfectly well.

Almost all gall-bladder disease is associated with stone formation. No one knows why stones form but it is thought that they result from too high a saturation of cholesterol in bile. This saturation level can be reduced by eating high-fibre foods (roughage) and this led researchers to ask whether gall-stones (present in a third of all seventy-year-olds and even more common in the obese) might not be a disease of western eating. Certainly, a high-fibre diet does reduce the level of cholesterol in bile but it is not yet known whether this is the total answer.

Whatever is found to be protective, gall-stones currently cause millions of gall-bladders to be removed each year so a cause is well worth looking for. Today the operation to remove the gall-bladder (cholecystectomy) is the commonest elective operation in the western world. More money is spent on removing gall-bladders in the US, for example, than on the whole of medical care in the continent of Africa.

The commonest symptoms of gall-stones are bouts of pain or gall-bladder infection. There may also be indigestion, a bloated feeling, excessive belching, an intolerance of fatty foods or more rarely sharp, knife-like, colicky pains in the

upper part of the abdomen which may shoot to the shoulder
on that side or through to the back. Sometimes a stone blocks
a duct completely, causes back pressure of bile and renders
the person jaundiced. The sufferer or her relatives notice that
the whites of her eyes are tinged with yellow and she may
pass dark urine. I say 'she' because very many more women
get gall-stones than do men.

Making a diagnosis is usually straightforward but the
pains may make the doctor think of heart disease or the
oesophageal regurgitation of gastric contents. Hiatus hernias
(see page 214) and gall-stones sometimes go together. The
diagnosis is finally confirmed by X-ray studies of the biliary
system. These are described in detail on page 422.

Many gall-stones are produced and are no doubt passed
into the bowel while they are very small. After a while though,
a stone (or stones) may become too big to pass out of the
gall-bladder. It then stays there and grows over the years.
Gall-stones vary in size from grit to large pebbles.

If a stone becomes caught in the duct from the gall-bladder
to the common bile duct, pressure develops and the gall-
bladder swells, becomes inflamed and tries to squeeze bile
past the obstructing stone. This is known as cholecystitis but
does not necessarily require an operation at once. Some
people pass a small stone or it may simply drop back into the
gall-bladder and the symptoms subside. At this stage bed rest,
plenty of fluids rather than food, pain relief and observation
are all that are needed. If the way in and out of the gall-
bladder remains blocked then it will stop working and more
trouble can develop.

Non-surgical treatment includes the management of
acute inflammation as described or the giving of anti-
spasmodic drugs and a low fat diet if the gall-bladder is
scarred yet has no gall-stones in it.

Today it is possible to dissolve some gall-stones using a
new drug, chenic acid (chenodeoxycholic acid). This was
first found in goose bile. Chenic acid makes up about 40
per cent of the bile acids present in human bile. The drug
probably reduces the production of cholesterol in the liver
and so allows the gall-stones to be slowly dissolved by the

body's natural dissolver – its own chenic acid. It is not suitable for many people with gall-stones though and certain conditions have to be met before its use can be considered. First, it is only effective on gall-stones made of cholesterol, because this is how it works and second, it can only work if the unsaturated bile it produces in the liver can get into the gall-bladder. This latter fact can be ascertained by taking special X-rays. Unfortunately, only about one in five of those coming to surgeons for removal of their gall-bladders falls into the treatable category as judged by these two criteria alone and there are other problems. Drug treatment cannot therefore replace surgery for most patients at the moment. Also, a single large stone is a poor candidate for treatment – many small stones do far better, partly because they have a larger surface area on which the chenic acid can act. Stones of less than five millimetres in diameter may dissolve completely within six to twelve months of therapy.

Because drug therapy with chenic acid has to be prolonged, it is necessarily very expensive. At the time of going to press the daily cost is one pound and because of this it has been suggested that a lower dose can be used provided the drug is taken at bedtime and a low cholesterol diet adhered to. Unfortunately, even once the stones have been dissolved, new stones can form if no preventive measures are taken. It is here that bran and a high-fibre diet can be useful because, as we have seen, high-fibre foods (especially wheat bran) reduce the concentration of cholesterol in the gall-bladder and so render gall-stone formation less likely.

## Why operate?
Surgery is usually necessary in the following circumstances: if an acute attack of cholecystitis can be definitely diagnosed very early in its progress (if it cannot be then surgery is delayed for a few weeks until the inflammation has settled); if the person has repeated attacks of pain caused by gall-stones; if there are other symptoms which make life unpleasant; if gall-stones are found as a chance finding (they are best removed rather than left, even if they are causing no trouble); and if medical treatment fails. In general, this means that if

gall-stones are present and causing symptoms the gall-bladder is best removed.

## How?

There is usually no special preparation for a cholecystectomy. If the operation is being done in the acute phase of cholecystitis then antibiotics, painkillers and intravenous feeding may be used. The operation is carried out under general anaesthesia through an incision below the right side of the rib cage. The incision, which is about 15 centimetres long, may be horizontal, vertical, or parallel with the rib cage. The gall-bladder is removed and often a radio-opaque fluid is introduced into the common bile duct to show up on X-rays (taken in the operating theatre) whether there are any stones in the duct. This procedure is called cholangiography. If there are stones present, the duct is opened and the stones removed.

The operation usually lasts about an hour.

## Post-operative progress

As after any major abdominal operation, the area itself is painful for a few days but most people are up and about the day after surgery. A drainage tube may be left protruding from a small (one centimetre long) incision so that there is no build-up of fluid in the operation area internally. This drain comes out after a few days and the person can go home after four to ten days.

Some surgeons think it wise to keep off fatty foods post-operatively for some months but this is by no means essential.

The success rate of the operation is very high. Almost 90 per cent of all gall-bladder patients are completely relieved of their symptoms and the once common second operation to find an overlooked stone is now very uncommon.

Surprising though it may seem, Man seems to be able to live perfectly well without a gall-bladder. People who have had their gall-bladder removed live normal lives and have no restrictions placed upon them.

# GANGLIA

**What are they?**
Hard swellings, usually found on the back of the wrists of
girls and young women. They can occur elsewhere but they
are always near a tendon or joint. No one knows why ganglia
occur but they are thought to be areas of degenerated
fibrous tissue, perhaps resulting from a minor injury.
Sometimes they occur after the repeated use of a joint or
tendon.

The swelling is so hard that it feels like bone. In fact, when
it is cut open at operation it has a tough outer shell of fibrous
tissue and a soft, gelatinous interior. Ganglia can be painful
and the pain (usually dull) comes on after using the affected
part.

Ganglia are completely harmless and are not related to
cancer in any way.

**Why operate?**
To remove the unsightly lump and to cure the symptoms it
produces.

**How?**
The classical medical method of dealing with small ganglia is
to hit them hard. It was always said that the family bible was
ideal for the job! This disperses the ganglion, often for good,
but should only be done by a doctor.

Larger ones, though, need an operation under general
anaesthesia. The whole structure and its deep attachment to
tendons are removed very carefully to try and ensure that it
does not recur but even so a few do.

**Post-operative progress**
The area is heavily bandaged for a week. Long-term results
are excellent and a complete cure is to be expected in most
cases. A few ganglia do, however, recur.

# GLAUCOMA

**What is it?**

A condition affecting the eyes in which the pressure inside them becomes raised. It is nothing to do with high blood pressure and is not catching. Glaucoma is a family of conditions, not a single entity, and there are acute and chronic forms. It is common, affecting one in 100 people over the age of 40. Glaucoma usually affects both eyes but one more severely than the other.

The acute form is dramatic but much less common than the slow-onset type. In acute glaucoma, the pressure rises inside the eye very rapidly and this produces pain in the eye and haloes which can be seen around lights and brightly lit objects. There may be redness of the eye and cloudy vision too. Vomiting occurs as the pressure rises further. Emergency medical help is essential because the eye can go blind within a very short time if not treated.

Chronic glaucoma is five times more common than this acute form but because of its slow, insidious build-up it can severely damage a person's vision before he seeks help. Glaucoma comes about because the circulation of the watery fluid in the eye becomes partly blocked. This causes a raised pressure in the eye. The pressure rise damages the nerves at the back of the eye and some loss of vision and eventually even blindness sets in. Signs include 'tunnel' vision in which the person sees things as if down a telescope.

Chronic glaucoma is a common disease as we have seen and can be inherited but skips a generation or two sometimes. It is about ten times as common in near blood relations as would be expected. Because of this, if it is found that you have glaucoma it makes sense for all your close relatives to be tested.

Although the surgeon cannot get back any lost vision he can by medication and surgery offer relief of symptoms and prevent further deterioration in vision. Chronic glaucoma is the cause of about 15 per cent of all blindness and every year thousands of people are blinded needlessly by the disease. If it is caught at the stage in which only peripheral vision is deteriorating, then vision can be saved with certainty.

Ophthalmic surgeons and ophthalmic opticians can measure the pressure of the fluid in the eye using a simple instrument called a tonometer. This test takes only a minute or two and involves the placing of a small, pressure-sensitive probe on the front of each eye. The operator then reads off the pressure inside the eye directly. This does not hurt because the sensitive front of the eye is anaesthetized first with a drop of local anaesthetic. Other methods of measuring intra-ocular pressure are now available.

Once *acute* glaucoma has been diagnosed, eyedrops and/or tablets, together with admission to hospital, alleviate the symptoms. Treatment can also halt the progress of *chronic* glaucoma. Drugs do not improve the drainage in the eye permanently, of course, but do prevent people having to have operations to improve the drainage and are a small enough price to pay for one's eyesight. These drops or tablets will have to be taken regularly for life. Once drainage is improved eye pressure falls to normal and the previous vision will get no worse.

Once you have reached this stage you will be able to play games, drive a car and go about your life in a perfectly normal way. If you want to wear *soft* contact lenses, seek advice first.

### Why operate?
Surgery is used when medical treatment proves inadequate and some people need to continue with medication even after an operation.

### How?
There are several drainage procedures a surgeon can use, and which is used depends on whether he is treating acute or chronic glaucoma. The operations are performed under a general anaesthetic and one (a peripheral iridectomy) involves cutting off part of the iris (the coloured part of the eye around the pupil). A crescent-shaped incision is made at the edge of the iris (where it joins the white) and this is closed with very fine sutures once the procedure is over. Eyedrops

will be put into the eye and a pad placed over it. You will be out of bed on the following day or even the same day and home within a week. Expect to be off work for three or four weeks.

This simple procedure cures almost all acute glaucomas and can be done as a preventive measure in an as yet unaffected eye in someone whose other eye is affected. Even if there has been an attack of acute glaucoma, vision is returned to normal by iridectomy. The operation is rarely done as an emergency in acute glaucoma because drugs are mostly used to tide the person over the acute crisis stage. An operation is performed later, if necessary.

# HAEMORRHOIDS

**What are they?**
Haemorrhoids (piles) are varicose veins in the mucous membrane which lines the anal canal. Doctors subdivide piles into *internal* (those which are not seen) and *external* (those which show). Often both are present.

No one knows for sure why we get piles but they are extremely common. Half the population over the age of 50 has piles and modern research suggests that this is because we eat a diet low in dietary fibre (roughage). Normally, when we in the West pass a stool, we strain to force the hard, craggy mass through the anal canal. In parts of the world where a high-fibre diet is the norm, the people never strain to pass a stool because their stools are soft like toothpaste. Recent anatomical research has found that normally there are special cushions of tissue that help keep the anal canal shut and that these are displaced when someone has internal haemorrhoids.

This kind of thinking has now revolutionized the whole subject of surgery for piles and countless thousands of people, who would have been operated upon even as recently as five years ago are now completely cured of their symptoms simply by changing to a high-fibre diet.

Having said this though, the most common signs of piles is

bleeding from the back passage and this is a sign that should not be ignored because it can also be caused by a cancer of the bowel. If you ever have rectal bleeding, you must see your doctor so that he can rule out causes other than piles or refer you to a surgeon who will do so. Once he has done so, unless you have large external piles with considerable tags of skin, you may well never need an operation at all.

Change your eating habits as follows. Eat wholemeal bread, high-bran breakfast cereals and plenty of fruit and vegetables. Do not eat foods made with white flour and cut down your sugar intake. You will know when you have got the balance right because you will be able to open your bowels with absolutely no effort. When you can achieve this, keep your fibre level up to maintain soft, easily-passed stools. This will relieve itching, bleeding and the other unpleasant symptoms of piles.

Having said all this, there will always be some people whose piles do not respond to dietary changes and who will need further treatment.

The symptoms of piles are usually bleeding, itching, irritation, a feeling of fullness in the back passage, or the presence of skin tags at the outside of the anus. A vein may become acutely swollen and extremely tender but this usually subsides with local heat (sitting in a hot bath, for example). A doctor may have to incise the tender area to relieve the pressure but this does not usually involve a stay in hospital.

Making the diagnosis is easy because all piles can be seen by a doctor either with the naked eye or using a proctoscope (see page 386). An accurate diagnosis is essential because it is crucial not to put rectal bleeding down to something simple like piles when in fact it is caused by cancer of the bowel higher up. A problem for doctors is that because piles are so common in middle age, it is easy to cure them and still miss a cancer of the bowel. Because of this you may be asked to have a barium enema X-ray examination (see page 422) and a sigmoidoscopy (see page 407) just to be sure. The survival rates from cancer of the large bowel are greatly improved if the growth is detected and treated early.

As well as changing their diet, some people benefit from local creams and soothing ointments to relieve the itching while the diet takes time to work (a week or two). Many surgeons offer injections for internal piles. These irritate the veins so that scar tissue closes them off. It is also possible to place tiny elastic bands around the base of the haemorrhoid so it falls away after two weeks. People who do not respond to dietary changes or these treatments need surgery but they are a *minority*.

## Why operate?
An operation is necessary if other more conservative measures fail; if there are unpleasant external skin tags; if the bleeding causes serious anaemia; or if large piles keep prolapsing ('coming down').

## How?
There are several operations for piles but the most common one involves actually removing the piles after tying them off at their bases and dissecting them away from the surrounding structures. This is carried out under general anaesthesia and takes about half an hour. Internal haemorrhoids can be treated with another technique known as rubber band ligation. In this, a latex rubber band is placed around the neck of the pile. It strangles the pile by starving it of blood and as a result it falls off after two weeks. This procedure is painless and does not require an anaesthetic – in fact it can be done as an out-patient procedure but may have to be repeated at two-week intervals.

The third method of treatment involves the use of an instrument which can deliver a cold burn to a tissue. This procedure is called cryosurgery and the cold literally burns the pile which then falls off in a week or two.

A fairly recent addition to the operative treatments for piles involves stretching the anal canal under a general anaesthetic. This is based on the reasoning that many people with piles have developed constricting bands of fibrous tissue. The surgeon stretches the anal canal and then inserts a sponge into the back passage. This is removed an hour later in the ward. Excellent results are claimed for this technique but some people are incontinent of faeces (leak) after it. This leaking is usually short-lived.

## Post-operative progress

After the common operations for piles there is pain for about a week but newer operative methods have reduced the amount of post-operative pain. Local anaesthetic creams, repeated bathing or sitting in warm water all help and it is vital to stay on a high-fibre diet so that the first stools passed are really soft and involve no straining at all. The person can get up the day after the operation, though sitting will be uncomfortable. He can usually go home within a week. On about the sixth post-operative day the surgeon will perform a gentle rectal examination with his finger to ensure that no narrowing is occurring. At this time he will also warn the person to expect a little bleeding as the stitches come away. After about fourteen days the area returns to normal and everyday activities can be resumed.

Haemorrhoids removed by this method do not recur in 90 per cent of those treated.

With the rubber band ligation method there is very rarely any discomfort or trouble once the bands are in place although the tied-off piles do give the sensation of the back passage being 'full' and an urge to open the bowels. Sitting for long periods can be uncomfortable and when the piles drop off there may be some bleeding. It if seems a lot, see your doctor. Other signs that might occur are a smelly discharge or a burning sensation.

After the stretching procedure you will be given a lubricating jelly or an anal dilator to use after a hot bath before going to bed. This should be left in place for a minute or two every evening for two weeks, on alternate days for the next two weeks, then once weekly for six months. Some faecal incontinence (leaking) is not unknown but is only temporary.

# HEART SURGERY

(See also Congenital heart disease; Coronary artery surgery; Pacemakers.)

Heart surgery has always been a more emotive subject than most other forms of surgery because of our innate feeling that the heart is more than simply a pump that pushes the blood round our bodies. Heart transplants, for example, have social and mystical overtones that are rarely, if ever, mentioned when livers or kidneys, let alone corneas, are transplanted.

In reality though the heart is simply a pump – a rather clever one but nonetheless still a pump and as such can be diseased and need surgery or complete replacement as can other body organs.

The heart is a muscular organ about the size of a fist which lies in the chest, slightly to the left of the breastbone. It is remarkably easy to get at surgically because the chest is easily opened and this reveals the heart clearly. It is far easier to get at than lots of the abdominal contents, for example. Depending on which part of the heart is to be operated on, the incision to reveal the heart is made in the left or right side of the chest or the breastbone is split and then wired up again afterwards.

All heart operations are done under a general anaesthetic and fall into two basic categories: closed heart surgery (in which the heart is not opened but continues to pump blood as normal); and open heart surgery (in which the blood circulation is taken over by a pump outside the body).

**OPEN HEART SURGERY** This is possible because a piece of equipment called a heart-lung machine takes over the heart's pumping action and the lungs' oxygen-giving function while the person's heart is stopped for an operation. Oxygen is put into blood taken from the big inflow vessels to the heart (which are closed off temporarily) and carbon dioxide is removed from it. A gentle pump then forces the blood back into the main arteries to supply the body. In addition, the blood can be cooled or passed through a heat exchanger. The most critical part of the whole procedure is the pumping mechanism because almost any commonplace mechanical pump would so damage the red blood cells that they would be rendered useless for carrying oxygen. In order to overcome this problem, special pumps that 'milk' the fragile blood around the system have been developed. Once the heart is empty of blood, an electric shock is given to render the heart muscle motionless and the surgeon has a bloodless, still organ on which to operate. Once the operation is over, the surgeon shocks the heart back into action after its blood supply has been connected back again. In this way the heart-lung machine gives surgeons an hour or so in which to complete their work. This method is now so well proven that it is used all over the world on a routine basis. The main drawback is its expense as a team of highly-skilled surgeons, technicians, nurses and anaesthetists is needed for such a procedure. It is these that make open heart surgery so expensive. Pre-operative assessment and post-operative aftercare are, however, also expensive for this group of patients.

The heart-lung machine has meant that several operations, previously impossible, can now be done with comparative safety. Some conditions can be treated by closed heart surgery if caught early or by open heart surgery if more serious action is needed. Mitral stenosis is a good example of this.

In order to understand heart operations we need to see how the heart works and what it does.

The heart is a four-chambered muscular pump situated in the left side of the chest. It is divided into two halves, left and right, handling oxygenated and deoxygenated blood respectively. Each side of the heart has an upper collecting chamber or atrium, a set of valves through which the blood passes to the lower pump chamber or ventricle and an outflow vessel. Blood can flow only from the upper chamber to the lower when the interconnecting (mitral and tricuspid) valves are open. These valves also prevent reverse flow.

Blood which has performed its oxygen- and nutrition-giving tasks in the body is collected by veins which open into big collecting veins known as the inferior and superior venae cavae. In this way all the venous blood from the body ends up in the right atrium. This chamber contracts and pumps the blood through the tricuspid valve into the right ventricle below. The valve then closes and the blood is pumped up into the vessel which takes it to the lungs to be re-oxygenated.

Once its oxygen had been replenished, the blood returns to the heart, entering by the left atrium. This contracts and forces the blood into the biggest and most muscular chamber of all – the left ventricle. The blood is then passed out into the aorta under pressure high enough to carry it round the body.

The heart is made of a very special type of muscle that beats spontaneously, even when outside the body. The beating is controlled by a sophisticated set of pathways in the heart itself. The heart is a remarkable organ. It contracts all our lives: that is over 100,000 beats a day for 70 years or 2,575 million beats in a lifetime. At birth the pulse rate is about 140 and falls to around 100 at three years. It goes on falling in rate until middle age when it is about 70 beats a minute.

Every single beat is controlled by the heart's pacemaker which disciplines the natural tendency of each part of the heart to contract at its own rate into a concerted effort. So it is that all four chambers and four sets of valves (two in the chambers and two in the outflow vessels) work with split-second accuracy to ensure that the body gets the blood it needs every minute of our lives. The pacemaker's activity is modified by the sympathetic and parasympathetic nerves of the automatic (autonomic) nervous system.

The heart is the most demanding muscle in our bodies and uses a great deal of the oxygen supplied by the lungs. The blood needed to provide oxygen and nutrients for the heart reaches its muscle via the coronary arteries. These come off the aorta and give the heart a high-pressure supply of blood even before the rest of the body gets its supply.

Heart disease requiring an operation is of two types. The first is called *congenital heart disease* because it is present from birth and the second *acquired*, because the conditions are the result of diseases acquired after birth.

Many thousands of children each year are born with congenital heart defects (see page 148) but countless millions of adults in the western world acquire some kind of heart disease, which is now the biggest killer in the West. As surgical techniques improve, more and more people are being operated on for heart disease with increasing safety. In fact, even open heart operations are now done routinely just as are operations on the abdominal organs. Let us look at some of the more common heart conditions and the operations used to treat them.

**MITRAL STENOSIS** This is a heart condition that can occur a long time after rheumatic fever. Rheumatic fever is increasingly rare today but was common until about thirty years ago. It is the group of people who suffered from the disease thirty or more years ago that comes forward to be treated for mitral stenosis today.

Rheumatic fever occurs as the result of a sensitivity to a certain streptococcal bacterium. Many thousands of children and adults get streptococcal sore throats but only a tiny minority get rheumatic fever as a result. Any streptococcal infection of the upper respiratory tract (tonsillitis, scarlet fever or otitis media) can cause rheumatic fever.

Although the disease is more common in certain families it is not known whether this is due to an increased exposure to streptococcal infections or to genetic factors.

Rheumatic fever is uncommon today, as we have seen, but as recently as 1928 it filled one quarter of all the beds in a London children's hospital. The improvement has come about because of better public health, improved living conditions, better food and the control of streptococcal infections with antibiotics.

The most serious effect of rheumatic fever is on the heart muscle and the heart valves, causing enlargement of the heart and heart murmurs. Death can occur (though rarely) from heart failure. The damage to the heart valves can last into adulthood. Today, with good treatment, the chances of a child getting heart disease after rheumatic fever are very small indeed.

Rarely, the brain is involved and jerky, unco-ordinated movements of the limbs and face occur (St Vitus's dance).

A child that gets rheumatic fever today should take penicillin by mouth daily (or by injection monthly) for several years to prevent further attacks. If your child has had rheumatic fever he should be 'covered' by penicillin every time he has dental treatment or any operation, however small. If you are in any doubt, ask your doctor.

Aspirin is the best treatment for acute rheumatic fever and is used in very high doses to relieve the pains and fever. Steroid drugs are sometimes used.

Thanks to penicillin, streptococcal infections are killed off if caught early and rarely go on to produce rheumatic fever. If ever your child has a sore throat or earache and complains of joint pains or does not seem to be recovering as you would expect after about ten days, see your doctor.

The arthritis of rheumatic fever does not last like the joint swelling of rheumatoid arthritis and is a totally different disease.

Mitral stenosis is much commoner in women than in men and the symptoms are made worse by pregnancy. In the adult, the remains of the childhood infection with rheumatic fever produce changes in the heart in which the leaves (flaps) of the mitral valve become thickened, hardened and stick together. The tethering fibres that are attached to the valve flaps also shorten and the end result is a funnel-shaped opening rather than a valve which closes off flat. Because the valve is narrowed this causes back pressure in the lungs and a poor output from the heart. The person becomes short of breath on exertion and needs propping up at night to get his breath. He may spit up blood and may also develop a disorder of the heartbeat known as atrial fibrillation.

A plain chest X-ray and a full clinical examination usually confirm the diagnosis already made from the person's story of old rheumatic fever and it is only rarely that other more sophisticated tests are needed unless surgery is contemplated.

When the valve is stenosed (too tight) it can usually be split at a simple operation that does not involve opening the heart. The surgeon inserts a finger and a special instrument into the wall of the left atrium. This yields excellent results if there is no leakage from the tight valve. If the mitral stenosis is severe, open heart surgery at which a new valve is sewn into place is the only answer.

Rheumatic fever can also cause damage to the aortic valve.

**AORTIC STENOSIS** is a condition in which the aortic valve flaps become fused together just as in mitral stenosis. In fact the two conditions are often seen together. Unlike people with mitral valve disease, those with aortic stenosis are often little affected until angina comes on.

**AORTIC REGURGITATION.** This is a condition in which the aortic valve leaks so much that blood pumped out of the heart does not effectively get round the circulation – much of it simply falls back into the heart through the ever open valve. Eventually, heart failure develops and the person finds it difficult to breathe as fluid accumulates in the lungs. These symptoms, in addition to chest pain on exertion and fainting (both caused by too poor a blood flow from the aorta), may necessitate an operation. Open heart surgery enables the valve to be replaced.

**RHEUMATIC HEART DISEASE** does not always need operating upon. Many people go through life coping effectively on drugs and whilst they will be checked up regularly by a doctor or heart specialist, they will probably never need anything surgical done at all. Unfortunately, facilities in the UK are relatively restricted for such major heart surgery and some people who could benefit from such an operation die on the waiting list before their turn comes around. For those who are operated on, though, results are excellent.

Open heart surgery is very major surgery. The operations can take up to four or five hours, depending on what is done, but the person will be out of hospital within two or three weeks. Much of the early post-operative period is spent in an intensive care unit (see page 51).

# HERNIA

## What is it?

A hernia is a condition in which some of the contents of the abdomen push through the abdominal wall, often to form a pouch or sac, visible on the outside as a lump.

In the normal, healthy person the abdominal contents slide against each other because they have a slippery covering called the peritoneum. The major organs inside the abdominal cavity are fixed in place but the intestine and large bowel hang freely and move over each other as their 20-odd feet contract and relax as food passes along. As the abdominal wall muscles contract every time we cough or strain they remind us that under everyday conditions they hold our abdomens in shape and keep all the organs inside where they belong.

Under certain circumstances though, weaknesses occur in tnis normally tough abdominal wall and it is through these weakened areas that the mobile, flexible intestines can protrude, especially when we raise the pressure inside the abdomen by coughing or straining.

There are several weak points that occur naturally in the abdomen. The first is where the spermatic cords (vasa deferentia) enter the abdomen from the testes; the second is around the navel; the third is where the veins from the legs enter the abdomen; and the fourth is where the oesophagus (gullet) goes through into the chest. Because nature has breached the strong abdominal wall at these points to let vital structures through, it is here that the intestine may nudge its way through and form a hernia.

Hernias can occur for many reasons but often no cause is found. A sudden strain can certainly open up an already weakened area; an operation scar can cause an abnormally weak area; pregnancy puts strains on the abdominal wall and raises abdominal pressure so predisposing to hernias; serious chest diseases cause prolonged coughing; longstanding constipation causes repeated straining; and many other factors can all contribute to the formation of a hernia.

Hernias are seen at any age. Babies tend to have umbilical (around the navel) hernias; women, femoral (top of the leg) hernias, and men inguinal (near the scrotum) hernias. Because inguinal hernias are by far the most common and are seen most commonly in men, men are more prone to hernias than are women.

Let us look at each type in turn.

## Inguinal hernias

These arise because there is an inherent weakness in the lower abdominal wall of men. In the male fetus the testes are in the abdomen until just before birth when they come down canals (the inguinal canals) at the bottom of the abdomen and travel into the scrotum. Partly because the canal through the layers of the abdominal wall is so oblique (the layers automatically shut behind the testis as the muscles contract) and partly because tissues grow to obliterate the canal, the path from the abdomen to the scrotum usually shuts off completely, except to allow the spermatic cord through. This might seem a strange piece of design but testes have to be kept at about two degrees Centigrade cooler than the rest of the body for sperms to develop properly and for this reason cannot stay inside the abdomen.

In some men the canal remains a weak spot and, after a provoking factor (outlined above), cannot keep the abdominal contents inside any longer. At first a tiny knuckle of bowel or fat pokes through into the weakened area, causing a small bulge in the groin. This can grow to be very large indeed. The lump often goes down at night and reappears during the working day or on coughing (especially among smokers) or straining.

The bulging causes discomfort so something has to be done or complications may eventually develop. This kind of hernia never gets better spontaneously so help of some kind is essential.

The simplest thing is to wear a truss. This padded leather object supports the weakened area and firmly presses over the hole in the abdominal wall through which the protrusion usually occurs. Many older people never have an operation on their hernias; they simply wear a truss and are quite content. However, there is a problem. Hernias are usually only a discomfort for the vast majority of people but they can become life-threatening. Most hernias have a wide mouth which allows the abdominal contents to move in and out freely. On rare occasions, though, this may not happen and the bowel inside can become trapped in the hernia and lose its blood supply. Then gangrene sets in. This is called a strangulated hernia, is very painful, causes obstruction of the bowel where the gangrene occurs and is fatal if left untreated. For this reason, if you ever get a painful swelling of your hernia, you must see a doctor *at once*.

Most younger people do best with an operation and one is always advisable if your hernia is too large for a truss. The operation is carried out under general anaesthesia, although local anaesthetics are sometimes used, expecially in the frail and aged.

The idea behind the operation is to push back the contents of the hernia and then to strengthen the abdominal wall where the weak area is. Through an incision eight centimetres long in the groin over the hernia, the sac containing the abdominal organs is dissected free of surrounding structures, its contents pushed back into the abdomen and the sac itself removed. In an infant, removal of the hernial sac is all that is needed but in most adults the abdominal wall is then buttressed with layers of strong, non-absorbable sutures. Many different procedures are used and some surgeons even stitch on patches of tough, synthetic material to further strengthen the wall.

The whole operation takes about half an hour, provided there are no complications. There are few post-operative problems. You will be allowed up the day after the operation and be home within a few days. The wound takes seven to ten days to heal. It makes sense to take things easy for four to six weeks post-operatively, until the abdominal wall is completely healed but after that you should be back to normal. Many people take the opportunity at this time to learn how to lift properly and to see whether they could change to a job that is less physically strenuous but there should be no need to change to a less active job after a successful hernia operation. There is a trend towards people staying in hospital after a hernia repair for a shorter time than ever was the case even a few years ago. Also people are encouraged to be more active sooner.

## Femoral hernia

This is a type of hernia seen almost exclusively in women in whom it shows as a lump at the top of the thigh. Unfortunately, because so many women are fat and because this type of hernia is so small (compared with an inguinal hernia, for example) it can go unnoticed and give trouble for the first time in a rather dramatic way as it becomes strangulated. There is no place for the use of a truss with a femoral hernia and as the risk of strangulation is so high an operation is always suggested.

If the operation is not an emergency, a small incision (eight centimetres long) is made in the groin over the hernia. The hernial sac is opened and its contents pushed into the abdominal cavity. The sac is then cut off after tying around its base and the weakened area is stitched over with a strong material.

## Umbilical hernia

This type of hernia is most often seen in young children, especially those of African origin. The majority of umbilical hernias never need an operation: they get better spontaneously after the age of one year and even very large ones disappear by the age of five or six years. An operation to close the gap in the abdominal wall is only done if the hernia shows no signs of closing by the age of five years; if it becomes larger after the age of one or two years; or if the child has any symptoms from it.

Strapping the hernia used to be advised but is now thought to be unnecessary and ineffective. An umbilical hernia is best left alone unless it cannot be pushed back through the gap easily, in which case a doctor should be told *at once*.

If surgery is needed, the navel is lifted, turned back as a

flap so that it can be replaced, the hernial sac removed, the muscles pulled together with strong non-absorbable stitches and the navel replaced.

### Incisional hernia

After most operations the abdominal wall heals very well and is as strong as before but occasionally, because of poor operative techniques, obesity or a post-operative infection, an operation wound may allow abdominal contents through to form a hernia. Most of these conditions are considerably worsened if the patient also smokes. Such a hernia can occur soon after an operation or even years later.

The repair involves re-opening the incision, removing the scar, re-stitching the deeper layers and possibly fixing a synthetic mesh over the area under the skin to hold it all together. The operation is usually successful because the person is healthier than when the original operation was performed and this leads to better wound healing. He will also have the opportunity to give up or cut down on his smoking and to lose weight, if necessary. Success may also be more likely because better materials today give improved results compared with those used many years ago when the original operation may have been done.

# HIATUS HERNIA

### What is it?

A hernia of the upper part of the stomach into the lower part of the chest through the diaphragm.

The diaphragm is a strong, dome-shaped sheet of muscle that separates the chest from the abdominal cavity. The oesophagus (gullet) passes through the diaphragm on its way to the stomach which lies immediately on its underside. In a person with a hiatus hernia the oesophageal opening becomes slack and allows the top part of the stomach to rise into the chest. This is a form of diaphragmatic hernia and occurs most commonly in women over the age of 50.

Hiatus hernias are very common and many people who have them go through life totally free of symptoms. When they do produce problems they typically cause pain and heartburn, sometimes together with a sensation of the stomach's contents regurgitating back up the gullet. This occurs because the inlet valve of the stomach lies in the wrong place as a result of the hernia and so exerts very little effect as a valve. Stomach contents thus wash in and out of the lower end of the oesophagus producing unpleasant symptoms, especially on bending over and lying down. Some people have severe symptoms with a small hiatus hernia and others have quite large herniations yet are perfectly well. It is now known that malfunctioning of the lower end of the oesophagus may be accompanied by a weakening of the outlet to the stomach (pylorus) so that bile refluxes from the duodenum and irritates the lower end of the oesophagus.

The pain of a hiatus hernia can mimic heart disease and often the diagnosis cannot be made with certainty until a barium meal has been performed. The crucial part of this X-ray examination (see page 421), when looking for a hiatus hernia, is the tipping of the person head down a little to see if the barium refluxes back up the oesophagus. This does not happen in normal people. More rarely a doctor will look directly for the hernia using a fibre-optic gastroscope (see page 387) inserted through the mouth. Sometimes a test is done in which acid like that in the stomach is run down a tube to contact the lower end of the oesophagus. This reproduces the pain suffered by the true hiatus hernia patient yet will not produce symptoms in those whose pains are caused by other conditions. This is often a useful test because so many other conditions can mimic the pain of a hiatus hernia.

## Why operate?

A hiatus hernia needs treating because the symptoms of pain, heartburn and acid regurgitation are so unpleasant and also because longstanding irritation of the lower end of the oesophagus can produce so much scar tissue that it becomes narrowed and eventually prevents swallowing. Sometimes an operation is necessary because the damaged bottom end of the oesophagus bleeds over a long period and causes anaemia.

Medical treatment cures the majority of hiatus hernia symptoms. Clearly, medicines and a change of life style cannot change the anatomical disorder but they do relieve the symptoms and make life normal again for the sufferer. Weight loss is the single thing that makes the greatest difference to symptoms though no one knows why. As most of the sufferers are middle-aged, overweight women, this simple cure works for many. Tight belts and corsets should be abandoned and smoking stopped completely. If you have a hiatus hernia you will have to find alternatives to situations that involve bending over but this is not too difficult. Raising the head of the bed (a couple of bricks under the top legs works well) or having plenty of pillows helps keep you upright during the night and so prevents reflux occurring. Simple stomach medicines help mop up acids, as do small, frequent meals. Constipation, if present, should be treated to prevent straining at stool which further worsens the condition.

Some women get all the signs of a hiatus hernia when they are pregnant. This type (which is caused by the increased pressure in the abdomen caused by the growing baby) only needs simple treatment with alkaline stomach medicines.

If after a few months of such a medical regime you are still suffering from your symptoms, your doctor will look for other possible explanations. Gall-stones sometimes mimic a hiatus hernia and heart disease may cause the trouble. Once these have finally been ruled out surgery may be offered as the only effective cure.

### How?

There are many operative techniques but they all achieve the same basic thing – getting the stomach back down into the abdominal cavity; reducing the size of the hole in the diaphragm so that the stomach cannot slip back up again; and restoring the normal 'valve' mechanism.

The operation is carried out under a general anaesthetic and takes about an hour and a half. The incision is made either in the upper abdomen or in the chest.

## Post-operative progress
As after any abdominal operation, you will remain in bed for as short a time as possible and you should be home in a week or ten days. The wound heals at about this time and then you can start bathing again. The scar varies with the type of operation performed but is usually about 20 centimetres long. Return to work is usual within four to six weeks.

Because the operation restores the disordered anatomy to what it was previously, results are very good and fewer than one in five people have a recurrence of their symptoms.

If the oesophagus has become narrowed it will have to be excised and a length of bowel brought up to replace it. Occasionally, dilating (stretching) the oesophagus can prevent such an operation being necessary. In older people a partial gastrectomy or vagotomy (see page 281), by reducing acid secretion, may relieve symptoms without more major surgery. Recovery from these procedures takes longer than from the simpler hiatus hernia procedures.

# HYDROCELE

## What is it?
A condition in which fluid accumulates around a testis. It can occur at any age and the cause is not known. Although many people worry that an enlargement of the testis might be a cancer, it is often easy for a doctor to distinguish the two because a light shone from behind a swollen scrotum containing a hydrocele is visible and lights up the swelling. Growths of the testis itself do not illuminate like this.

## Why operate?
To reduce the swelling and hopefully to cure the condition completely.

**How?**
Treatment takes two forms. The first involves the repeated removal of fluid through a large-bore needle inserted into the bag of fluid. It does not cure the problem. The second involves an open operation to remove the (fluid-producing) wall of the sac. The operation is carried out under general anaesthesia, is over in half an hour, and the man is home within a few days. There are no after-effects but it may take several months for the scrotum to return to a normal size.

# HYDROCEPHALUS

**What is it?**
'Water on the brain'. The brain and spinal cord are bathed on their outer and inner surfaces with a nutrient, watery fluid called cerebrospinal fluid. This is produced in the cavities of the brain and circulates around the outside of the brain and spinal cord. It not only supplies the brain with essential nutrients but acts as a hydraulic buffer against the knocks of everyday life so that the brain does not sustain injury as we jolt about.

**Why operate?**
If for any reason the circulation of fluid becomes blocked, then it builds up inside the brain and distends it. In children in whom the skull bones are still soft and not yet fused, this causes an enlargement of the head. In adults, the situation is much more serious because the skull cannot 'give' and the pressure damages brain cells and can kill very quickly. Children with this condition sometimes also have spina bifida (see page 303).

**How?**
Many ingenious methods have been devised to shunt cerebrospinal fluid from the high pressure area in the skull to the venous circulation of the body and these are now performed in children with great success. A small burr hole is made and a tiny plastic tube inserted into the cerebrospinal

fluid-containing ventricular cavity of the brain. This tube is then passed under the scalp and inserted into the jugular vein in the neck. Results are excellent but the child may need another tube if the original one becomes blocked for any reason.

# HYSTERECTOMY

**What is it?**
The surgical removal of the uterus (womb).

In women over the age of 25 hysterectomy is the second most frequent operation after a D and C (see page 166) and in the US more than a quarter of a million women lose their uterus each year. In other countries the medical profession is not quite so ready to perform the operation but it is nevertheless very common indeed.

**Why operate?**
There are many indications for a hysterectomy. The signs and symptoms of fibroids (see page 182) may only be curable, if severe, by removing the whole uterus and sometimes persistent, heavy bleeding only responds to a hysterectomy. Sometimes a D and C reveals a pre-cancerous state which can be controlled by removing the uterus and of course uterine cancer itself may entail removing the uterus (see page 337). More rarely and hardly at all in the UK, hysterectomy may be performed as the ultimate in contraception. This is not at all advisable as the risks of a hysterectomy operation, whilst not high, are much greater than those associated with other sterilization procedures.

**How?**
There are two ways in which the uterus can be removed. The first involves its removal via an abdominal incision and the second via the vagina.

The abdominal type of operation is preferred when the uterus is enlarged because of a tumour or when it is stuck to other organs in the abdomen. An incision about 15 centimetres long is made low down in the abdominal wall, running from side to side across the abdomen. The uterus is then removed with or without the cervix. The fallopian tubes and ovaries are usually left in place so that the woman does not suffer an artificial menopause.

The vaginal operation involves the removal of the uterus through an incision made deep in the vagina. This is a good method of removing the uterus in women who are older or who have a prolapse (see page 285) because the vaginal walls can be repaired and strengthened at the same time. As this is not an abdominal operation in the true sense of the word, there are fewer post-operative problems than are associated with abdominal surgery in general but, even so, the procedure is a major one and the woman should take just as much care as if she had had an abdominal operation.

Almost always a general anaesthetic is used but a spinal or epidural anaesthetic can be used and the operation lasts about an hour.

## Post-operative progress

There is usually very little pain after a vaginal hysterectomy but the abdominal operation occasionally results in considerable pain and sometimes distension of the bowels with gas. After the vaginal type of procedure a urinary catheter may be needed for a few days if the woman does not pass water spontaneously. If buttressing and strengthening procedures have been carried out then a catheter will be needed for several days. In certain circumstances a catheter may be placed into the bladder through the lower abdominal wall. This helps to establish normal urination.

Most women get out of bed a day or two after the operation and stay in hospital for seven to fourteen days. As the vaginal tissues heal there is often a discharge and even some bleeding but this is normal and should not cause concern. It is probably wise not to bathe for four to five days after the operation. Showering or a good wash down are preferable during this time. After about eight weeks the vagina is completely healed and intercourse can safely be resumed.

Hysterectomy is a successful operation which cures all of the conditions outlined above in almost 100 per cent of cases. Early cancer is curable too.

Most women (and indeed their husbands) worry about sex after a hysterectomy but there is no change in a couple's sex life worth talking about. Women's reactions to losing their womb vary enormously. Some are so pleased to be rid of the unpleasant and debilitating symptoms the condition gave them that they become new women and this is reflected in their sex lives. Others who feel their womanhood has been taken away can become depressed, may overeat and get overweight. These women may suffer a reduction in sexual pleasure and activity. This complication is, however, less likely to occur if the woman has received pre-operative counselling.

One of the greatest practical advantages of having a hysterectomy is that contraception is no longer a problem. Menstruation, of course, ceases but ovulation carries on (if the ovaries are left as is usually the case in the younger woman) and a woman continues as normal until her menopause sets in.

It is often difficult (except in cancer cases) to decide whether a hysterectomy is absolutely necessary. Many experts feel that too many women have their uteri removed too readily and that we do not understand all the implications of this for their future lives. You may feel that a second opinion is desirable if you are at all unsure. After all, some of the non-cancerous conditions respond very well to other treatments and you may feel these are worth a try.

# ILEITIS (REGIONAL ENTERITIS OR CROHN'S DISEASE)

**What is it?**
An inflammatory condition of the last part of the small intestine (the ileum) that occurs in young adults and especially commonly in Jews. Ulcers and sometimes abscesses form in the affected parts of the ileum. The diagnosis can

often only be made at an operation. It has become more common in recent years but no one knows why.

The signs and symptoms of the condition are weight loss, poor appetite, a low fever, colicky abdominal pains, loose, frequent stools and even malnutrition. It is a long-term, recurring illness and there can be a flare-up of the inflammation which resembles acute appendicitis.

No one knows what causes this rather strange condition but complications are, unfortunately, quite common. Abscesses can form, loops of ileum can stick to one another and produce a fistula (a hole through to another organ) and sometimes these fistulae open on the skin, where they are particularly unpleasant for the sufferer. Peri-anal fistulae are examples of this and may have to be operated on separately.

The diagnosis is usually confirmed with a barium enema X-ray or a 'follow-through' from a barium meal (see page 420) and has to be made with certainty before treatment is started. Colonoscopy (see page 386) can also be helpful in making the diagnosis. Once the diagnosis is made medical treatment is started. Although this helps it does not cure the condition and even the surgical cure rate is only about 70 per cent. Medical treatment is worth a try first though and bed rest, steroids (as tablets and enemas), various other drugs and medication to improve the appetite and the person's sense of well-being are worth a try. Reducing the number of bowel movements helps the person to feel better and also means he will absorb more nutrients from his food as it passes more slowly through the bowel.

Some people respond well to this kind of regime but others need an operation.

## Why operate?
Although a small percentage of people with regional ileitis have a single acute attack and then get better, for most the disease is a long, smouldering inflammation that may eventually require surgery. Surgery will, of course, have to be done for any blockage of the bowel causing obstruction and for fistulae. Sometimes the sufferer presents such a classical appendicitis picture that the surgeon will operate for that –

even though as soon as he opens the abdomen he will suspect ileitis. The appendix is removed if the caecum is normal.

## How?

The operation, carried out under general anaesthesia, lasts about two hours though the time clearly depends upon the severity of the condition once the surgeon sees what is going on. Quite simply, the diseased parts of the ileum are removed and the next healthy area re-connected to the colon. Some surgeons bypass the diseased parts by bringing a loop of ileum directly into the colon, leaving the diseased area in situ. The idea behind this is that with no food going through, the bowel will heal. Today's operations are rather more conservative than those of the past and it is rare for large sections of bowel to be removed. It is now known that the removal of large sections of the bowel does not prevent a recurrence of the condition and can produce side-effects in its own right.

If the person is fit, there is no special preparation before the operation but disturbances of fluid balance caused by vomiting and diarrhoea are corrected by an intravenous drip (see page 396) and a nasogastric tube is passed to empty the stomach (see page 403).

## Post-operative progress

After surgery the person has intravenous fluids and has a nasogastric tube down for several days post-operatively. The time at which these are removed varies according to the magnitude of the operation and how ill the person was before the operation.

The scar is about 20 centimetres long and is to the right side of the navel. Healing usually occurs uneventfully in about two weeks. However, because so many people come to surgery in such a bad state with this condition, hospital stays can be long and two months is not uncommon for the worst cases. Similarly, although a few people go back to work soon after leaving hospital, many need weeks or even months of further convalescence before being fit to work.

In the long term there are very few problems. Most

sufferers are left with more than enough small intestine to absorb food normally and can live just like the rest of us.

# ILEOSTOMY

**What is it?**
A surgical procedure in which a spout-like aperture is formed on the abdominal wall to let bowel contents pass out of the body. An ileostomy is made in those people in whom some of the bowel has had to be removed for ulcerative colitis affecting the colon and rectum. After removal of the large bowel, normal ridding of the body waste is impossible, so clearly another way out has to be found for food residues. As ulcerative colitis is increasing in frequency, larger numbers of people are likely to need an ileostomy in the future.

For details of the operative procedures that result in an ileostomy, see ulcerative colitis, see page 331. Also see page 147 for a comparison of ileostomy and colostomy.

Learning that one has to have an ileostomy is one of the most emotionally upsetting pieces of news that most people have to face in hospital and some fear that life will be unbearable with one. This is far from the truth, especially today as modern technology has made the bags and appliances so easy and pleasant to use. Of course, it is still something most of us would rather be without, but the alternative is all the long-term suffering that goes with ulcerative colitis. A surgeon will never lightly create an ileostomy: it is always performed after the most extensive consideration of each patient's clinical problem.

Most surgeons spend a good deal of time explaining what an ileostomy is and how it will alter your life *before* actually doing the operation and this is time well spent because if you feel happy about it before you have it done, the chances are that you will cope better afterwards.

The Ileostomy Association of Great Britain, 23 Winchester Road, Basingstoke, Hants, has useful leaflets and through its visitors can give valuable pre-operative counselling. Do not be afraid to ask your surgeon if you would like to meet someone from this Association – he will probably be only too pleased. Many larger hospitals now have a stoma nurse whose job it is to help people with an ileostomy or a colostomy before and after their operation. These sisters are full of useful information on practical matters but cannot offer the ileostomists' point of view as can a member of the Ileostomy Association.

It is an anxious time before an operation to create an ileostomy and many questions will come to mind. Will the ileostomy smell; will it be noticeable to others; will it be dangerous in any way; will it mean a special diet and a score of other questions will need answering. A book such as this cannot cover all these in depth but here are a few general facts.

An ileostomy is a spout of ileum (small bowel) that protrudes from the abdominal wall. It produces liquid motions all the time and does not open daily like most people's bowels do. Because the fluid is irritant to the skin it must be kept off it so that ulceration and inflammation do not occur. An ileostomy is usually odourless.

The first ileostomy appliances and dressings you will need are supplied by the hospital in which you have the operation, but on returning home you can get everything through your family doctor. He will prescribe them on a special form and will give you stocks to last a suitable time. You can apply for exemption from paying a prescription charge if you are an ileostomy patient.

Once home you will be looked after by your family doctor and if you get any problems at all with your ileostomy, talk to him. Ileostomy Association members will get in touch with you (if you ask them to) and they too will be a mine of useful information, especially on day-to-day things you might feel unwilling to bother the doctor with. There are several different types of appliance on the market so, if one does not suit you, ask your doctor or specialist about another. The 'appliance' is basically a plastic bag with a special adhesive for making a comfortable, leak-proof joint to your skin. When the bag is full it needs to be emptied or replaced depending on its design.

Ileostomy appliances do not show under clothes and even women with fairly close-fitting dresses can wear their appliance without embarrassment. The appliance needs changing from once a day to once a fortnight, depending on the individual, and a change takes only a few minutes.

In practical terms the only day-to-day problem is keeping the skin around the ileostomy clean and free from soreness. Your doctor and Ileostomy Association member will give you tips on how to achieve this. Generally, an ileostomy is odour-free but if it begins to smell, there are ways round the problem.

Most people with ileostomies eat and drink everything just as before. Too much fibre (roughage) in the diet early on can make the motions too liquid and common sense must, as always, rule the day. If you find certain foods make your ileostomy run, then omit them completely or eat only small amounts of them. It is almost never necessary to come off certain foods altogether. Most ileostomists find that their diet is less restricted than it was when they were suffering from the condition for which the operation was performed.

People with ileostomies can marry just like others but surveys have found that they tend to have more sexual problems than would be expected. Researchers have found that ileostomists get used to their stomas quickly and that any embarrassment is only temporary. It is interesting that the partner adapts to the ileostomy sooner than does the ileostomist himself. Women with ileostomies conceive and bear children normally and sexual desires and appetites are not altered (except, perhaps temporarily because of embarrassment). The ileostomy itself is not fragile and will not be damaged during love-making. Couples find their own love-making positions that are most suited to them and soon adapt to these changes. The operation to remove the colon and rectum can itself cause a loss of sexual potency in some men but this is less frequent with newer operations and complete recovery is now usual.

There are thousands of people walking about with an ileostomy though others are unaware of it. Most people go back to their old jobs and a change is only ever considered if you do very heavy work indeed. Except for those who do boxing, wrestling or judo as sports, ileostomists can return to their hobbies and sports even if they need to protect the ileostomy in rough sports. Even swimming is perfectly possible.

Just before having an operation at which an ileostomy will be created, most people are naturally bewildered and anxious. After all, most of them have been ill for some time and are looking for a way out of their problems, not a way of creating new ones. In contrast, the vast majority of ileostomists actually live perfectly normal lives and hardly give their condition a second thought.

# IMPOTENCE OPERATIONS

Until recently, impotence, the inability of a man to obtain or sustain an erection, was managed by medical means. These included assessments of the glandular and urinary systems of the body, sex counselling and psychiatric evaluation. And all produced disappointing results.

In the light of such failures, doctors turned to surgical answers to the problem and started designing penile prostheses from silicone and rubber, acrylic, cartilage and bone and polythene rods. In 1973 a new method of penile splinting was developed involving the implanting of two semi-rigid, moulded silicone shells with sponge-filled interiors. Results were good but the penis remained semi-erect all the time and this was less than ideal for the men treated.

Over the last five years a team from Houston in the US has had excellent results with two inflatable silastic cylinders implanted in the penis, connected to a pumping mechanism implanted in the scrotum. When the scrotal bulbs are pumped, fluid stored in a reservoir behind a stomach muscle enters the cylinder and produces an erection. A release valve allows the fluid to return to the reservoir on demand.

Clearly, this implant does not make the man ejaculate but it does give him an erection so that intercourse is possible.

Results seem to be good provided the men are carefully selected for the operation. Ironically, research on those living with the older type of prosthesis has found that many had not used their implants for months and that in many cases their wives were unaware that they had them.

# INGROWING TOENAIL

**What is it?**
A condition in which the outer edges of a toenail (usually the big toenail) bite into the tissues at the sides of the nail, causing inflammation and considerable pain. There is also a discharge of watery fluid or pus.

Ingrowing toenails are most often seen in young people who cut their nails too short, let their feet get dirty and wear badly-fitting shoes, especially soft shoes such as running or tennis shoes in which the toes are jammed into the toe of the shoe. The inner side of the big toe is most often affected because the tough nail on this toe, if not cut properly, soon irritates the soft adjoining tissue.

**Why operate?**
To cure the pain and infection.

**How?**
There are many different procedures. The simplest is non-surgical and involves pushing a small piece of cotton wool under the nail to hold the soft tissues away from the projecting nail spike so that it can be cut and allow the tissues to heal.

Simple removal of the toenail can be completed under local anaesthesia in ten minutes but leaves a painful toe for several days. The nail grows back because the germinal tissue that actually makes the nail is left intact in this procedure.

A more extensive operation, done under local anaesthesia injected into the toe, involves removing the nail and part of the nail bed too. This produces good results quickly. According to one study, after one week, 79 per cent of people having this operation were back in their normal shoes and after three years only two per cent had had a repeat of their trouble. In general, toenail removal is painful (after the operation itself – not at the time) and the soreness can last for weeks.

If none of these procedures helps, the whole nail bed can be removed at an operation under general anaesthesia. After this, the nail does not re-grow.

### Post-operative progress
Walking can be painful for a week or so after these procedures but the simpler the procedure done, the sooner healing occurs. Frequent baths, preferably with salt added, help healing and soothe the pain.

Prevention is, of course, better than cure. Always be sure to cut toenails straight across and ensure that there are no spikes of nail at the sides, especially of the big toenail. The feet must be kept very clean. At the first sign of trouble, cut off the nail as best you can and soak your feet twice a day in hot water. Dry them thoroughly and keep them from getting too hot and sweaty by wearing wool or cotton socks and well-fitting shoes made of natural fabrics or leather. Do not wear tennis shoes or other soft shoes until your toe has completely healed.

# INTESTINAL OBSTRUCTION

### What is it?
A condition in which the intestine (usually the small bowel) becomes obstructed, so stopping the passage of food. Sometimes the bowel is totally obstructed by disease conditions and at other times only partially so. The signs and symptoms also vary according to whether the large or small bowel is affected.

Large bowel obstruction usually makes itself known slowly. Vomiting is uncommon and there may be little pain.

Slowly the abdomen becomes distended as the bulky colon blows up on the near side of the obstruction. If obstruction is only partial, diarrhoea may alternate with constipation but with complete obstruction, no stools or wind come through at all.

The small intestine produces very different signs when it becomes obstructed. There is often central abdominal pain which is cramp-like and very unpleasant. Vomiting is an early sign, the abdomen blows up and no stools or wind are passed from the back passage.

The diagnosis of small and large bowel obstruction is usually straightforward because the doctor hears 'tinkling' sounds as he listens over your abdomen with a stethoscope. These noises are characteristic of bowel obstruction. A plain abdominal X-ray shows swollen loops of intestine with levels of fluid in them and a barium enema X-ray (see page 422) may be used to find the exact site of the obstruction of the colon.

There are many causes for intestinal obstruction and one of the commonest is an adhesion. Adhesions arise as a result of a previous operation or infection in the abdominal cavity and produce bands of fibrous tissue which 'glue' loops of the bowel or other organs together in the abdominal cavity. Normally, all the abdominal organs slide over each other and so never become twisted but with adhesions, fixed points occur and sliding is hampered. It does not then take much for a loop of intestine to twist and so obstruct.

Another common cause of obstruction is a hernia. Millions of people have a hernia at any one time (see page 210) but in most cases the neck of the hernia is either so narrow that abdominal contents do not get through into the hernia itself or is so wide that the contents slide in and out of the hernia easily. In between these two states the neck of the hernia (where it enters the abdominal cavity) may be large enough to let a loop of bowel through but not large enough to let it out easily. The piece of bowel then becomes trapped and obstructed. If the blood supply to the trapped bowel is jeopardized, the bowel becomes strangulated and is in danger of permanent damage. An operation is essential as an emergency in this situation.

The large bowel can twist on its supporting tissues and produce a condition called a VOLVULUS. This is much more common in the elderly and is always considered as a possible cause of bowel obstruction in this age group. At the other end of the scale, children under three suffer from a condition called INTUSSUSCEPTION in which a part of the small bowel (the ileum) telescopes into a part of the large bowel (colon) and causes obstruction.

## Why operate?

Surgery is often the only answer for intestinal obstruction, even when it is only partial, and speedy intervention may be essential. The longer the bowel is left obstructed, the more likely it is that gangrene will develop. Also, the obstructed bowel can rupture, causing peritonitis and making the person severely ill. Any of these complications will call for instant surgical intervention.

## How?

The nature of the surgical procedure used depends upon the underlying cause of the obstruction. The abdomen is opened using an incision at least 15 centimetres long that extends equally above and below the navel to the right. Simple adhesions causing small bowel obstruction can be divided and the bowel saved, if caught early. If the surgeon is in any doubt as to the viability of the piece of bowel affected by the obstruction, he will wait and watch to see if it regains its colour and if motility returns to normal before he closes up the abdomen. If the bowel is irreparably damaged, the affected segment will have to be removed. The healthy ends above and below are then joined together.

If a hernia has been the cause of the obstruction, the bowel loop is freed and its viability assessed as above. If gangrene has set in, the loop has to be cut out and the healthy parts stitched together. The hernia is also repaired. A volvulus is more difficult to treat because it is so likely to recur. Various tethering procedures can be used to fix the loop of large bowel so that it does not twist again but some surgeons play safe and remove the loop altogether. This obviously reduces the chances of the problem recurring but is a more serious operation.

A child with an intussusception can be cured completely if caught early simply by pushing the telescoped small bowel out of the large bowel like toothpaste from a tube. If left though, the small bowel part becomes gangrenous and has to be removed. The condition does not usually recur.

If the obstruction is in the large bowel it is often caused by a tumour or diverticulitis, especially in the middle-aged and elderly. Some of these people may not be well enough to undergo major surgery because of a combination of their age and the problems created by the obstruction. In these cases an emergency colostomy (see page 147) is created simply to take the pressure off the bowel by creating an opening of the colon on to the skin of the abdomen. This allows the passage of stools and gas, so enabling the abdominal swelling to subside. The person can then be nursed back to better health until ready for an operation on the underlying colon trouble some weeks later. Some surgeons leave the colostomy open after removing the affected bowel segment so as to give the newly stitched bowel a rest. A few weeks later they re-operate to connect things up as they were and to remove the colostomy.

A temporary colostomy may not take more than half an hour to perform but the more major procedures described take from two to four hours, depending on what is done.

As usual with major abdominal procedures, a tube is passed into the stomach (see page 403) and an intravenous drip put up to replace fluid lost and to allow drugs to be given. Some people need blood transfusions down this drip too.

## Post-operative progress
The simplest of operations (dividing an adhesion) leaves the person well enough to be up the day after the operation. The more serious procedures keep the person in bed for a few

days, on an intravenous drip (see page 396) and with a nasogastric tube (see page 403) for about five days. As after most abdominal procedures, the doctors wait for evidence of normal bowel functioning before allowing food to be taken by mouth. This takes a variable length of time depending upon what was done at the operation, but may well be a week. In the meantime the person is fed intravenously.

Recovery times vary enormously as well but someone having a multi-stage procedure could be in hospital for two months. The operations are very successful though, thanks to safe anaesthesia, antibiotics, blood transfusions and a knowledge of the body's fluid balance. Intestinal obstruction is a potential killer, so the quicker it is caught the better, because the more minor the surgery then has to be. Surgeons are very aware of this and always operate if in doubt so that major surgery can be prevented if possible. The greatest 'at risk' group are the very old and the very young but with modern surgery even these do well.

There are no long-term effects of having intestinal obstruction treated. Even if a piece of bowel is removed, there is plenty more for normal digestion, so there is no problem.

# IUCD INSERTION

### What is it?
The insertion of a intra-uterine contraceptive device (coil, loop, IUD) is a simple and usually trouble-free procedure in good hands. There is no room in a book such as this to go into the advantages of the coil as a means of contraception but suffice it to say that for many women it is ideal. It is especially suitable for women who have had their families and do not want any more children. There are basically two types of coil – the first generation of simple, inert, plastic devices and the second generation of devices that are either coated in copper (the copper-7 for example) or impregnated with hormones. The insertion method is much the same no matter which device is being used.

**Why operate?**
To prevent conception.

**How?**
An intra-uterine contraceptive device should only ever be
inserted by a trained person because putting something into
the uterus is a skilled, though simple operation. An
experienced operator will also know how to get the woman to
relax, which is very important if the procedure is to be
successful. The woman is placed on a couch with her legs up
in stirrups or lying on her left side and the vagina is swabbed
with a mild antiseptic. The doctor does a vaginal examination
(see page 414) to ascertain that everything is normal and
inserts a speculum so that he can see the cervix (the opening
to the uterus). He then inserts an introducer, from which the
IUCD will pass into the uterus. This introducer is very
narrow and does not stretch the cervix nearly as much as
does a D and C, for example (see page 166). Most women do
not need any local anaesthetic around the cervix but if the
procedure is painful, it can easily be given.

Once the introducer is in position the plunger on the end
is pushed. This discharges the coil from the end of the
introducer into the cavity. The natural elasticity of the device
springs it open and keeps it in the uterus. The introducer is
withdrawn gently and the string or the protruding 'tail' of
the device is cut to the right length. There has to be a tail or
string protruding from the cervix into the vagina or the
device cannot easily be removed. The introducer and the
speculum are removed from the vagina and the procedure is
over.

**Post-operative progress**
Bleeding, mainly as heavy or prolonged periods, is the main
after-effect of the coil. Sometimes bleeding even occurs
between periods. Nearly one in ten of all coil users has to
have it removed in the first year for this reason alone.
Prolonged bleeding can be caused by too big a device or by
the right device slipping out of position. Unfortunately, some

women have to have several devices fitted until, by trial and error, they find one that suits them.

Recent research has shown that the copper-containing devices cause less bleeding than the larger devices but if bleeding persists and the woman is very keen to carry on with an IUCD, drugs can be taken to stop the flow. This, however, negates one of the main reasons for having a coil – *not* going on long-term medication. The newer hormone-impregnated IUCDs do not seem to produce as much bleeding but here again the body is absorbing small doses of hormones over a long time and some women do not like the thought of this.

The coil is especially suitable for women whose cervix has been enlarged by giving birth but today there are coils that can be inserted through the relatively tighter cervix of women who have had no children. Pain may be a greater feature among these women and they may indeed expel the device altogether. If this happens, it is probably better to try another method of contraception until after the first baby. Most women feel some period-type pains after the insertion of an IUCD but this is usually easily cured with simple painkillers.

The most unwanted side-effect of all is, of course, another pregnancy – so how does the coil perform? The Lippes loop (one of the simple plastic types) has a pregnancy rate of two or three pregnancies per 100 woman years and the copper-7 a rate of 0·7–2·2 per 100 woman years. As a figure of 2·4 per 100 woman years can be obtained with a condom and spermicide (properly used) one could be forgiven for thinking the coil might be a waste of time, but this is not so. IUCDs have the advantage that once they are satisfactorily in position they can be forgotten (which cannot be said for condoms and spermicides). Having said this though, any woman using an IUCD must realize that it is possible to get pregnant either with it in place or because it has accidentally been expelled unknown to her. Some women use spermicides too as a safety measure and it is always a good idea to feel inside the vagina every month after your period to check that the tail or strings of the device is still there.

IUCDs are still in their relatively early days, so the long-term effects of irritating the lining of the uterus for several years are as yet unknown. Studies looking for increased cancer rates have as yet proved negative. When pregnancy occurs with an IUCD in place there is a greatly increased chance of spontaneous miscarriage though it is possible to remove or retain the device without damaging the fetus. With more and more chemically-impregnated devices coming on to the market it makes sense to ask how these might affect the fetus but at the moment no evidence points to abnormal babies being born to coil users.

There are a few serious complications that can occur with the coil. First, because of poor insertion techniques the device may inadvertently be pushed right through the uterine wall and into the abdominal cavity. This is obviously undesirable and the device will have to be removed at an open abdominal operation or at laparoscopy (see page 398). Second, in the presence of an IUCD a pregnancy may occur in the fallopian tubes that lead from the ovaries to the uterus. If you ever suspect that you are pregnant with an IUCD see your doctor at once. Lastly, infection can occur in the uterus or fallopian tubes in a coil wearer. This is uncommon but if you have a history of pelvic infections you should tell your doctor and he will not put a coil in in the first place. IUCDs probably do not themselves produce infection but may activate old infections.

# JOINT REPLACEMENT

The use of artificial joint surfaces or structures to replace damaged or diseased natural ones. Several joints can now be replaced if they are damaged by arthritis but by far the commonest to be replaced is the hip.

The size of the clinical problem, and hence the cost involved, is enormous. It is estimated that over 30,000 people fracture their hips each year in England and Wales and although some die as a result of the injury, many benefit from a replacement hip joint. In addition to fractures people may wear out their hips and it has been calculated that simply to cope with the number of hip joints needing replacement in the increasingly aged population we should need a new 300-bedded hospital every year for the population of Britain alone. As technology improves and other joints become readily replaceable, even greater financial stress will be put on the health care systems of the West as more people clamour for new joints.

## Hip joint

Although attempts were made to make a hip prosthesis (artificial joint) in the last century, the vast majority of progress has been made in the last 30 years. In the early days of hip joint replacement it was reserved for old people with osteoarthritis. Today, younger people and those with other disease conditions also enjoy the benefits of the operation.

The problem with any joint replacement is that it is going to be in the person's body for a very long time. Because of this it has to be almost totally wear-resistant and must not corrode in the body's fluids. In addition to this, the material of which the joint is made has to be very strong so that even with the whole of the body's weight on it, it will never crack or fracture. Early attemps led to the use of a stainless steel ball as a replacement for the ball-shaped head of the thighbone but such balls tended to work loose.

Perhaps the greatest breakthrough in this field was made in the late 1960s when a British surgeon, John Charnley, started using polymethylmethacrylate cement to bond the artificial joint to the skeleton. This technique is now almost universally used to fix artificial joints of all kinds.

Metal to metal joints proved unsatisfactory in the body's fluids and in 1962 Charnley switched to using a high molecular weight polythene as the material from which to make one of the two components an artificial joint.

Basically, in a hip replacement operation the head of the thigh bone is replaced with a metal ball on a stalk that is embedded and cemented into the the thigh bone (after removing the natural head). The socket part of the joint (in the pelvic bone) is replaced with a polythene cup to receive the metal head. There are numerous variations on this theme, each of which is held to be superior by its followers but, whichever is used, the operation to replace the hip results in a comfortable, mobile joint on which the person can carry out all his usual activities without pain. Provided the hip is not infected pre-operatively, almost every hip can be replaced successfully regardless of the underlying medical condition. Unfortunately, the operation involves considerable damage to healthy bone but newer techniques are being perfected to get around this.

There are now scores of thousands of people all over the world with replacement hip joints and results continue to be excellent. The operation takes about two hours and after the first three days the person is allowed to walk. Recovery is very quick and the stay in hospital is only about three weeks.

## Knee

The knee has been replaced for about as long as the hip. Early joints were simple hinges but these soon became unpopular because the early results were not encouraging and because in order to insert them too much good bone had to be sacrificed, making a later fixation of the knee (as a last resort) difficult. In the early 1970s new designs became available, designs which consist of several unlinked parts, all of which replace certain areas of the normal knee joint. There are now more than two hundred different types of artificial knee joint but they all fall into one of four different categories. The first are modified hinges lined with high molecular weight polythene; the second are modified hinges without an axle; the third replace the whole width of the knee but the upper and lower components are not linked mechanically; and the fourth are devices that replace the joint surfaces with artificial materials.

Very severe knee disease lends itself to the use of the first two types of knee joint but they do have the drawback of removing a lot of healthy bone in order to place them. Less severe conditions can benefit from replacement of the natural joint surfaces with polythene and metal ones.

As there are so many different designs available and

because so few have been in use for long it is difficult to be as certain about the long-term outcome of knee joint replacements as it is about hip joints. At the moment, results are not quite as good as those with hip replacements but things are improving quickly.

## Ankle
The ankle was first replaced in 1972 in Britain and Germany, since when various other devices have been used in other countries. It is too early to tell whether the operation is better than fixing the joint rigidly and anyway the numbers of people involved are very small compared with the hip.

## Fingers
Because the hands can be so seriously affected with rheumatoid arthritis and because we feel the loss of our dexterity very greatly, finger joint replacements should have a real place in improving the quality of life for those with severe rheumatoid arthritis. The first implants used were hinges but these tended to work loose and were abandoned. Silastic joints followed but have not proved very satisfactory. The poor success rates with these joints probably reflect the serious local damage done by the rheumatoid arthritis itself, damage which extends to tissues outside the joints themselves. There is hope for the future as better joints are being devised along the lines of current artificial knee joints.

The shoulder, elbow and wrist can be replaced with artificial joints but rarely need to be because conditions affecting them respond well to drug therapy and to other surgical procedures.

## Why operate?
The indications for surgery to replace joints with artificial ones are simple – the person has to be sufficiently disabled to be sure that the advantages of major surgery outweigh having to endure his longstanding disability.

## How?
Operations to replace joints are (for the hip and knee

anyway) major procedures lasting two hours or more. There are three major problems that can occur at or after such surgery. The first is a blood clot in the deep veins of the legs. This seems to be especially common after hip replacement. The use of low doses of heparin reduces the risk but it is still a factor to be reckoned with. Infection is the second possible problem. This may not show itself in the immediate post-operative period but only years after the operation. It arises from bacterial contamination at the time of the surgery or may be carried in the blood to the joint area at some time after surgery. Unfortunately, this infection is almost impossible to eradicate with the prosthesis in place and the cure involves removing the prosthesis with a loss of all that was gained. The third possible problem is a loosening of the components of the new joint. Fewer than one in 20 joints do become loose, so this is not a great problem. If this occurs the joint can be re-cemented into place.

All in all then, joint replacement generally and hip replacement in particular is a valuable procedure which is expensive but provides real benefits to the recipient. The majority of people can go about their daily lives more effectively after receiving such a joint; some can resume work after many years of unemployment; and drugs can be reduced or eliminated altogether. A successful outcome, which is the norm, also greatly benefits the relatives of the sufferer and reduces the demands he makes on social and medical services.

# KIDNEY TUMOURS

## What are they?
As with any organ, tumours of the kidney can be benign or malignant. Benign tumours of the kidneys are usually cystic and can be difficult to distinguish from malignant ones without full investigation or an operation. Ultrasound (see page 410) and computerized tomography (see page 424) are helping greatly to increase diagnostic certainty in this field.

Cancer of the kidney occurs at both age extremes. It is one of the commonest tumours in children (when it is known as a Wilm's tumour) and is also seen in old people.

Kidney tumours may produce no symptoms at all for months or years but when they do they give rise to kidney (loin) pain or blood in the urine. Sometimes there is a fever for which no other cause can be found. A child's Wilm's tumour may first show up as a lump in the abdomen but usually this is accompanied by vomiting, loss of weight, pain over the affected kidney and a fever.

Modern diagnostic tools enable a surgeon to be very sure what he is dealing with before the operation. Intravenous urograms (see page 423) are widely used and isotope studies of kidney function can also tell whether the tumour has destroyed working kidney tissue. An arteriogram (see page 419) may also be done. Sometimes, if such studies show little remaining kidney tissue, it is better to remove the whole kidney (the operation is called a nephrectomy).

## Why operate?
Kidney tumours are removed to cure the symptoms they produce and to relieve pressure on the remaining kidney tissue so that it can function properly.

## How?
Cysts of the kidneys can be removed leaving the rest of the kidney intact but malignant tumours necessitate the removal of the whole of the kidney.

A nephrectomy is carried out through an incision starting in the small of the back and running forwards to the abdomen. The operation is a major one, lasting up to three hours but children seem to do well after it and are home within two weeks and playing normally again within six weeks or so. A child can live quite normally with only one kidney and the cure rate of Wilm's tumours caught early is very high indeed. If the growth has spread beyond the kidney, anti-cancer drugs and radiotherapy are used to try to cure the condition.

# LAPAROTOMY

**What is it?**
An exploratory operation in which a surgeon takes a look inside the abdomen of a patient who has an otherwise undiagnosable abdominal problem.

Some surgeons also use the word loosely when they in fact know what the operation is for. Until the last few years, laparotomies were fairly common operations because there was no other way of seeing what was happening to the abdominal organs. Today though, surgeons and physicians use various endoscopic techniques to visualize the insides of abdominal organs and a laparoscope (see page 398) can be used to see the outside of many abdominal and pelvic organs. Modern X-rays combined with computerized tomography (see page 424) and ultrasound (see page 410) methods also add to the surgeon's armament and all of these help save people from having to have abdominal 'look and see' operations.

**Why operate?**
As we have seen, a common reason for doing a laparotomy is to make a firm diagnosis in a person who has trouble which cannot otherwise be sorted out. The two commonest sorts of trouble in this context are fevers of unknown origin and undiagnosed abdominal pain.

A laparotomy is a fairly useful procedure for finding out the cause of undiagnosed fevers. Between 50 and 80 per cent of cases end up being diagnosed at operation after all else has failed. The condition most often found is some kind of inflammatory process, including inflammation of the liver, a liver abscess, tuberculosis of the peritoneum and kidney inflammation. Sometimes an abdominal cancer can cause an undiagnosable fever.

A small number of people complain of longstanding abdominal pain for which no cause can be found but the place of laparotomy in helping such people is not clear cut. Many research studies show that little is found at operation and in one series of 40 patients no useful findings were revealed by the operation. In this series, three quarters of the patients had complex emotional problems and many doctors are understandably loath to advise any surgery for long-standing abdominal pains as in many the cause is emotional or psychological rather than physical. This clearly puts the surgeon in a very difficult position because he will not want to operate unnecessarily yet will also feel he has to do all he can just in case there *is* an underlying physical cause for the pain. The problem seems to be most common in young women and one survey of 427 patients with longstanding undiagnosed abdominal pain found that there were many women who had had a psychiatric admission during the period of investigation. Appendicectomy did not seem to help in this series and the re-admission rate for women who had had their appendix removed was still high. Other researchers have found that such recurrent abdominal pains were triggered by a bereavement or other major life upheavals and that the sufferers tended to come from larger families than normal. Many of the women in this last series were found to be depressed and, once this was treated, they were free from further abdominal pains.

At the other end of the scale are the emergency situations in which a laparotomy is absolutely essential. After an accident involving the abdomen a surgeon will often have to look for internal bleeding if there is clinically any doubt. Serious abdominal pain of sudden onset could come from a perforated peptic ulcer, atypical appendicitis, gangrenous diverticulitis, an intestinal obstruction or a host of other conditions, all of which must be ruled out or treated as an emergency.

**How?**

A long vertical incision (about 20 centimetres) is made to the left or right of the midline, thus giving the surgeon the best possible view of the abdominal contents. The operation is carried out under general anaesthesia and takes upwards of an hour, depending on what is found.

Once the abdominal cavity is open the surgeon works his

way around the organs, inspecting them all systematically. If the appendix has not been removed and all else seems normal, he may remove it to prevent trouble in the future. Any condition he finds will be treated there and then, if possible, but there may be conditions that do not need a special procedure, in which case he closes the wound and treats the condition post-operatively.

**Post-operative progress**
This depends entirely on what is found. See individual conditions for details.

# LARYNGEAL OPERATIONS

The larynx is at the top of the trachea (windpipe) through which air passes down to the lungs. It is also known as the voice box. It produces a lump in the throat visible from the outside as the Adam's apple. Inside the larynx are two folds of membranes called the vocal cords which have muscles attached to them. Air expelled from the lungs passes over these cords, which are altered by the contraction and relaxation of the muscles to form notes which are modified by the mouth, tongue and lips to produce speech.

The larynx can be affected by benign and malignant growths but both produce one key sign – hoarseness.

BENIGN TUMOURS. These form the majority of growths of the larynx and are really excessively overgrown areas of mucous membrane on the vocal cords and laryngeal lining. If the swelling is very severe, there may be difficulty in breathing as well as hoarseness.

The diagnosis is easily made because an experienced surgeon can look down into the larynx using a special mirror held in the back of the throat. Once the surgeon has seen that there is a growth he will then advise the person to come into hospital to have a special instrument (a laryngoscope) passed under general anaesthesia so that he can have a more detailed look at the larynx. Benign growths can be operated on through a laryngoscope and, if an operation is done, the person will stay in hospital for a few days. The only post-operative precaution is *not* to talk for a week so as to allow healing. This seems like a long time at the time but, if it is any help, just bear in mind that people were asked to remain speechless for months when tuberculosis of the larynx was common.

If you find yourself having to remain speechless for a week, get a substantial, rigid block of paper, preferably on a board, and a felt tip pen. Write all your instructions or other messages out for people. You can even prepare a few standard cards with phrases you use a lot which you can bring out at the appropriate time. People usually find this very amusing but it is no joke for you. If you have just had a laryngeal operation you will *have* to rest your larynx – it is certainly not a game.

**LARYNGEAL CANCER.** This affects middle-aged people, many of whom have been heavy smokers. Hoarseness is the first sign, and it should always be investigated thoroughly when it occurs because if laryngeal cancer is caught early, cure rates are high. If you ignore the hoarseness for months, the chances are that the growth will spread.

In the UK, about 90 per cent of people with laryngeal cancer are treated first with radiotherapy. If this fails, surgery is resorted to. There are two types of operation, a partial or a total removal of the larynx.

A **PARTIAL LARYNGECTOMY** is carried out under general anaesthesia. A vertical incision is made from the tip of the Adam's apple downwards for about eight centimetres, the laryngeal cartilage is split open and the growth excised. If the procedure looks like being difficult or taking a long time, a tube is inserted into the trachea five centimetres or so below the larynx. This provides an open airway throughout the operation (and immediately afterwards) and can be removed easily a few days later when the operation site has become less swollen. The hole into the windpipe where the tube was seals off on its own and does not need stitching.

Post-operatively there are few problems, though there may be some difficulty in swallowing. In some cases a nasogastric tube (see page 403) may have to be used to overcome any feeding difficulties, particularly if the person suffers from pain on swallowing. This tube can usually be removed after a few days. Stitches come out in a week and the person goes home a few days later. With a partial laryngectomy the voice is not lost but the patient is always 'gruff' after the operation.

A **TOTAL LARYNGECTOMY** is a much more serious procedure. At this operation the whole of the larynx is removed, so removing the connection between the lungs and mouth. After such an operation the person breathes through an opening in the neck made by stitching the cut end of the windpipe to the skin. Intensive care may be necessary after a total laryngectomy to protect the airway and to let the person get over a major (two- to four-hour) operation on the neck which may be combined with a local dissection of other tissues too. Usually though, immediate post-operative recovery is straightforward and the person goes home in about two to three weeks.

Clearly, after this operation the person can no longer 'speak' in the normally accepted sense of the word, because he has no voice box. This can be extremely daunting for the sufferer but with proper pre-operative preparation (by meeting others who have had the same operation) and support from a speech therapist after the operation, the patient can learn to produce what is known as oesophageal speech.

In the early days there is a lot to get used to. The tracheal opening in the neck has no natural valve over it and so can easily take in water when bathing if the person is not careful. In everyday life a small dressing over the hole makes it less conspicuous and many sufferers get used to wearing a roll neck sweater or similar garment. Before the new type of speech is learned, the person needs a notebook in which he can write all his messages to people and this can be very tedious at first. Most people get used to using sign language and soon develop a system of signals that the family understands. However, the more you rely on writing things down and making signs, the less incentive there is to learn the new type of oesophageal speech.

Once the neck area has healed, the person can start to learn his new method of speaking. Basically this involves swallowing air and belching it up to make sounds. The column of air resonates rather like that in his old larynx and pharynx and after some weeks the person can make noises which are distinguishable as 'words'. Once this has been mastered, the person can go on to learn how to produce the more difficult elements of speech which involve using the tongue and lips to modify sounds made in the pharynx and the back of the mouth. This new form of speaking sounds a little gruff, but with practice it improves and becomes acceptable. This is a substantial improvement on the oesophageal variety of speech and is a very adequate way of communicating. A very few people find that they cannot master oesophageal speech and for them electrical vibrators are available that produce a single sound tone. Such a gadget is held against the neck as the person forms words with his tongue, mouth, palate and so on as he used to. The result is a rather robot-like 'voice' all on one tone but it is at least comprehensible.

All of these methods need considerable motivation and perseverance if there is to be anything approaching normal speech but many people rise to the challenge and do very well. Perhaps the electronic future will provide a more sophisticated answer to their unpleasant dilemma but only time will tell. In practice earlier diagnosis and better treatment are improving the outlook year by year so perhaps new gadgets will not be needed.

Many patients with cancer of the larynx now receive anti-cancer drugs. Because these can have unpleasant side-effects, they are often given as an in-patient.

# LIPOMAS

### What are they?
Harmless overgrowths of fatty tissues in the skin. No one knows why they occur but they are quite common and can occur anywhere on the body. They are painless and, apart

from looking unsightly, cause no problems at all. Many people leave them alone and never have anything done but if they are in an embarrassing position or occur in an area where clothes continually rub or press, it is worth having them removed. Lipomas occasionally enlarge quickly. If this occurs, see your doctor.

### Why operate?
To remove the unsightly lump.

### How?
Lipomas are very superficial and can easily be removed under local anaesthesia. The lump is cut out and the skin re-stitched. There are no side-effects.


# LIPS AND MOUTH

The lips are often affected by benign, non-cancerous tumours, most of which are wart-like. They are easily removed with low temperature equipment (cryosurgery), electric current burning equipment (diathermy), radiation therapy or by surgery.

CANCER OF THE LIP usually occurs on the lower lip of men in late middle-age. It grows very slowly and, because it is noticed early, is treated easily. Some of these cancers respond well to radiation treatment but surgery may be needed to excise the growth. The growth is excised widely to remove all the malignancy and the lip re-stitched. The cosmetic result is excellent.

LEUKOPLAKIA is a pseudo-cancerous disease which shows as white, thickened patches on the lining of the mouth, lips, tongue and gums. The patches may be painful and often become actually cancerous. It is thought that long-term irritation, such as a life-time's smoking or ill-fitting dentures that rub on the gums, is the cause of this cancer. The condition is mostly seen in the elderly.

The cure involves removing any obvious causes and a dental opinion is always worth seeking. White patches can be removed by a diathermy needle under local anaesthesia and repeated sessions may be necessary.

**TONGUE CANCER** is a disease of middle-aged and elderly men and occurs at the tip or the sides of the tongue. If caught early, treatment is successful and relatively simple, so all tongue ulcers should be seen by a doctor. If it is left, the lymph nodes in the neck become involved and very serious surgery is then required. Small tumours can be removed easily, leaving most of the tongue intact. Speech is obviously altered more as larger proportions of the tongue are removed. When a large amount of the tongue has been removed, swallowing becomes difficult and food has to be liquidized.

As with many other cancers, radiation therapy may be used instead of or in conjunction with surgery but this will depend on the practice in the centre you go to. Rarely, the cancer may have spread to involve the jawbone which will then have to be removed. It can be rebuilt with a bone graft or with a synthetic alternative.

# LIVER OPERATIONS

The liver, the body's largest organ, lies beneath the right side of the chest at the top of the abdominal cavity. It has extremely complex functions including the production of bile, the storage of sugar (as glycogen), the production of essential substances (such as cholesterol), the detoxification of drugs and some body chemicals and the production of a substance called prothrombin which is essential for blood clotting.

Food, once digested, goes via the portal vein to the liver which produces and stores certain foodstuffs as body building blocks, ready for when we need them.

Liver surgery is not often undertaken because, apart from cirrhosis which is very common but is not usually treated surgically, the liver is not often the seat of disease in the western world.

A **LIVER BIOPSY** is sometimes done to obtain a sample of tissue to look at its structure in conditions such as cirrhosis and hepatitis. This is usually carried out under a local anaesthetic as a needle is inserted between the ribs or via the abdomen. An inner needle is then inserted through the outer one and a tiny sample of liver tissue removed.

A **LIVER ABSCESS** is now uncommon except with the tropical disease amoebiasis. Drugs cure this condition and an operation is usually unnecessary.

In the past, infection sometimes spread to the liver after appendicitis, cholecystitis (inflammation of the gall-bladder) or abdominal surgery but antibiotics have reduced this danger today. Even when there is a liver abscess, surgery is by no means essential and antibiotics may cure the condition. If an operation is necessary, an incision is made either in front (over the upper right part of the abdomen) or behind (over the lower part of the back of the chest) and the abscess is opened and drained. There are few complications.

**CIRRHOSIS** of the liver itself is a condition which rarely calls for surgery but its secondary effects may be reduced by surgery. In cirrhosis (which is caused not only by excessive alcohol consumption but by viral diseases and severe malnutrition) the liver becomes knobbly, hard and infiltrated with scar tissue. Because all this restricts blood flow, back pressure builds up in the veins of the liver which causes varicose veins around the bottom of the oesophagus (gullet). These can bleed very severely and may be life-threatening, so a shunting operation may be done to relieve the venous pressure. Whichever of several alternative methods is used, the idea is to shunt some of the blood coming from the intestine (all of which normally goes to the liver) to another part of the circulation. It is a major procedure lasting up to five hours and is done under general anaesthesia. Such heroic surgery can help about a quarter of severely cirrhotic people but many are too unwell even to attempt operating upon.

**LIVER TRAUMA** is surprisingly common and is often seen today as a result of car crashes. The liver is so rich in blood vessels that even a small tear can bleed profusely so an urgent operation is necessary to stitch the bleeding area. Sometimes, a special foam material is used to help stop the bleeding. The foam is later absorbed by the body. Special stitches have been developed for this purpose too. A drain may well be left in the abdomen to let out any small leakage of blood that continues even after stitching. On occasions a very long hospital stay may be needed because there are often other injuries as well.

**PRIMARY LIVER TUMOURS** are relatively uncommon. Secondary cancer deposits often find their way to the liver via the blood stream from other cancerous organs but unless there are masses of secondary deposits the liver seems to continue serving its owner well. A primary tumour of the liver can occasionally be removed at an abdominal operation lasting about one or two hours. The incision is made in the upper right abdomen and the person may be in hospital for weeks. The liver has great powers of regeneration and this means that nearly 80 per cent can be removed before the person's body cannot cope.

For a discussion of liver transplants see page 325.

# LUNG ABSCESS

**What is it?**
A collection of pus in the lung, usually caused by the inhalation of infected material, food or vomit which first causes a localized pneumonia and then an abscess. Lung cancer sometimes first shows up as an abscess.

The affected person has a high temperature, a cough with foul sputum, may have chest pain and feels generally ill. X-rays of the chest will show an opacity and may demonstrate a fluid level where the pus lies in the abscess. Bronchoscopy using an endoscope (see page 388) may help with the diagnosis but it is not often required.

More than three quarters of people with a lung abscess can be treated with antibiotics and a rigorous programme of physiotherapy aimed at draining the pus from the abscess. If a foreign body is responsible, it can be removed via a bronchoscope without having to have an open operation on the chest. A really deep-seated foreign body may have to be removed after opening the chest, but this is uncommon.

## Why operate?
An operation is necessary only if medical treatment fails.

## How?
The abscess is opened through an incision in the chest and left to drain while antibiotics get to work on the causative bacteria. The best treatment after the failure of the non-surgical approach is to remove the whole of the affected lobe of the lung. If many abscesses are present, a whole lung may have to be removed. These operations are major ones taking from one to three hours but recovery is good.

## Post-operative progress
Even when a complete lung is removed, the person recovers very well post-operatively and lesser operations are very safe indeed. The incision is usually long but heals quickly, enabling the person to be out of hospital in two weeks. If a part of one lung is removed, the remainder expands to fill the rest of that side of the chest. When a whole lung is removed, nothing regrows but the person can cope with all but the most vigorous exercise using his one remaining lung.

# LUNG CANCER

## What is it?
A cancer of the bronchial tree (airway) inside the lung affecting many more men than women, although women are quickly catching up. Well over 40,000 people a year die from lung cancer in the UK and Scotland has the highest death rate from this disease in the world.

Cancer of the lung is the commonest cancer in the western world and it is certainly linked to heavy cigarette smoking. Although smoking is by far the biggest cause of lung cancer, there are other causes. Air pollution by coal smoke appears to raise the risk and men in certain occupations (working with asbestos dust, chromates, nickel, arsenic, mustard gas and radio-active materials) run an increased risk of developing this cancer, especially if they are also smokers.

There are several different kinds of lung cancer recognized by doctors but they are all very dangerous. Most lung cancers spread via the blood stream and the lymphatic system to the bones, brain and liver. The growth can also invade tissues locally, blocking off an airway completely, eroding into the oesophagus (gullet), or involving nerves and blood vessels.

A cough and spitting up blood are common signs – in fact in half of all sufferers a cough is the first symptom. Later there may be breathlessness or difficulty in breathing. Any of these signs in a middle-aged person should make him think of cancer of the lung and seek medical help at once. Less commonly the lung cancer patient starts off with pneumonia, hoarseness, bone pains or even an enlarged lymph gland in the neck.

X-rays of the chest may confirm the diagnosis and a bronchoscopy (see page 388) can allow the surgeon to see the growth directly in many instances. At this procedure he can also take a sample (biopsy) to examine under the microscope. The type of cells he sees can help him plan the best treatment for that particular cancer type. Sputum may also be examined to look for cancer cells. By the time the average person goes to his doctor the growth will have spread outside the lungs and it is this that produces such a poor outlook for the disease.

**Why operate?**
To prevent further growth of the tumour and to relieve symptoms.

**How?**
Surgery is the treatment of choice for lung cancer but only about a quarter of people with the condition go to a doctor early enough, while the cancer is still localized. An intensive course of radiation therapy may make the tumour operable when it was not before and radiation therapy may be used after the operation too.

If the cancer is reasonably well confined to one area of the lung, either the affected lobe or the whole lung can be removed. The operation is carried out under a general anaesthetic through an incision made on the back over a length of about 25 centimetres and the whole procedure takes about two hours.

## Post-operative progress
The person is out of bed within two or three days and the vacuum drains are removed from the chest a few days later when they have collected all they are going to. The person who has no complications can go home in about two weeks.

The management of lung cancer is still very unsatisfactory, partly because it is such a rampant tumour. Recent statistics suggest that people unwilling to undergo major surgery may fare just as well if treated only with radiation therapy. Post-operatively the surgeon may use radiotherapy or, more rarely (as most lung tumours seem to be resistant to them), anti-cancer drugs but even with the best treatment, fewer than one in ten people are alive five years later. Doctors and nurses therefore spend most of their time making the lung cancer patient comfortable and free from pain.

Most people with cancer of the lung are dead within three years of the diagnosis being made.

These very depressing figures can be influenced. There is no doubt that the incidence of lung cancer can be dramatically reduced if people do not smoke. It has been calculated from a British study of doctors who gave up smoking that smoking increases one's chances of dying from lung cancer by as many times as the number of cigarettes smoked each day. Someone smoking 20 a day increases his risk of death from lung cancer 20-fold compared with a non-smoker.

One distinguished UK statistician has examined these mortality figures meticulously and has come up with the following dramatic conclusion. Of every 1000 young smokers, one will be murdered, six will die in road crashes but 252 will die from smoking-related diseases, including lung cancer. If you smoke at all, you lose on average between ten and fifteen years of life.

Lung cancer is now by far the commonest cancer in men in the western world. Ironically, other cancers have become less common in the UK since the turn of the century but the incidence of lung cancer has gone up so enormously (recently among women as well) that overall cancer death rates have risen.

When discussing the subject of lung cancer with smokers the question of whether or not to inhale comes up time and again. Amongst light and moderate smokers, those who say they inhale have a higher risk of lung cancer than those who say they do not. In several studies though it has been found that among *heavier* smokers, those who inhale have a slightly lower risk than those who do not. This apparent anomaly can be explained because other research has found that almost all heavy smokers inhale and that their opinions as to whether they do or do not can be shown to be very inaccurate.

The risk of lung cancer is greater in those who start smoking young; in those who take more puffs per cigarette; in those who keep the cigarette in their mouth between puffs; and in those who re-light half-smoked cigarettes.

Stopping smoking is well worth while. Several studies have shown that the ex-smoker of ten years' abstinence reduces his risk of getting lung cancer to that of the man who has never smoked.

# MASTOIDECTOMY

Before antibiotics were available, infections of the middle ear often used to spread to involve the cells of the mastoid bone behind the ear. Today, this is very uncommon but a chronic infection of the mastoid bone can still arise as a result of longstanding middle ear infection.

A mastoidectomy operation before the advent of antibiotics used to involve opening the cells of the mastoid bone and leaving them open to drain. Today, this simple type of operation is rarely necessary. Infections in the mastoid bone are dangerous and should be treated thoroughly because they can spread to involve the brain and nerves nearby inside the skull. If they cannot be controlled adequately with antibiotics a more radical mastoidectomy operation may have to be performed. At this operation the surgeon not only tries to produce a safe, uninfected ear but also tries to save or even improve the hearing by some sort of repair procedure, often of the drum (myringoplasty). Some surgeons replace the entire eardrum and chain of bones in the middle ear with tissues from the patient's own body.

This intricate operation is performed under a microscope. It is carried out under a general anaesthetic through an incision inside the ear canal or behind the ear itself. With today's techniques it is safe, leaves an almost invisible scar and the person is home within a week.

# MOLES (PIGMENTED NAEVI)

### What are they?
A mole is a pigmented, flat mark; skin-coloured or brown swelling; or a frondy tag of skin, each of which may be hairy or hairless. Many children develop moles in the first few years of life but they rarely give trouble or cause embarrassment. Most are completely harmless and are best left alone. If a mole bleeds, ulcerates, becomes tender, has an extension of pigment around its base or enlarges, the person should seek medical help.

### Why operate?
Usually for cosmetic reasons, but rarely to examine a growing or painful mole under the microscope to see if it has become malignant. These malignant melanomas, as they are called, tend to develop more often from moles on the lower legs and feet than from elsewhere.

### How?
Under local anaesthesia the mole is excised and the area stitched up. Because malignant melanomas tend to recur in the nearby skin, a wide area of skin is excised under general anaesthesia and a skin graft used to cover the area.

# MYRINGOTOMY

**What is it?**
An operation on the ear which involves an incision in the eardrum to allow drainage of fluid from the middle ear behind it.

Children are particularly prone to infections of the middle ear after common infectious illnesses because the tube that connects the middle part of the ear to the back of the throat (the eustachian tube) is especially short and horizontal in children and allows infection to spread very easily. Middle ear infections are commonly preceded by tonsillitis, colds, 'flu, scarlet fever, whooping cough and measles. They are especially commonly seen in children with infected adenoids, tonsillitis or sinusitis and occur most often in children aged from five to seven years. Such infections sometimes produce a thick, glue-like fluid in the middle ear cavity.

**Why operate?**
A surgical puncturing of the eardrum (myringotomy) is done to drain fluid from inside the middle ear so that the condition causing the build-up of fluid can heal. Because of the early and widespread use of antibiotics it is rarely done for acute ear infections today but is done to remove the sticky fluid that accumulates in a condition known a 'glue ear' (see below).

**How?**
Myringotomy is a simple procedure carried out under general anaesthesia. As soon as the surgeon makes his tiny (2–3 mm long) incision in the eardrum, fluid flows out if there is an acute infection. More usually it is too thick to flow and has to be sucked out. The drum heals of its own accord and no stitches are needed.

Myringotomy is most often performed today for 'glue ear' in which there is sterile (non-infected), glue-like fluid in the middle ear which does not drain down the eustachian tube.

Almost ten per cent of all schoolchildren have some degree of hearing loss and glue ear is by far the commonest cause of this. Fluid in the ear is a poor sound conductor (unlike the air that is usually there) and because of this some degree of deafness is common. Enlarged adenoids are sometimes the cause of glue ears because they block off the openings of the eustachian tubes in the back of the throat, but adenoids are not always the culprit. In two thirds of children with glue ear the adenoids have already been removed or are small. The child feel a sense of fullness in his ear and it may click when he swallows or moves his jaw. Some doctors believe that glue ears are more common than they need be because too many children are given inadequate doses of antibiotics when they suffer from an acute middle ear infection. This only partly eradicates the pus and causes the glue-like fluid to build up.

It is important to treat glue ears because some experts believe they can cause permanent deafness. If initial treatment with antibiotics, decongestant medicines, nose drops and the treatment of any underlying allergy do not improve the symptoms in six weeks, an operation will have to be performed.

The operation is called a myringotomy. Under a general anaesthetic the surgeon makes a tiny incision in the eardrum as outlined above and sucks out the glue-like fluid. He may insert a tiny plastic drainage tube with a flange at either end through the hole in the drum. This grommet, as it is called, is left in the drum so that fluid can drain down the external ear canal and so allow the inner ear to heal. The grommet usually falls out of its own accord at some time between two months and two years after. Some surgeons remove the adenoids at the same operation if these are blocking off the openings of the eustachian tubes in the back of the throat.

**Post-operative progress**
Myringotomy rarely needs to be performed for an acute infection but when it is it cures the symptoms at once and allows the middle ear to heal, perhaps with the aid of other treatments. In the days before antibiotics, this was often all

that was done for middle ear infections and they did very well.

After myringotomy for glue ear some children show a temporary improvement only to become deaf again. Six months after the operation there is no difference in hearing whether a grommet was put in or whether the fluid was simply sucked out, though the hearing is better during the six months after an operation if a grommet has been inserted and this is a long time for a child to enjoy improved hearing. Some experts feel that the short-term advantages of a grommet are counterbalanced by the disadvantages of the thickened eardrum it can cause in the long term as this may, in itself, lead to hearing loss.

Children with grommets should be allowed to swim only if they have a snugly-fitting earplug or the middle ear may become inflamed after irritation by chlorine-containing water or sea water.

A child who has simply had a grommet inserted will be allowed home the following day but if the tonsils and/or adenoids have been removed, the stay will be governed by these operations.

# NASAL POLYPS

**What are they?**
Swellings arising from the mucous membrane lining the nasal cavities. No one knows why they arise but they may come about as a result of allergies. They are non-cancerous but are troublesome because they produce difficulty in breathing through the nose and a sense of fullness, excessive nasal discharge and sometimes headaches.

**Why operate?**
To relieve troublesome symptoms.

**How?**
Polyps are usually removed under a general anaesthetic but the procedure can be done under a local anaesthetic. It is

usually quick and simple and the person can be home the day after the operation. To control bleeding the surgeon may pack the cavity of the nose with ribbon gauze which is usually left in for some hours or until the next morning.

# NASAL SEPTUM DEVIATION

### What is it?
A condition in which the tissue that forms the partition between the left and right sides of the inside of the nose is bent (deviated). Many people have this deformity and it gives them no trouble but others have problems with breathing through the nose as it becomes partially closed off. Half of all those suffering with this condition complain of nasal obstruction of the *opposite* side of the deviation. This is caused by a compensatory overgrowth of tissues locally. The septum may be so badly deviated that it impedes drainage and ventilation of the maxillary sinus on that side, resulting in repeated sinusitis.

### Why operate?
To improve breathing through the nose and help prevent sinusitis.

### How?
The operation to cure this condition is called a SUBMUCOUS RESECTION and involves removing the tissues that are bent. Because this is done in such a way as to leave the mucous membrane intact, the person still has a central division inside his nose. This operation is becoming less popular as surgeons are learning how to re-position the bone and cartilage. Such a procedure is called a SEPTOPLASTY.

When you awake after the general anaesthetic your nose will be packed with gauze, which can be uncomfortable. Ask for painkillers if you need them. The packing comes out after a few hours and you may be allowed home in a few days.

# OBESITY

Even after strict dieting and the use of appetite-suppressant drugs some people are still grossly obese and look for a more dramatic way out of their dilemma. Surgery can offer such a way out, though only in a very few, carefully selected cases.

The main anti-obesity operation is one in which a substantial length of small bowel is bypassed so that food is not absorbed. The length to be bypassed is critical. If the surgeon leaves too much, the person will not lose weight, yet if too much is removed the person will have diarrhoea and far too great a weight loss.

As well as losing weight, there are numerous other reported benefits of small bowel bypass operations to the obese person. These include a reduced blood pressure; improved respiratory function; reduced blood lipids (such as cholesterol); and even psychiatric recovery.

Large Danish studies have found that those operated on had a much improved quality of life but that some of them also had unpleasant side-effects – especially diarrhoea – which could be persistent. In one study a substantial proportion of people were still passing between five and fifteen stools a day a year after the operation. Also, there is evidence that bone formation is impaired several years after the operation and there is a higher than normal incidence of gall-stones among this group than would be expected. Sometimes liver function deteriorates and the bowel has to be reconnected as before to prevent liver failure and death.

Dental splinting (wiring up the jaw so that the person cannot open his mouth to eat) has also been tried in severely obese people either alone or as a forerunner to a small bowel bypass operation. Unfortunately, many people have teeth that are so poor that the method cannot be used and others go straight back to their old eating patterns directly the mouth is unwired. Newer and more experimental surgical approaches to obesity include partitioning off part of the stomach with a stapling device and vagotomy (see page 281). Both produce good weight loss but the long-term results are unknown.

# OESOPHAGEAL ATRESIA AND TRACHEO-OESOPHAGEAL FISTULA

## What are they?

Atresia means the absence of the cavity of a tube. In the condition known as oesophageal atresia, a baby is born with a blocked-off oesophagus (gullet). Below the level of the blockage the oesophagus usually communicates with the windpipe through an abnormal opening. About one in every 3,000 babies is affected by this condition.

The signs that are suggestive of trouble start in pregnancy when the mother has too much liquor (fluid) in her uterus. The baby may be of low birth weight, chokes when feeding is attempted and may also have attacks during which he goes blue.

The diagnosis is made by the doctor trying to pass a nasogastric tube down the gullet into the stomach. Because of the blockage the tube will not go down more than a few centimetres. X-rays confirm the position of the end of the tube.

## Why operate?

To remove the obstruction in the gullet and repair the other defects so that normal eating and breathing can take place.

## How?

Once the baby has been diagnosed as having this condition, nurses keep his saliva from running into his windpipe by regular suction.

The operation is carried out through an incision in the chest. The gullet and windpipe are separated from each other and stitched up to form normal channels for food and air. If the cut ends of the gullet cannot be brought together to reform a new tube, the top end is brought out and stitched to the skin of the neck to allow the collection of saliva and a tube put into the stomach through the abdominal wall so that the baby can be fed. Between six and twelve months of age the baby is operated on again to bring up a piece of colon or a tube of stomach as a bridge between the two short ends of gullet. Normal eating and drinking are then possible as the anatomy is returned to its proper state.

## Post-operative progress

The sucking out of the baby's mouth continues post-operatively for a day or two as the newly-constructed gullet will not allow saliva down. Physiotherapy helps keep the lungs clear and thus reduces the likelihood of pneumonia developing. The chest wound in drained using a tube inserted into the chest at the operation.

A nasogastric tube for feeding is inserted down the length of the oesophagus at the operation but for the first 24 hours post-operatively the baby is fed intravenously. One week after the operation the baby can start having proper feeds by mouth.

If there are no complications the baby can go home two weeks post-operatively. The only common long-term complication is a narrowing of the gullet where the join is made. This occurs in about a third of all babies having the operation but the constricted area can be widened without another operation.

Assuming there are no other abnormalities, 95 per cent of babies undergoing surgery for this condition survive but, as many of them have other things wrong too, the overall survival figures fall to about 65 per cent.

Tracheo-oesophageal fistulae are operated on in the neck as the abnormal connecting passage between the gullet and the windpipe usually occurs very high up. The fistula is identified and divided and apart from tube feeding for five days post-operatively there is no special management of the baby. Recovery is usually uneventful.

# OESOPHAGEAL CANCER

**What is it?**
Cancer of the oesophagus (gullet) is a disease of old age. The commonest sites are the lower end of the oesophagus in men and the upper end in women. It is especially common in Japan, possibly because of the food they eat.

Difficulty in swallowing, pain or a sense of food 'sticking' and a loss of weight are the main symptoms. Most people can point to the level of obstruction caused by the growth and they are usually accurate. Unfortunately, many people ignore the symptoms until they are coughing and spitting out lots of saliva because the oesophagus is so obstructed they cannot swallow the litre or so of saliva they produce each day.

The diagnosis is easy to make. X-ray studies involving swallowing barium (see page 420) and endoscopy (see page 385) both offer excellent views of the trouble. If endoscopy is performed, a sample of the cancer can be obtained and examined in a pathology laboratory.

**Why operate?**
If the growth occurs in the upper two thirds of the oesophagus, radiation therapy is used but if it is lower down an operation is better, if the person is otherwise fit.

**How?**
Unfortunately, many people with oesophageal cancer are old and frail and cannot withstand a major operation well. For them, one of several lesser procedures is carried out. These involve the insertion of rigid-walled tubes to allow food through the centre of the growth.

Removal of the growth itself is done under general anaesthesia and is a major operation. In the early stages the growth may be confined to the oesophagus alone but later it spreads and a much wider removal of the tissue is needed. This major procedure means a long incision which opens both chest and abdomen on the right or left side, following the line of the eighth rib around the chest.

If the section of oesophagus to be removed is very large, the far end of the stomach or a piece of small bowel is brought up into the chest and stitched to the healthy lower part of the oesophagus. If the growth is so large that removal is impossible, a loop of small bowel is brought up to bypass the cancerous area completely and the stomach itself may even have to be removed. Some surgeons replace the section of diseased oesophagus with a piece of colon (large bowel) mobilized from the abdomen and swung into the chest.

### Post-operative progress
After such major surgery the person has a chest drain and will need pain relief for several days. Feeding is carried out via an intravenous drip and the person is in hospital for a month. Some centres use radiation therapy with very good results and this can sometimes prevent an operation or shrink a tumour down so that it can be operated on later.

# OESOPHAGEAL DIVERTICULUM

### What is it?
An oesophageal diverticulum is a pouch-shaped deformity or 'blow-out' produced when the lining of the oesophagus (gullet) ruptures through its muscular wall. It usually occurs in the neck part of the gullet but can occur anywhere along its length.

The classical symptom of an oesophageal diverticulum is a sensation of fullness in the neck immediately after eating, as food collects in the pouch. Eventually, if left that long, it causes pressure on the gullet and makes swallowing difficult.

An X-ray after swallowing barium usually confirms the diagnosis.

### Why operate?
To cure the unpleasant symptoms.

## How?

Under general anaesthesia an incision about ten centimetres long is made in the neck at the level of the Adam's apple. The pouch is dissected out and removed and the opening into the oesophagus tied off.

## Post-operative progress

The operation is not a major one and the person is out of bed the following day and home within a week. Pain may hamper swallowing for several days but fluids can be taken by mouth and food taken after about a week when healing has occurred.

# OTOSCLEROSIS

## What is it?

A condition in which the tiny joints between the bones that conduct sound to the inner ear become fixed. Normally, three little bones form a chain which conducts sound from the eardrum to the innermost parts of the ear but if they become fixed, the result is deafness and ringing in the affected ear (tinnitus). Otosclerosis is twice as common in women as in men and pregnancy and childbirth are known to lead to a deterioration of otosclerosis in many cases.

There are two main types of deafness. When the nerve that takes sounds as nerve impulses to the brain is diseased, deafness is almost always permanent. This is called nerve (sometimes perceptive or sensori-neural) deafness. The second type of deafness, conductive deafness, comes about when the conduction of sound waves from the air to the ear nerve is impaired. Otosclerosis is one of the causes of conductive deafness.

## Why operate?

To improve hearing and hopefully to cure the tinnitus.

## How?

The innermost bone of the three in the chain described above is called the stapes and the operation to cure otosclerosis involves its removal and replacement with another structure. This operation (stapedectomy) is done under a general or a local anaesthetic and takes about an hour. The eardrum is flapped open, the stapes bone removed and the opening into the inner ear (which comes away with the stapes) is re-formed with a piece of vein or synthetic material. A piece of synthetic material is then used as a strut to bridge the gap between the middle of the three bones and the inner ear opening (the gap that used to be filled by the stapes bone). The new bone link is then tested and, if it is working well, the eardrum is replaced. The whole procedure is carried out under an operating microscope which enables not only the surgeon but also assistants or students to see all that is going on under magnification.

## Post-operative progress

Immediately after the operation you will be asked to lie with your operated ear on a pad or dressing on a pillow. This enables any blood to drain away and so helps healing. You will be in hospital for a day or two and then allowed to go home. There may be some giddiness during the first day or two but drugs can be given to control this.

By the time you see the surgeon for the first follow-up at two weeks post-operatively, you will be hearing again if the operation has been successful. He will clean out any crusts from the external ear canal and if the drum has healed you can go about your normal life. Unless you are a window cleaner or an aeroplane pilot, that is. A lot of people suffer temporarily from vertigo (dizziness) and violent air pressure changes can actually displace the prosthesis. Patients are often advised not to fly for at least six weeks.

Results are very good indeed. Over 85 per cent of those having a stapedectomy report an improvement in hearing. The bad news though is that two people in 300 will lose all hearing in the operated ear, even with a hearing aid. If the condition affects both ears a successful outcome will see the person going back for his other ear to be done but most surgeons are loath to operate sooner than six months after the first operation and many surgeons advise against operating on the other ear.

People who had normal hearing nerve function before the operation (and this can be tested accurately) will probably have normal hearing after the operation and can throw their hearing aids away. Should there be an impairment of auditory nerve function (nerve deafness), the outcome is less good but is still a great improvement on the pre-operative condition. If the nerve has degenerated badly, then the operation will improve things sufficiently to make a hearing aid useful. Unfortunately, many of those coming for such surgery are elderly and have too little auditory nerve function to make the operation of practical value. Most of those having the operation are back at work in three weeks.

# OVARY OPERATIONS

The ovaries can develop cysts or tumours (benign and malignant) and the ovaries may be removed to control the growth of a hormone-dependent tumour, as can occur in the breast for example.

## Cysts
Several sorts of cyst can develop in the ovaries. Normally each month a 'cyst' (follicle) forms around an egg which is then released at ovulation when the follicle bursts. Sometimes, for reasons we do not understand, the follicle enlarges without bursting and may have to be operated upon. Rarely, a follicle grows to an enormous size, filling much of the abdomen and even making the woman wonder if she is pregnant. Unfortunately, such a large cyst often damages the ovary. Clearly this type has to be removed at an abdominal operation.

Infertility can arise as a result of a condition known as polycystic ovaries but the trouble can often be cured with a drug (clomiphene) or by removing a wedge of ovary. No one knows why the operation works.

**Tumours**

Just as other organs, the ovaries can develop benign or
malignant tumours. These tumours may produce pain in the
groin or lower abdomen or menstrual abnormalities.
Malignant tumours (now the fourth commonest cause of
cancer death in women) often produce no signs or symptoms
at all. Cancer of the ovary is becoming more common as
cancer of the cervix becomes less so. Women with cancer of
the breast have twice the standard risk of subsequently
developing cancer of the ovary and women with a cancer of
the ovary are three to four times more likely to develop a
separate primary cancer of the breast. Ovarian cancer also
seems to run in families.

Often an enlarged ovary is discovered by chance at a
vaginal examination done for some other reason. For these
women an exploratory operation (a laparotomy or a
laparoscopy) is usually done to decide what sort of treatment
is needed. Often the ovary is removed and an immediate
microscopy examination of the tissue carried out so that the
other ovary can be removed if the first is malignant.

**How?**

The removal of an ovary (oophorectomy) is a straightforward procedure. Under general anaesthesia a 10–14
centimetre long incision is made in the lower abdomen. The
ovary is easily removed because it hangs on a fairly thin
'stalk' of tissue. The operation usually takes less than an
hour, depending on what has to be done. If there is simply a
cyst, the surgeon removes this alone and tries to retain as
much of the rest of the ovary as possible, if the woman is still
of childbearing age. When ovarian cancer is the condition
being treated then, providing it is possible, the other ovary
and the uterus are also removed.

**Post-operative care**

Pain is much as for any abdominal operation and there are no
particular precautions that have to be taken. The woman is
out of bed within a day or so and out of hospital within a
week. Normal life can be resumed within a month and sex

after six weeks.

Almost all cystic conditions of the ovary are completely cured by removing the affected ovary and early cancer also has a good chance of a cure. Unfortunately, as many as 70 per cent of those with ovarian cancer go to their doctor late in the growth of the tumour. A woman like this will live on average eight months from the time of the diagnosis.

In the medium and long term there are no effects after removing one ovary or part of one, provided that the other is normal. Ovulation will still occur each month. If both ovaries have to be removed, the woman develops symptoms of the menopause unless she is treated with drugs which replace the hormones normally produced by the ovaries.

Sometimes painful intercourse (dyspareunia) can be caused by a low-lying or prolapsed ovary which is situated low in the pelvis. This can be cured by repositioning the gland on the side wall of the pelvis. The operation is called an orchidopexy.

# PACEMAKERS

### What are they?
A pacemaker is a piece of electronic equipment that generates an electrical pulse to 'trigger' the heart into contracting at a given rate. Under normal circumstances the heart's muscle contracts spontaneously under the influence of a special area of the heart called the sino-atrial node. The impulses generated by this node travel firstly in a special bundle of conducting tissue and then all over the heart muscle to make the heart contract in a specific and well-coordinated way.

Should disease damage this mechanism, muscular contraction becomes slow and often uncoordinated and the pumping action of the heart becomes less effective. This state can be temporary or permanent but if the reduced blood flow causes signs of poor blood supply to the brain (giddiness, fainting or convulsions) then something has to be done to make the heart pump normally again.

Drugs may be the answer to certain kinds of heart block (as this blockage of conduction is called), but usually drugs cannot produce an acceptable outcome and the heart must be paced electronically.

An artificial pacemaker is a small electronic impulse generator about the size of a matchbox. It has a wire coming from it which is attached to the heart in some way. There are two ways of doing this. Either the electrode can be attached to the heart directly or it can be pushed along a vein in the shoulder or neck until it reaches the heart.

In the second type of operation to implant a pacemaker, a wire is fed down a vein in the shoulder or neck and thus into the right side of the heart. This is usually done under a local anaesthetic. The wire lead is tethered where it goes through the skin and subsequently attached to a pacemaker situated under the skin (see below).

In the first method (the transthoracic approach) the person's chest is opened under a general anaesthetic and the electrode is attached directly to the outside of the heart muscle. The pacemaker itself is fixed under the skin either on the abdomen or on the uppermost part of the chest. It stays in place permanently, but may be removed after a variable number of years to replace the batteries. This is a simple procedure carried out on a day-stay basis. Newer pacemakers can be recharged and do not need removing. Both the placing of the electrode on the heart and the implanting of the pacemaker are carried out at the same operation which lasts about two hours. This transthoracic method is now not used unless the chest is being opened anyway to perform surgery on a heart valve or when the venous sites have been used up.

Both operations allow the person to be up and about within a day or so and home within a week.

Electronics has come a long way since the early pacemakers which fed a standard rate heart beat to the heart to which they were fitted. Today's are more sophisticated and are made to switch off automatically when the person's heart is beating normally and switch on when it is not. So good are modern pacemakers that they keep people alive for years who would otherwise suffer from crippling symptoms or even die. With the miniaturization of components, pulse generators are now very much smaller than they used to be and are thus more comfortable for the person. Rechargeable batteries, nuclear batteries (with a predicted life of 20–40 years) and a host of other developments are on the way, especially in the US where the number of people with pacemakers is growing. Today's best pacemakers can be 'reprogrammed' without another operation on the patient because they have a mini computer inside.

Pacemakers go on working with no trouble in the vast majority of people for years but there are several hazards to some pacemakers (some of which are being overcome as technology provides answers). The commonest are library book detectors, faulty domestic appliances (those with motors), microwave ovens and airport weapons detectors. Such devices produce interference with the electric 'heart' of the device and should be avoided by anyone wearing a pacemaker. Some airports have notices warning pacemaker passengers but many do not, so keep a look out for the door-like apertures you will be asked to walk through to screen for guns.

A pacemaker, whatever its type, goes on working as long as its battery. The early batteries were mercury ones which lasted for 2–3 years. Today's lithium battery gives a pacemaker a life of six to twelve years. Periodic checks have to be made of the pacemaker battery but as technology improves, these checks are now few and far between.

As well as using permanently implanted pacemakers, a cardiologist will use temporary ones too. If the person's condition is only a temporary one (the heart's conducting system is sometimes temporarily depressed after an anaesthetic or after a heart attack, for example,) a venous electrode is used coupled to an impulse generator beside the bed. No operation is done for this temporary pacing.

# PAIN SURGERY

Although the vast majority of pains can be treated successfully with drugs or even with unorthodox but increasingly popular methods such as acupuncture, some people continue to suffer pain which is completely untreatable by any method other than surgery.

*Causalgia* is the medical name given to a continuous burning pain which follows the incomplete division of a nerve, usually after trauma. The nerves in the armpit, the nerve to the hand or the sciatic nerve in the leg are most commonly involved. All of these nerves contain large numbers of sympathetic (autonomic nervous system) fibres. Because damage to one of these nerves alters the pain mechanism so severely, changes take place in the skin supplied by the nerve and serious ulcers can form. Most people who suffer from causalgia get better spontaneously over months or years but a small proportion only get relief if the sympathetic nerve supply to the affected area is cut. This operation is called a **SYMPATHECTOMY**. It is successful in most people.

Persistent pain is a very difficult subject because each person is so different in his perception of pain and in his ability to put up with it over long periods. The pain that can remain after shingles, for example, can be so bad that the sufferer cannot face life without increasingly large doses of painkilling drugs. This can, in the most severe cases, lead to addiction.

People with secondary cancer deposits in their bones suffer pain which can be relieved in a variety of ways but in a few there is considerable long-term pain. Certain nerve diseases can be distressing for the same reason. Serious *neuralgia* can be cured by cutting away a section of the nerve supplying the painful area but this procedure is only used if the person can manage without the nerve to supply muscles. Usually, nerves contain sensory (pain, temperature etc) fibres as well as motor (supplying muscles) fibres, so cutting a nerve causes paralysis in addition to pain loss.

A **RHIZOTOMY** is a procedure in which sensation nerves are cut or rendered non-functioning by injecting alcohol around them as they go into the spinal cord. This is not quite as simple as it sounds because there is a considerable overlap of pain nerves and several sensation nerves may have to be operated upon to achieve the desired result.

A **CORDOTOMY** is an operation at which pain-carrying fibres are interrupted in the spinal column on their way to the brain. It is usually carried out in the chest region of the spinal cord.

**LEUCOTOMY**. Very rarely the brain itself has to be operated upon. If so, the operation performed is a leucotomy.

Electronic technology is also providing some answers to the problem of longstanding pain and experiments with electrical impulse generators implanted into pain-carrying areas of the spinal cord are proving useful. The affected person can turn on his equipment when his pain is severe and so reduce his dependence on drugs.

Operations for pain will always be much less common than drug treatment. Recent research is helping us understand even better how we feel pain and the discovery of naturally-occurring, morphine-like substances in the brain has led to the manufacture of even better, more naturally-acting painkilling drugs.

# PANCREAS OPERATIONS

The pancreas is a gland which lies deep in the abdomen, behind the stomach and across the back wall of the abdomen from the right side to the left kidney. Most of the gland consists of cells that produce a digestive juice which is delivered to the duodenum via the pancreatic duct. In between these cells are others which produce insulin to control blood sugar. This hormone is passed directly into the blood and circulates to every cell in the body.

The commonest disorder of the pancreas is pancreatitis – an inflammation of the gland. There are two types, acute and chronic, and they are very different indeed.

**ACUTE PANCREATITIS** may be of unknown cause but some sufferers have gall-stones or are heavy drinkers. A small gall-stone may block the opening of the pancreatic duct into the duodenum, thus causing a back pressure of pancreatic juice and hence inflammation. The person (usually an obese woman with a history of gall-stone trouble) suddenly gets severe upper abdominal pain which goes through to the back. There is usually shock; she may look pale; may have cold, damp hands and feet; a fast pulse and a low blood pressure. An emergency blood test (serum amalyse, see page 368) confirms the diagnosis but if there is any doubt, an emergency laparotomy is performed to look and see (see page 242).

Surgery for this condition involves doing nothing but draining the abdominal cavity of any inflammatory fluid and closing up the incision. The gall-bladder is drained if it contains stones. The person is given powerful painkillers and muscle relaxant drugs which help the pancreatic duct to open up and to drain pancreatic juice into the intestine.

The stomach is kept empty by suction up a nasogastric tube and the person is given fluids intravenously. An antibiotic may also be given. Acute pancreatitis is a serious condition and about a quarter of the sufferers die from it. If there are gall-stones, the gall-bladder should be removed at a later operation.

**CHRONIC PANCREATITIS** is a different condition entirely and is seen more commonly in the US than in Great Britain. It is more common in men than in women and about a third of the people involved are chronic alcoholics, though no one knows which comes first. Such people suffer from frequent attacks of upper abdominal pain with nausea, wind and constipation. These repeated attacks damage the pancreas permanently and cause diabetes and serious disorders of digestion.

There is no certain cure for this condition. If gallstones are present, the gall-bladder is best removed and if the pancreatic ducts are full of stones they too are removed. If all this fails, a large part of the pancreas can be removed but as many of these patients are mentally sick or addicted to drugs by this stage, results are often poor. Fortunately, this is a rare disease in Great Britain. Medical aid in the meantime takes the form of a high-carbohydrate, low-fat diet; vitamin B supplements; painkillers; the treatment of diabetes, if present; and, in some cases, the use of pancreatin, a preparation of pancreatic juice extracts.

NON-MALIGNANT TUMOURS of the pancreas can rarely affect the insulin-producing cells to produce a condition in which excess insulin keeps the blood sugar very low, leading to weakness, sweating, trembling, mental confusion, seemingly 'drunken' behaviour and even convulsions. These tumours can be removed quite safely.

CANCER OF THE PANCREAS is increasing in frequency in all western countries. It has trebled in frequency in the US since 1930 and doubled in the UK over the same period. No one knows what causes it but there is an association with cigarette smoking if more than ten to fifteen cigarettes a day are smoked. Smokers also get the disease ten to fifteen years earlier than do non-smokers. Diabetics are more than twice as likely to get cancer of the pancreas as are others and the development of diabetes in a middle-aged person with no family history of diabetes is rarely caused by an underlying cancer of the pancreas. Between 50 and 80 per cent of people with cancer of the pancreas have pain as their first sign that anything is wrong. It is usually dull and boring in nature, steadily progressive and often worst at night. Up to a third first complain of back pain. Weight loss and jaundice are also common complaints.

Making the diagnosis is not simple but is being made easier as CT scanning and ultrasound (see pages 424 and 410 respectively) pick up more cases than was previously possible. There is a need for much better diagnostic methods of detecting the disease.

Surgery is unfortunately rather unsatisfactory because only rarely can the tumour be removed. About 20 per cent of those operated on die as a result of the operation and only two per cent survive for five years. Operations for pancreatic cancer are long (lasting from four to six hours) and are very major from the patient's point of view. Because of this, many surgeons confirm the diagnosis at laparotomy (see page 242) and perform a simple by-pass operation. This gives good relief of jaundice, though the patient will get more trouble later. At least it gives a further period of good health.

# PARKINSON'S DISEASE

## What is it?

A condition of unknown cause affecting mainly elderly people that produces shaking, rigidity, repeated movements of the fingers and weakness. Parkinson's disease can arise after encephalitis, in which case the symptoms and signs are seen before the age of 40, but the usual type is probably caused by arteriosclerosis (hardening of the arteries). The same signs and symptoms can be caused by certain drugs (usually the phenothiazine group).

Treatment is mainly medical, as opposed to surgical, and there are many drugs for today's physician to choose from. Unfortunately, some have unpleasant side-effects and are not well tolerated by the patient.

## How?

Surgery is aimed at destroying brain cells in the areas known to be affected. Unfortunately, these lie so deep inside the brain that they cannot be approached by open incision, otherwise too much normal brain tissue would have to be cut. Very fine needles can be inserted under X-ray guidance, and electric currents, very low temperatures or burning used to destroy the areas in question. The tremors and rigidity are helped by the operation but the slowness of movement is little improved. A combination of surgery and drugs is probably the answer for those people in whom drugs alone produce poor results. Unfortunately, nothing yet can be done actually to *cure* Parkinson's disease.

# PEPTIC ULCER

**What is it?**
An ulcer is a breach in one of the body's lining tissues. An ulcer in the stomach or lining of the duodenum is known as a peptic ulcer. The word peptic comes from pepsin, the enzyme in stomach juice that starts off protein digestion.

Peptic ulcers are common, occurring as they do in about 1 in 20 of the population at some time in their lives. About 80 per cent of ulcers are in men. They are most common between the ages of 20 and 60 and occur four times more often in the duodenum as in the stomach. Peptic ulcer craters vary enormously in size though size does not necessarily have any bearing upon the severity of the symptoms. A small, penetrating ulcer can erode a blood vessel and cause serious bleeding, yet a large, superficial one may be present for months and cause only vague pains.

Peptic ulcer symptoms vary a lot but classically the pain is in the upper part of the abdomen and is relieved by eating something. Some people wake at night with a gnawing upper abdominal pain which can only be relieved by eating or drinking. Heartburn and belching are also common and the person may bring up a watery, acid fluid into his mouth. This is known as waterbrush (stomach juice regurgitating back up into the gullet from the stomach).

The diagnosis of a peptic ulcer can often be made confidently from a person's story alone but to be sure that there is not another condition causing the problem, an X-ray is usually advised to make a positive diagnosis. Unfortunately, X-rays do not reveal an ulcer in all of those who in fact have one and so the doctor may recommend an endoscopic examination so as to make a definite diagnosis. For details of the X-ray procedure involved, see barium meal page 420; for details of the endoscopic procedure, see gastroscopy, page 387. Between these two procedures nearly all of those who have peptic ulcers are positively diagnosed, which means that treatment can be started with confidence. In the past, great stress was placed on studies of the acidity of the gastric contents but today it is considered less important and you may never have such tests done at all.

A book such as this is no place to go into all the theories as to the cause of peptic ulcers and anyway no one really knows for certain what causes them. They seem to be getting less common than they were but again no one knows why.

Treatment is either with drugs or surgery and most people with a peptic ulcer get better without surgery. Medical treatment aims to reduce the amount of acid produced, neutralize that which is there and on occasions to tranquillize the patient if it is thought that worry or anxiety are the cause of his ulcer. Diets were all the rage until the last decade when all ulcer diets were shown in large trials to be useless. Regular, frequent, small meals are helpful in soaking up acid and ensuring that the stomach does not remain empty for too long but apart from this and avoiding any specific foods that give pain, dietary regimes are a waste of time. Drugs and sensible eating usually prove to be a satisfactory remedy within a week or two but the ulcer can take weeks to heal completely. Several new ulcer-healing drugs have been developed in recent years, culminating in a particularly powerful one which reduces acid secretion. This seems to be reducing the number of operations done for ulcers very considerably at present.

## Why operate?
Surgery is needed in those people who do not respond to medication; in those whose ulcer becomes complicated in some way; and in those in whom malignancy is expected. Malignancy never occurs in duodenal ulcers. Today, with fibre-optic gastroscopy so widely available, most people with a gastric ulcer have their ulcers looked at directly and biopsied to see if they could be malignant.

Complications of peptic ulceration are perforation, bleeding, obstruction and penetration.

**PERFORATION** occurs when an ulcer erodes through the wall of the stomach or duodenum, allowing gastric juice to irritate the peritoneum lining the abdominal cavity and causing severe pain. Emergency hospital admission and operation are necessary to sew up the burst area. An operation to cure the underlying ulcer problem may be done at the same time.

**BLEEDING** can and frequently does occur from peptic ulcers, usually because a tiny blood vessel is eroded. Even small ulcers can leak blood on a long-term basis and make the person anaemic without a massive bleeding crisis. Such a crisis will occur though if a blood vessel of any size is breached. The cause of bleeding from the upper end of the intestinal tract can now be found in almost every case using endoscopy.

Blood can be vomited up or passed on down the bowel. Blood in vomit need not necessarily be red and this can confuse a person who has never vomited blood before. Altered (partly digested) blood is brown and can have the appearance of coffee grounds. Of course, fresh, bright red blood may also be vomited. Blood which goes through the intestine colours the stools black and can make them tarry. In either case the person may feel weak and dizzy and may even faint from the lack of blood in his circulation.

Medical management, including transfusions to replace the lost blood, often cures the condition. Surgery, if necessary, consists of sewing over the area to shut off the bleeding and doing an operation to reduce acid production.

**OBSTRUCTION** can occur from duodenal ulcers at the outlet of the stomach (pylorus) as a result of long-term ulceration and its resultant scarring. The person usually vomits persistently and has evil-smelling belching because stale food is trapped for long periods in the stomach by the constriction of the outlet. Surgery is needed to widen the outlet to the stomach or to make another way out.

**PENETRATION** can occur when an ulcer goes right through the wall of the stomach or duodenum and extends to the pancreas or other neighbouring organs. If the pancreas is involved, the character of the ulcer pain changes: it becomes more constant and goes through to the back.

## How?

Operations for peptic ulcers are a subject of considerable

medical controversy and several give very good results. Which operation is chosen depends on the size, position and type of the ulcer, and the presence or not of complications. Obviously, where there are several operations available, the one you will end up having depends on your surgeon's personal experience and preference. Basically there are two main types of operation.

A **VAGOTOMY** is a procedure in which some or all of the vagus nerves which supply the acid-producing cells of the stomach are cut. The ulcer is not touched at all and does not need to be because simply reducing acid secretion allows it to heal spontaneously. Because cutting the vagus nerves also produces a tightening of the muscles around the pylorus (the outflow valve) of the stomach, many surgeons perform a widening operation of this valve at the same time. This is known as a pyloroplasty, so you may well be told that the operation you are to have is a vagotomy and pyloroplasty.

Vagotomy is a well-tried and safe operation with side-effects in only about 10 to 15 per cent of people. The incision is made in the upper part of the abdomen and is about 20 centimetres long. Some surgeons combine a vagotomy with a partial gastrectomy (see below). A variation on the vagotomy theme is to do a 'highly selective vagotomy' in which only some of the nerves to the stomach are cut. This avoids the need for a pyloroplasty or gastro-enterostomy. It is a less major procedure but has a rather higher recurrence rate so not many surgeons advise it.

A **PARTIAL GASTRECTOMY** involves the removal of more than half of the stomach – the half containing the acid-producing cells. The stomach is then either joined back to the first part of the duodenum or to a loop of the next part of the small bowel – the jejunum. Partial gastrectomy is the operation of choice for gastric ulcers and entirely removes the ulcer itself along with the rest of that half of the stomach. Some surgeons, especially in the US, remove the furthest third of the stomach and also do a vagotomy as a treatment for duodenal ulcers. When the stomach is joined back to the duodenum, the person suffers fewer post-operative symptoms than when it is joined to the jejunum and this is one reason why surgeons favour the former operation. The incision for any of these procedures is made vertically in the upper abdomen and is about 20 centimetres long.

All these operations are performed under general anaesthesia and last from one to three hours, depending on which is done.

Before the operation the preparation you will have depends on how seriously the ulcer has affected you thus far. If it has been bleeding, blood will be transfused so that you go into the operation in a strong condition and, similarly, if you have been vomiting a lot, the body's chemical balance will be out and you will have a drip containing the right chemicals to correct this. You will almost certainly have a nasogastric tube passed (see page 403) so that the stomach can be emptied before the operation. This is especially important if the pylorus is narrowed and the stomach is emptying poorly on its own.

## Post-operative progress

Operations for peptic ulcers are major procedures but most patients are not in a great deal of pain even immediately following the operation.

Because the stomach and upper bowel need resting for a few days after these operations you will have to be 'dripped and sucked' as surgeons call it. The intravenous drip gives you the fluid you will need and the sucking (up the nasogastric tube) removes secretions produced by the stomach. Most people are up the day after the operation and can go home within a week or two. The scar is usually quite long (about 20 centimetres) and can be in one of several places, according to the choice of the surgeon and the nature of the operation done. Some surgeons use an incision which runs from the bottom of the breastbone to the navel; others a similar length to the left or right of the midline, and others one which runs across the top of the abdomen.

The wound heals well enough to have a bath within two weeks and you can eat normally by this time too. Before this it is advisable to keep to small meals of soft, easily digested foods taken frequently throughout the day.

Although most people feel well enough to go about their normal lives when they get home from hospital, you will not be able to go back to work full-time (especially if you have a job that involves physical work) for about six weeks after the operation.

Operations on the stomach and vagus nerves do produce side-effects and some of these can be unpleasant or annoying. The 'dumping' syndrome consists of nausea, palpitations, sweating, a sense of flushing after meals and weakness and is seen in five to ten per cent of people who have had partial gastrectomies. This occurs because the stomach no longer holds on to the food as it previously did but shoots it straight into the duodenum or small intestine. This is what gives rise to the unpleasant symptoms a few minutes after eating. They last for about half an hour. Frequent, small, dry meals are the answer for most sufferers and lying down for a while after each meal helps. Sugary drinks should be avoided as they seem to make matters worse. The symptoms tend to disappear with time.

Many people lose weight or fail to regain their pre-operative weight after a gastrectomy. No one knows why this occurs but it is possible that the bowel never again absorbs the whole of the food properly because the rate at which food is passed down the intestine is speeded up. Diarrhoea is not a problem after a gastrectomy but it is seen quite commonly after a vagotomy and pyloroplasty. A small number of those who have had a vagotomy find that diarrhoea is a serious problem which needs further treatment but it tends to settle in time.

Apart from these bowel symptoms, most people are well pleased with their operations. The ulcer symptoms (for which the operation was performed) are greatly improved. Unfortunately, about ten per cent of those operated on get another ulcer but this will not necessarily mean another operation.

Even though removing a substantial piece of stomach can produce problems in the short term, the remainder of the stomach seems to enlarge over the years to accommodate more food and so act more like it used to. Certainly there is no evidence to suggest that after such operations a person's life span or health outlook is altered adversely.

# PILONIDAL SINUS

### What is it?
A pilonidal ('nest of hairs') sinus is a troublesome condition first seen in people in their early twenties. There is a little opening (or possibly more than one) in the midline of the body in the crease between the buttocks at the very lowest part of the back. This hole is very liable to become infected and to form an abscess.

Children often have a little pit in this position but this is not the same condition at all. A pilonidal sinus is only ever seen after hair grows (at puberty) and it is thought that a hair (or hairs) grows into the skin and causes irritation. It is most commonly seen in dark-haired men.

### Why operate?
An operation is necessary to remove the irritating, painful area under the skin containing the hairs.

### How?
Under a general or local anaesthetic the surgeon inspects the area to see the true extent of the problem. He looks for the pits and then identifies all the tracks that are discharging pus. The idea then is to remove all the affected tissue. Usually, a fairly wide area of skin is removed and left open to heal from the bottom up.

If an abscess has formed in a sinus it is drained and left to quieten down before further surgery is done.

### Post-operative progress
Surgical after-care is almost more important than the operation itself. The operation usually leaves a surprisingly large cavity but this heals quite quickly with good supervision. Usually the area is packed each day by the nurse following your bath. Gradually the hole fills up from the

bottom and is healed in three to six weeks. During, and indeed for some weeks after this time, it is important to keep the area shaved.

This whole procedure has recently been simplified by the use of a sialastic dressing. The surgeon sees you each week and after the shaving you have a special 'stent' made to fit exactly into the hole. You can then take this out and bathe twice a day without the nurse having to do the dressing. Although healing is no quicker it is all a lot more comfortable.

Expect to be in hospital for a week and to be back at work in three weeks. Some people find it difficult to open their bowels for a few days (although the bowel has not been touched, of course) and yet others have difficulty passing urine. Talk to your doctor about these if they occur. You can have a bath even though the wound has not healed over completely, starting from the end of the first week.

# PROLAPSE OF THE UTERUS

### What is it?
The downward displacement or rupture of the uterus with or without the vaginal walls, usually resulting from a weakening of the supporting ligaments during and after childbirth.

In a normal healthy woman the uterus sits in the pelvis above the pelvic floor muscles and is held in place by ligaments and other tissues. During pregnancy the uterus grows in size to contain the growing fetus, but in addition to the uterine growth all the ligaments and other pelvic support structures soften and elongate under the influence of pregnancy hormones and under the sheer mechanical tensions and pressures. If labour is of normal duration and well supervised, the baby is born without undue damage to the birth canal and its surrounding structures and all is well.

However, prolonged labour, the birth of especially large babies and indeed repeated normal births can all stretch the elastic tissues of the supporting muscles and ligaments in the pelvis so that they never really regain their original elasticity.

This is rather like stretching an elastic band too much – the band never returns to its original size and elasticity again.

Prolapse of the uterus and vagina can also occur because of the withdrawal of oestrogen from the body after the menopause. It may rarely be due to a congenital weakness of the supporting structures and it can occur like any other rupture as a result of prolonged coughing (as in chronic bronchitis) or straining (as in constipation). It is very difficult to know which factor is most important in any one woman and it is probable that sometimes several of these factors interplay to produce a rupture of the uterus into the vagina.

Any part of the vagina and uterus can be affected and each produces particular signs and symptoms according to the organs drawn down with the prolapse. A prolapse is actually felt as a 'lump down below' or 'something coming down', which is exactly what is it. A woman complaining of predominantly urinary symptoms may need to have some simple investigations carried out pre-operatively to rule out certain other conditions that mimic prolapse but are in fact of urinary origin. The diagnosis is usually very simple though, and no special tests are needed. The doctor performs a vaginal examination (see page 414) and, using a speculum, examines the vagina as the woman coughs, strains and bears down. Nearby organs may prolapse along with the uterus. If the bladder prolapses, this is called a CYSTOCELE and can cause stress incontinence (a loss of urine on sneezing, laughing or coughing). A cystocele can be present though without any stress incontinence. The rectum too may sag, producing a RECTOCELE.

Prevention is obviously better than cure in any condition and prolapse of the uterus is a particularly good example of this principle. The judicious use of episiotomies (see page 178) and of forceps prevents the damage done by prolonged pushing in the later stages of labour, and post-natal exercises to strengthen the pelvic floor muscles also help greatly. Rest for several days after birth also seems to be of protective value against future prolapses.

## How?

There are two simple operations for prolapse. They both involve the removal of the redundant vaginal skin and a buttressing of the supporting muscles and tissues. In some cases the treatment may be a vaginal hysterectomy together with a tightening up of all the tissues concerned; or the cervix and the supporting ligaments may be shortened. In women who intend to have more children or the elderly and frail, a polythene ring pessary can be inserted into the vagina. This holds back the floppy tissues and means that in a young woman an operation can be postponed until her family is complete. Such a ring has to be replaced every three months. Most women with a prolapse eventually end up having an operation because it is the only way of providing a permanent answer to their problems.

## Post-operative progress

As repair operations for prolapse are all vaginal there are no serious side-effects in the vast majority of cases. There may be some urinary problems, in which case a catheter is used. The woman gets up a day after the operation and can go home a week later. Because the woman's vaginal wall is now so firm and her uterus is back in the right place, intercourse may be more pleasurable than when she had the prolapse. If she has had a hysterectomy she will be unable to have more children but this can bring dividends at a sexual level because any fear of pregnancy has gone. Because a prolapse can be so unpleasant with its urinary symptoms, incontinence on laughing or coughing, unpleasant sensations of a lump in the vagina, backache and a disrupted sex life, a repair often comes as a great relief.

# PROSTATE CANCER

## What is it?

A cancer of the prostate gland usually occurring in men in their 60s and 70s. Rather as with benign enlargement of the prostate, there may be no symptoms at all for some time.

Later, as the gland enlarges with the growth, there will not only be increasing difficulty in passing urine but also blood and pus in the urine and all the other signs of benign prostatic enlargement (see page 289). If the cancer has spread to involve the bones of the spine and pelvis, there may be bone pain.

The diagnosis is usually easy to make. The enlarged prostate gland (felt rectally) feels hard and knobbly to the surgeon and X-rays of the spine and pelvis may show a spread of the tumour to the bones. A biopsy of the gland provides a definite diagnosis but a blood test can also give very useful suggestive evidence of cancer. The serum acid phosphatase level (see page 369) can be diagnostic but the blood specimen must be taken before a rectal examination is performed as the massaging of the prostate gland by the examining finger can cause the blood level of this enzyme to rise. Some surgeons massage the prostate to milk some fluid out down the urethra. They collect this as it drips from the penis and look for cancer cells in it.

**Why operate?**
To relieve symptoms and to reduce complications.

**How?**
In many of the men affected with prostate cancer, their age and general condition makes an operation undesirable. By the time that many men see their doctor, the condition is so advanced that surgery would anyway not be able to cure the condition. About 70 per cent of tumours have already spread by the time they are first seen. These men are given female hormones in the form of oestrogens, which are usually extremely effective. With hormone treatment the gland shrinks in size and even secondary deposits in the bones may heal. Many men have a prolongation of life as a result of this treatment. Prostatic cancers seem to fall into two groups – those that are highly malignant and those that are not. The former do very badly but, of the latter, 80 per cent are still alive five years after the diagnosis.

If the malignancy is confined to the gland itself, prostatectomy (see page 290) can be successful in removing the cancer, as can radiation treatment. If the trouble has spread too far then hormone treatment is the only hope although some surgeons use anti-cancer drugs and radiation with some success.

# PROSTATE OPERATIONS

The prostate is a gland about the size of a walnut that lies at the base of the bladder and produces fluid which is added to the sperms from the testes to form semen. Because the gland encloses the first part of the urethra as it leaves the bladder on its way to the penis, any enlargement can shut off the urethra and cause a build-up of urine in the bladder.

As men age, their prostate glands enlarge. No one knows why the gland enlarges though there are many theories. Most men of 60 or more have some enlargement of the prostate and one in ten men in the West will have their prostate gland removed surgically. As the gland enlarges, passing urine becomes more difficult and the stagnant urine in the bladder easily becomes infected. The back pressure of urine in the bladder may be bad enough to travel back up to the kidneys which can be permanently damaged by it. This damage can cause a build-up of waste products (which would normally be lost in the urine) in the blood or a raised blood pressure. As the months and years go by the man has to pass water in smaller and smaller amounts with increasing frequency. Getting up at night to pass water becomes a major feature of the disease and there may be dribbling of urine and a difficulty in starting. Many affected men say they feel like passing water most of the time, even immediately after having done so.

The diagnosis is made from the person's story and by a doctor feeling the enlarged prostate gland rectally. A rectal examination usually detects an enlarged gland in affected men but parts of the gland that cannot be felt rectally may be enlarged. These enlarged areas can be diagnosed either on X-ray (a urogram, see page 423, or a cystogram, see page 424) or on cytoscopy (see page 163).

Treatment is not always surgical and in fact only a quarter of men need operating upon. Many respond well to the treatment of their urinary infections and some men can go on for years even if they have to have periodic catheterization (see page 372) to relieve the pressure of built-up urine. Trouble at night can be greatly reduced simply by restricting fluid intake during the evening.

### Why operate?
An operation is definitely needed if the symptoms persist and are unbearable for the sufferer; if there is any evidence of kidney function becoming jeopardized; or if there has been more than a small number of acute bladder shut down attacks in which passing urine is impossible.

### How?
There are several types of prostatectomy (operations to remove the prostate).

**TRANSURETHRAL PROSTATECTOMY**. Today the vast majority of prostates are removed down an operating cystoscope. This operation, called a transurethral prostatectomy, requires no abdominal operation as the procedure is carried out via an operating cystoscope (resectoscope; see page 163) passed down the urinary passage (urethra). Under general or spinal anaesthesia the surgeon can see the enlarged prostate down the operating cystoscope and can cut away pieces of the enlarged prostate gland little by little using an electric knife. The pieces are washed out down the operating cystoscope and any bleeding areas coagulated with an electric current. Once all the enlarged part of the gland is removed, a catheter is inserted into the bladder, where it is left for several days. The man gets up out of bed the day after the procedure and, all being well, should be home within seven to ten days.

A **RETROPUBIC PROSTATECTOMY** is performed through an incision in the lower abdomen under general anaesthesia. The prostate gland is shelled out of its fibrous capsule and a catheter left in the bladder via the urethra for a week or so while healing takes place.

A **SUPRAPUBIC PROSTATECTOMY** is also performed under a general anaesthetic. An abdominal incision allows access to the bladder which is opened. The surgeon then removes the enlarged prostate through the urethral opening from the inside of the bladder. The man is left with drains from the abdominal wound and a catheter to rest the bladder until healing has occurred a week or so later.

### Post-operative progress

Today, with most prostatectomies being done through an operating cystoscope, many elderly men fare better than they would with an open abdominal operation. The operation causes very little pain post-operatively (the abdominal procedures are, of course, as painful as any other abdominal procedure, post-operatively) and the cure rate is very high.

Bleeding can be a problem a few days post-operatively but this can usually be stopped by irrigating the bladder repeatedly and giving blood transfusions, if necessary. Many men have difficulty retaining their urine for several weeks post-operatively, but very rarely does this problem become permanent. Men over 80 may take longer to regain urinary continence. Sexual performance is not necessarily reduced although many men are less potent after the operation.

# PSYCHOSURGERY

### What is it?

A little-practised branch of brain surgery that aims at altering a person's psychological state. It is a surgical approach to psychiatric disease. The earliest of the procedures (lobotomy) involved cutting the brain's frontal lobes but although this produced some good results it also had its problems. Since the lobotomy era drugs have come a long way and today very few people are operated on for psychiatric illness.

There has always been opposition to psychosurgery, rather as there has been to ECT (electroconvulsive therapy, see page 380), mainly because it is difficult to prove that it works. This efficacy is all the more difficult to prove as there are so many different procedures that it is difficult, if not impossible, to assess them adequately. Studies of the studies have found that too many variables were being left uncontrolled and that it was impossible to tell whether changes in drug treatment, intensification of psychotherapy or even social rehabilitation had brought about the positive improvements supposed to have been due to the psychosurgery.

Controversy rages over such procedures being carried out on prisoners and compulsorily committed in-patients in mental hospitals. In the US the patient must be able to give rational consent before such a procedure can be done and legal restrictions in the UK also provide considerable safeguards for patients.

It is unlikely that psychosurgery has much of a future in the light of improving drug therapy. Surgery will always be an expensive alternative for a tiny minority of people with psychiatric illness.

# PYLORIC STENOSIS

**What is it?**
A condition in which the pylorus (outflow valve of the stomach) becomes narrowed. There are two types of this condition. The first occurs in adults as a result of longstanding peptic ulceration in the region of the pylorus, resulting in scar tissue formation which slowly closes off the outflow from the stomach. More rarely it can be caused by a cancer in this part of the stomach. The second type is seen exclusively in infants. They are entirely separate conditions and will be considered separately here.

**ADULT PYLORIC STENOSIS** usually starts with dyspepsia (heartburn, upper abdominal pain and indigestion) which can go on for months or years. Eventually, bouts of vomiting take the sufferer to his doctor. The vomit is large in amount, contains undigested food and smells foul. Often, the contents of several meals are brought up. The vomiting results in a loss of weight and a barium meal confirms the diagnosis.

Treatment starts with making the person well enough to withstand an operation. The stomach is washed out before the operation itself. The surgical procedure employed is either a partial gastrectomy (see page 281) or a vagotomy and gastroenterostomy (see page 281) – the latter being favoured if a duodenal ulcer is the cause. Post-operative and other details can be found under Peptic ulcer, page 278.

**INFANTILE PYLORIC STENOSIS** is an entirely different condition brought about by an overgrowth of the muscles surrounding the pylorus. The condition affects five times as many boys as girls and the narrowing does not produce symptoms until about two to three weeks after birth. The child starts vomiting, becomes constipated and weight gain slows or stops. Classically, the vomiting is said to be 'projectile' – that is, it travels a considerable distance. The child is very hungry yet vomits much of what he eats.

This condition can be very serious because the repeated vomiting causes imbalances in the body's chemicals and the child becomes dehydrated. The diagnosis is confirmed by a doctor feeling the swollen lump of pylorus in the abdomen. This hardens and softens as the baby feeds. An X-ray may be necessary if the diagnosis is not obvious.

A medicine can be given to help the muscle of the pylorus relax but usually an operation is necessary. The procedure is simple. A small incision is made in the upper right part of the abdomen through which the surgeon operates to make a split in the pylorus muscle, leaving the lining intact. The split is left just as it is and heals on its own. The operation is often over within half an hour. The child can be fed within a few hours of the operation and the condition does not recur. After a few days the infant can go home and the wound is usually completely healed in seven to ten days at which time he can be bathed.

There are no after-effects from this operation and as no part of the bowel has been opened, recovery is quick.

# RECTAL CANCER

**What is it?**
A cancer of the back passage (rectum) that is readily
diagnosed. The vast majority of rectal cancers can be felt by
the doctor's examining finger.

The commonest sign is rectal bleeding and there may also
be a change in bowel habit too. The diagnosis is straightforward. A lump found on digital examination can be
biopsied as an out-patient and an operation done later to
remove it.

The cause of rectal cancer is not known.

**Why operate?**
To remove the mass; to prevent its spread; and to increase
the survival chances of the sufferer.

**How?**
Under general anaesthesia the whole tumour is removed.
Just how this is done depends on the position of the growth.
The rectum is only about 14 centimetres long. If the growth
is in the upper half of the canal, it can be removed and the
bowel joined back to the lower half of the rectum, so
preserving the sphincter which controls the opening and
closing of the anus. If the growth is in the lower part,
sphincter function cannot be preserved and a more major
procedure called an abdomino-perineal resection is carried
out. Whereas the former operation simply involves an
abdominal incision, the latter involves cutting away the
affected tissue both via an abdominal approach and through
an incision around the back passage, to remove it. The whole
rectum is removed and the area closed up completely. The
cut, healthy end of the colon above the rectal tumour is
brought to the skin surface on the abdomen as a colostomy.
This now becomes a permanent opening on the abdominal
wall (see colostomy, page 147).

The procedure is complex and takes about two to three

hours. Before the operation the bowel is washed out and antibiotics are given to reduce the chances of infection spreading from the cut bowel.

## Post-operative progress

For the first few days there is pain both in the abdomen and in the area behind the genitals. Slowly, over a few days, bowel function returns to normal but in the meantime you will have an intravenous drip and have the stomach fluids removed via a nasogastric tube (see page 403). The colostomy will not work for a few days but once things seem to be on the mend you will be allowed to eat soft foods, gradually building up to a normal diet. Many hospitals have experts in colostomy care who will explain how the bags for collecting stools work and how to look after your colostomy (see page 147). Remember that a colostomy does not necessarily smell and no one will know you have it. Sometimes a temporary colostomy is made and this will be closed after a few weeks.

Of course if the growth was removable without a colostomy, none of this will apply to you. You will recover as after any other major bowel operation.

The success rate of operations for rectal cancer is fairly good. Half of the sufferers will still be alive three years later and just under 40 per cent ten years later. Rectal cancers detected very early can be treated better and three quarters of people with such early tumours will be alive three years later.

There may be some sexual difficulties after major surgery in this area, as some local nerves are damaged.

As with any cancer, you will need help and support from both professionals and your family.

# RECTAL PROLAPSE

## What is it?

A condition in which the mucous membrane lining the rectum or the whole lower end of the rectum appears outside the anus (back passage). In children the mucosal type is the one most often seen and in old people the whole of the lower rectum comes down.

In childhood, rectal prolapse, when present, is usually only seen when the child passes a stool. The treatment is non-surgical as many of these children are fussy over food and are constipated. The first thing to do is to improve the child's diet so as to include a lot more dietary fibre (roughage) in the form of wholemeal bread and flour products, high-bran breakfast cereals and plenty of fruit and vegetables.

When it comes to treating the actual prolapse the procedure is as follows. After each bowel motion the parent covers his finger with a disposable tissue and inserts it into the child's back passage, pushing the prolapsed bowel back up as he does so. He then gently removes the finger, leaving the paper tissue inside to come out with the next motion. Even if the parents do nothing more than this the condition cures itself within a year or two.

If these measures do not prove successful, the rectal area can be injected with phenol which causes scarring and tethers the mucosa in place. Alternatively, a ring of catgut can be inserted just under the anal skin. This leaves a small opening for stools to emerge and by the time the catgut has dissolved spontaneously (in about a month), the prolapse has often healed.

## Why operate?

Adults need an operation because the condition is more serious and distressing than that in children and because there may be an underlying problem that needs treatment anyway. Many adults with a rectal prolapse have piles; others are very old, have no control over the anal sphincter or may have a large prostate gland.

## How?

Under a general or local anaesthetic one of two operations is currently performed. A single strand of nylon can be inserted to support the anal sphincter; or, via an abdominal incision a special kind of sponge can be used to fix the rectum from above. The former is the less serious operation but the latter often gives the better result.

After all of these procedures you will have to ensure that your stools are kept very soft and easy to pass and this can easily be done by increasing the amount of dietary fibre in your diet.

### Post-operative progress

The simple operation produces no side-effects or long-term problems, provided that the stools are kept soft. The more major operation has the after-effects associated with abdominal surgery.

# SALIVARY GLANDS

### What are they?

There are three pairs of glands around the face that produce saliva. The largest of them are the parotids which lie just in front of and below the ears and it is these that become enlarged with mumps. Saliva produced in these glands passes down fine ducts that open inside the mouth opposite the second molar teeth on the inner sides of the cheeks.

The submandibular glands lie under the lower jaw bones and a pair of sublingual glands lies under the tongue. These four glands deliver the saliva into the floor of the mouth via short ducts.

Saliva keeps the mouth moist, lubricates food and starts off the process of digestion as it contains a substance called ptyalin (an enzyme which converts starch to sugar). Saliva is produced automatically at the sight, smell and taste of food and there is more than enough tissue in all six glands for one or more to be removed if diseased, yet still provide enough saliva for healthy digestion.

The most common problem occurring with the salivary glands, apart from infection with mumps (in which surgery has no part to play) is STONES. These can form in any of the glands but most often occur in the submandibular ones. A stone forms for reasons which are as yet not clear, blocks off the duct from the gland and causes back pressure and swelling of the gland. If the stone is in one of the ducts at the front of the mouth it can sometimes be felt but usually a special X-ray (a sialogram) has to be carried out to locate it. In this, X-ray-opaque material is injected into the duct's opening in the mouth and X-ray pictures taken to show up the blockage. Once the site of the stone has been ascertained, an incision is made under general or local anaesthesia directly over the stone. If the gland is permanently damaged and remains swollen or if the stone cannot be reached in the duct, the gland may have to be removed but this is not a major operation and the scar is almost invisible after about a year.

**SALIVARY TUMOURS** are not common but of all the glands the parotid is most commonly affected. Almost all of the tumours are non-malignant and grow very slowly. Removal is carried out through an incision across the gland. This is a tricky operation for the surgeon because the facial nerve runs through the gland and any damage to this nerve could paralyse that side of the face. A malignant tumour may already have damaged the nerve which will anyway have to be cut to remove a malignant parotid tumour.

After the removal of the tumour the person can get up the following day and is allowed home in under a week. It will be painful to chew for up to a week so a fluid diet is advised but otherwise recovery is uneventful.

# SEBACEOUS CYSTS

**What are they?**
Fluid-filled benign growths in the skin caused by a build-up of the natural fluid (sebum) that normally lubricates hairs. When the duct of a sebaceous (sebum-producing) gland becomes blocked, the fluid cannot escape and produces a tense, swollen mass.

Sebaceous cysts can occur anywhere there are glands that produce sebum. They are most common on the scalp, back and scrotum and are never seen on the palms or soles. They may be single or multiple.

The cyst is firm to the touch, is not fixed to structures underneath and may be present for years without causing any trouble. Sebaceous cysts can become infected, so their removal is worthwhile for this and cosmetic reasons.

### How?
Under a local anaesthetic the cyst is removed intact, if at all possible. If it bursts it is more difficult to remove completely and regrowth may occur.

# SINUSES

### What are they?
The sinuses are cavities within the bones of the face and skull which help to give resonance to the voice. They connect with the nasal cavity and are lined with mucous membrane in continuity with that of the nose. In sinusitis this mucous membrane becomes inflamed and swollen so that the communication between the sinuses and the nose is blocked. This causes pus and secretions (mucus) to build up and the resulting pressure produces pain. Irritant vapours, allergy and infections are the commonest causes of sinusitis and by far the commonest of these are the common cold viruses. The intense pain, fever and malaise can be best treated with painkillers, inhalations, local warmth and bed rest but antibiotics may be necessary if these simple measures produce no improvement after two days. Some doctors also prescribe decongestant medicines or nose drops to shrink the mucous membranes and so allow accumulated pus to drain from the sinuses into the nose.

### Why operate?
If none of these procedures works or if there is evidence of persistent pus in a sinus, surgical drainage may be necessary.

## How?

The sinuses that most often need surgical drainage are the facial (maxillary) ones in the cheek bones. Because these sinuses lie just above the roots of the upper teeth, one surgical approach is through the mouth and involves making a hole above the roots of the upper eye tooth under the gum. Working through this opening, the surgeon clears all the infected material from the sinus and then makes another opening from the sinus into the nose so that drainage is continuous and will also be effective in case of future infections. It usually means a stay in hospital of six or seven days. Swelling of the soft tissues of the cheek may occur after this operation and there may be slight discoloration of the skin.

A simpler procedure involves piercing the wall of the sinus with a stout needle through the inside of the nose. This is done under a local anaesthetic as an out-patient and is usually tried a few times before the more major procedure is carried out.

All such surgery is usually done by a specialist ENT (Ear, Nose and Throat) surgeon.

# SKIN CANCER

## What is it?

A very treatable cancer commonly seen in sunny countries among white-skinned people. Fortunately, if caught early, it is almost never fatal.

Skin cancer shows itself in many different ways, so if you have a sore that does not heal, a wart or mole, birthmark or scar that changes in any way – do see your doctor. He will take a tiny sample (a biopsy) or refer you to someone who will. If the lesion is a small one it may be considered wise to excise it all and then to examine it under a microscope. The only dangerous form of skin cancer is a MALIGNANT MELANOMA (see Moles, page 256).

X-ray therapy is the answer to most skin cancers (except

malignant melanomas) and treatment is nearly 100 per cent successful. Growth that cannot be treated in this way can be excised and skin from another part of the body grafted to make up the deficit if necessary.

A **RODENT ULCER** is a particular type of skin cancer which occurs on the face above the level of the lips, but can rarely occur elsewhere. It is seen equally often in men and women and is unusual under the age of 40. The main sign is an ulcer which crusts over and bleeds and typically has a pearly edge. This ulcer can be removed surgically or treated with radiation therapy, both of which produce good results.

# SKIN GRAFTING

## What is it?

A surgical procedure in which skin is used from another part of the person's body (or from a donor) to replace lost skin somewhere. Although many people think of skin grafting as a purely cosmetic pursuit, this is not the case, even though cosmetic surgeons do, of course, use the techniques (see page 159). The majority of skin grafting is done by surgeons who want to restore the continuity of a person's skin after an accident, a burn or the surgical removal of skin during another procedure.

An area from which skin has been lost can be left to heal over of its own accord but the result is the formation of scar tissue, not new skin. Scar tissue is more fibrous (harder), whiter and less elastic than normal skin, so a scarred patch always looks and feels very different from the surrounding skin. To overcome this, skin can be placed over the affected area and left to grow there. Any *large* area of skin loss or that across a joint *must* be grafted because as the fibrous scar tissue grows it causes the area to contract. This can produce severe disfiguration and even a loss of use of the area concerned.

Skin from a 'bank' or from another person provides

temporary (about six weeks) success only. Skin grafts must be from the person himself if they are to provide a permanent answer.

## How?

Grafts are of two kinds. They can be full-thickness or partial-thickness and they can be 'pedicled' (see below) or not.

**PARTIAL-THICKNESS GRAFTS** are the most commonly used as they will 'take' even on infected surfaces such as those occurring after a burn (the commonest reason for skin grafting). Such grafts are not very good cosmetically though because they are applied in patches and the joints between the patches show permanently.

**FULL-THICKNESS GRAFTS** heal much less readily than do partial ones and are often taken from the abdomen or from behind the ear. The skin is stitched into place very carefully with fine sutures and pressure applied to prevent bruising. Flaps of skin can be swung from nearby healthy areas to be attached to the area to be grafted. In this way the graft retains a blood supply.

A **PEDICLE GRAFT** is less often used but can enable a surgeon to transfer skin a long way on the person's body without initially completely removing the piece of skin to be grafted and so destroying its blood supply. In this procedure a bridge of skin is raised but left attached at its ends. The cut surfaces are stitched to form a tube and the raw surface underneath grafted with partial-thickness grafts. After about three weeks one end of the tube is opened and joined to the area to be grafted. After several more weeks, if the tube is healthy, the other end is severed and the skin then moulded to the size and shape required for the damaged area. In this way a pedicle graft from an arm can be used to repair a face, for example. This is awkward for the person as he has to have his arm in a position close to his face for a long time but provides his only hope of a really good outcome.

All but the simplest of skin grafting is done under a general anaesthetic. In a partial or split-thickness graft, skin is taken from the donor site (often the thigh) using a special shaving instrument and is laid as a single piece or as postage-stamp-sized pieces. The donor site regrows back to normal again without much scarring because only the most superficial layer of the skin has gone. Full-thickness grafts leave gaps in the skin which do not heal but which can be repaired with split-thickness grafts from elsewhere.

Burns are one of the great 'consumers' of skin grafts and as scores of thousands of people are burned each year in the UK, it is no surprise that this is so. In the early stages of a severe burn, shock is the greatest problem doctors have to treat. The burned area loses fluid as tissue fluid seeps out. This fluid needs to be replaced if the person's circulatory system is to be kept topped up and so prevent shock.

The second problem with burns is infection. As such a large area of the body's surface is breached by a serious burn, infective organisms can easily enter the body. Both shock and infection can be helped or even overcome entirely by adequate skin grafting. Temporary grafts may be used until the person's condition improves sufficiently to undergo more permanent surgery.

Severe burns present such formidable problems both to the surgeon and patient alike that great patience and skill are required. Your plastic surgeon will make a plan which might run over months or even years with staged operations, often not even starting until months after the original burn so as to allow you to recover fully before further operations.

Small grafted areas heal within weeks and, if well done, are hardly visible within a year or so. Make-up can be used to cover any remaining blemishes.

# SPINA BIFIDA

**What is it?**
A defect, present from birth, in which one or more of the bony arches encircling the spinal cord is absent or defective. Spina bifida is one of the commonest of the serious birth abnormalities in the UK and the UK has one of the highest occurrence rates of spina bifida in the world. Every year

nearly a thousand babies are born with the condition in Britain – more girls than boys.

In the most serious type of spina bifida there is a skin defect and part of the spinal cord (normally covered by a transparent membrane representing the meninges) is exposed on the newborn baby's back. The exposed nerve tissue is called a meningomyelocele and the extent of the disorder depends on the amount of the spinal cord exposed. Usually, the defect is low down on the back where the lumbar and sacral regions of the spine join. The trouble is not always this obvious though, and there may be normal-looking skin over the affected area.

Spina bifida may cause paralysis of the legs, incontinence of urine and faeces, club foot and dislocation of the hips, depending on the level of the cord affected. Nine out of ten children with spina bifida also have hydrocephalus (see also page 218) because of a defect in the base of the brain. About half are mentally retarded to some degree.

No one knows what causes spina bifida but because it tends to run in families a genetic factor has been suggested. Environmental factors may also play a part because the condition is so much commoner in certain geographical areas than others.

### Why operate?
To close the defect in the back and to prevent infection entering the nervous system.

### How?
Pre-operatively the affected area is kept moist with a sterile saline dressing covered with a plastic sheet. The degree of muscle control in the legs and arms is assessed and the skull measured. X-rays are taken of the back to see the extent of the trouble. If at all possible the operation to close the defect is done within the first 48 hours after birth. This helps prevent infection entering the spinal cord and causing meningitis when it ascends to the brain. If the defect is large, the skin locally is loosened and pulled over to cover the gap. If this is done, vacuum drains are inserted at the time.

## Post-operative progress

Particular care is taken to keep the temperature of these babies normal both before and especially after the operation as they are susceptible to cooling which lowers their temperature to unacceptably low levels. The suction drains are removed after 48 hours and the stitches taken out at ten to twelve days.

If there is paralysis of the lower limbs, a physiotherapist puts them through their full range of movements at regular intervals. This reduces the degree of deformity. If deformities develop, strapping or splinting may be necessary and further surgery may be needed at a later stage to correct them. A close watch is kept on the baby's head size and treatment started if it enlarges too rapidly because of a build-up of fluid inside (see page 218).

Routine urine samples are taken to ensure that no infection is developing. These children often have abnormalities of their urinary systems and so need extra special care. Operations may be needed on the urinary tract.

Mortality rates are high. About a third of affected children die in the first year and even those that live often present considerable problems to both parents and doctors. Approximately half die before their fifth birthday. Active treatment can, however, improve the outcome and many spina bifida sufferers now live into adulthood and hold down jobs.

One of the greatest problems when a baby like this is born is deciding what to do. The situation throws considerable stress on to those parents who feel that they do not want the doctors to try too hard to save the life of the baby. Others react in exactly the opposite way and are determined to do all they can to produce as normal a child as possible from such a poor start. To some extent the outcome depends on the severity of the condition to start with but perhaps the most important factor in developing the child's optimum potential is the teamwork of the paediatricians, physiotherapists, surgeons, general practitioners and parents. There is no denying that a child with anything but the most minor of spinal defects presents both parents and the medical profession with formidable short- and long-term problems. There is no easy way out of this situation.

Unfortunately, spina bifida and its related condition anencephaly run in families so parents who have had one baby with either condition should seek genetic counselling before considering having another baby. Amniocentesis (see page 352) enables doctors to test for a special substance, alpha-fetoprotein, in the fluid surrounding an affected baby in the womb. This substance can also be detected in the mother's blood. In this way spina bifida and anencephaly can be detected early and the parents offered an abortion if the fetus is known to be affected. An ultrasound scan (see page 410) early in pregnancy can also detect anencephaly and some cases of spina bifida.

## SPINAL CORD SURGERY

The spinal cord runs down the canal inside the back bones (vertebrae) starting at the base of the skull and ending about half way down the back. From then on the central canal in the vertebral column is filled with nerve roots. The back wall of the bony canal is formed by a series of bony plates called laminae. These may have to be removed over the section of cord to be operated on. This procedure is called a laminectomy.

More than half of all tumours affecting the spinal cord arise from the meningeal coverings of the cord and are not cancerous. They produce symptoms because of the pressure they exert and are treated with complete success in most cases. If a tumour occurs actually inside the spinal cord, the chances are higher that it will be malignant. Such a tumour is difficult to remove without damaging nervous tissue.

The spinal cord can, of course, be injured just like any other organ. It can take quite a lot of punishment though, partly because it is encased within bone and partly because, being surrounded by fluid (the cerebrospinal fluid), it is buffered from trauma to a great extent. Severe damage to the spinal column can force pieces of bone into the cord which is then cut through to some degree. Unfortunately, a cut cord does not regenerate so the chances of recovery are small. If after an accident there is no movement or sensation in a part of the body, the outlook is bad but if either is present it is possible that pressure is the problem and that this can be relieved by surgery. After serious spinal column damage, bone grafts (either from the person himself or from a bone bank) may be used to fuse the spine in the damaged area to fix it rigidly. While this bone is healing the person may be placed in a plaster cast or immobilized in other ways.

Perhaps the best-known operation on the back is that for a **SLIPPED DISC**. This is indeed a relatively common operation but should only be carried out when there is good evidence that the person's problems are in fact caused by disc trouble. There are many causes of back pain, including pain of psychological origin and, as a result, a fair proportion of those operated on for a disc lesion are not improved by the operation and continue to suffer from their old trouble.

Between the body of each vertebra is a roughly circular disc of cartilage and connective tissue. Each disc is quite thick and acts as a shock absorber between adjacent bony vertebrae so that when we walk or jump, bone does not crunch against bone in the spine. Trouble occurs when the strong outer covering of a disc breaks, allowing the soft inner part to rupture. If this rupture presses on a nerve, pain is the result.

The symptoms of a ruptured disc vary according to the site of the disc affected but by far the commonest one to rupture is that between the last lumbar vertebra and the first sacral vertebra. This causes 'sciatic' pain which runs down the leg to the foot. The pain may be followed by pins and needles and weakness of the legs and there may be back pain. There are scores of causes of back pain and only a small proportion is caused by prolapsed intervertebral discs but when the combination of signs just described is present, the chances are that a disc is at fault. The diagnosis of a ruptured disc is made clinically and with a special X-ray (a myelogram) in which a radio-opaque fluid is injected into the spinal cord. Today, computerized tomography (see page 424) is sometimes used to give excellent pictures and so save the person from a possibly unpleasant myelogram.

The operation to remove a prolapsed disc is done through a 12 centimetre long vertical incision over the affected area. Sometimes a laminectomy is done in order to get at the disc but most often it can be reached without removing bone. Some surgeons enlarge the canal through which the nerve leaves the spinal column at the same time, to relieve any pressure there might be. Although the operation is a major one (taking two hours or more) the person is up and about in a few days and home within two weeks though some surgeons keep their patients in bed for three weeks. It is sensible not to do heavy manual work for a few months but your doctor will advise on this, according to what was done at the operation.

If the spine has to be immobilized (for pain, for example) it can be fixed rigidly over a given length. Chips of bone are used either from the hip bone of the person himself or from a bone bank to stimulate natural bone growth in the area to be immobilized. The bone graft dies and only acts as scaffolding over and through which new bone cells grow. This is rather akin to the healing of a fracture by new bone formation. Just as with fracture healing, the spine may have to be immobilized in a plaster cast to allow healing to occur and this can take months.

The outcome of disc surgery varies greatly according to the certainty of the diagnosis before the operation. Today, surgeons are very wary of operating on backs unless they are sure of their diagnosis and, because of this, results are very good. Increasing numbers of people are keen to try conservative measures first, even though they can take months, rather than resort quickly to surgery. In general, pain in the legs (caused by a protruding disc) responds well to an operation but back pain responds less well. A recent survey of 323 disc operation patients found that 86 per cent of the men and 79 per cent of the women were freed of all symptoms but that 9 per cent and 15 per cent respectively had some persistent back pain. Of those people treated in another survey, but this time with non-operative measures, 57 per cent had a recurrence of the disc trouble within five years of the start of the treatment.

# SPLEEN OPERATIONS

The spleen is an organ about the size of a clenched fist that lies under the lower end of the rib cage in the front on the left side of the chest. It forms blood in the fetus but in adults destroys red blood cells when they wear out. It also produces antibodies to fight infection.

Rather like the gall-bladder and the appendix, the spleen seems to be disposable because many hundreds of people have lived and are living perfectly well after their spleens have been removed.

Normally, the spleen cannot be felt because it lies tucked under the rib cage but in certain blood diseases and tropical diseases it enlarges greatly. When it is very large it becomes more susceptible to knocks which can cause severe and, rarely, fatal internal bleeding.

The spleen may have to be removed for one of several reasons. Rupture after a car crash or other trauma means it has to be removed and in the rare event of the organ being the seat of a tumour it will also have to be excised.

Certain kinds of splenic enlargement cause anaemia, jaundice and blood clotting problems and these can be completely cured by removing the overactive spleen.

The spleen is usually removed as a 'cold' (as opposed to an emergency) procedure. Obviously, a ruptured spleen calls for emergency surgery but usually the whole thing is planned over a long period of treatment by haematologists (specialists in blood diseases).

Under general anaesthesia an incision about 20 centimetres long is made in the upper left abdomen. The spleen is then removed along with any accessory spleens which may enlarge once the main organ has been removed. The operation takes about an hour. Post-operatively there is very little trouble. A nasogastric tube may be left down to keep the stomach from becoming distended with gastric juices and air. The person is up the day after the operation and home within two weeks. He can go back to work in about eight weeks.

There are no long-term complications apart from the person being a little more susceptible to infections. The functions of the spleen are taken over by the other tissues and people without a spleen fare perfectly well. Removal of the spleen is usually completely curative for the condition for which it is performed.

# SQUINT

**What is it?**
A condition in which the eyes are not directed together at the object a person is looking at. Squints are much more common in children and most surgery done for squints is performed in childhood.

In the earliest weeks many babies squint simply because their eyes have not become coordinated one with another. However, any child over the age of three months with a squint probably has an imbalance of the muscles moving the eyeballs and needs medical attention. This is more likely to occur if either parent squinted in childhood.

Squints must be taken seriously because a child with a persistent squint may lose the sight of the eye. This comes about because the brain cannot cope with the double image of the world it is fed by two 'independent' eyes and so suppresses one image permanently. A child with an alternating squint – one in which both eyes squint from time to time – is less likely to lose the vision of one eye but still needs expert supervision.

Treatment need not be surgical and starts with simply covering the good eye, thus encouraging the squinting eye to work properly by re-educating or 'exercising' those parts of the brain that have become underactive because of the squint. Surgical operations can be carried out to alter the length of the eye's muscles to rebalance the eye.

Squints can be associated with short sight, long sight or

astigmatism inadequately treated. Measles, meningitis and a few other diseases can also produce a squint.

Wise parents take their children for routine checks at the health clinic or to their family doctor. These places check for squints (which may not be obvious) and test the eyesight in both eyes separately.

## Why operate?
In some cases exercises for the eye and other measures fail, leaving an operation as one way of saving the vision in the affected eye. Even after the operation (which simply re-aligns the eyes) the affected eye will have to be re-educated to see normally and this will need further trips to the hospital. Surgery can be done at any age and even within the first year.

## How?
The basic principle behind this surgery is to shorten eye muscles that are too long and vice versa. This is achieved by removing the attachment of the muscle to the eyeball and re-attaching it somewhere else, according to the effect required.

The whole operation takes place outside the eyeball – which is not opened. Because of this there is no danger to the child's vision at all. Under general anaesthesia an incision is made in the white of the eye to get at the affected muscles. If both eyes are affected (usually only one is) either one or both can be operated upon at the same session. Strictly speaking a squint is not a one-sided condition – it affects both eyes, at brain level anyway. Because of this it does not matter which eye is operated upon so long as they both end up being approximately in line again.

## Post-operative progress
Eyes are not bandaged today and the child is usually up and about almost immediately after the operation. The operation leaves little or no pain post-operatively and the child can be back at school within a week or so.

Although a seriously damaged eye cannot be given new visual powers, most eyes are successfully straightened by these operations, even if a second one is necessary to achieve this. Even if the eyesight has been largely lost, the child is usually grateful (and will be so especially later in life) to have a normal-looking face without a squint.

# STERILIZATION

### What is it?

A permanent method of birth control. We will consider here only the female methods. Vasectomy (male sterilization) is discussed on page 344.

The legal situation varies around the world but in many countries today sterilization is legal once proper permission has been given by the woman. Many clinics and hospitals also require the husband's permission in writing before his wife is sterilized because, after all, it is an operation which affects their marital relationship and cannot be reliably reversed. Although, as we shall see, sterilization *can* be reversed, reversal operations are not yet reliable. To all intents and purposes, a couple embarking on sterilization *must* consider it irreversible. This makes it a difficult decision because the relationship may break up and the woman may want children with a new husband, or all the existing children may be lost in a tragedy of some kind and she will be unable to 'replace' them.

The way to prevent pregnancies with certainty is to stop the eggs produced in the ovaries from getting to the uterus and sterilization does just this.

### How?

Almost all sterilization procedures in women involve doing something to the fallopian tubes down which eggs travel from the ovaries to the uterus. These two fine tubular structures, one on each side of the pelvis, are so delicate that their cavities are no wider than a bristle from a brush. The simplest sterilization procedure involves cutting the tubes. Through a small abdominal incision made under a general anaesthetic, the surgeon takes each fallopian tube, ties it in two places and cuts out a section about two to three centimetres long between the two ties. The skin incision is closed as usual and the patient is discharged home in two to three days.

A second type of sterilization procedure involves the use of a laparoscope (see also page 398). This is an instrument that can be inserted through a one centimetre long incision in the abdominal wall just below the navel. The instrument not only has a telescope and light which enables the surgeon to look directly into the abdominal cavity but has a tubular cavity down which fine instruments can be threaded so that operations can be performed inside the abdomen without opening it up. Laparoscopic sterilization is simple, safe and quick but is highly skilful and needs an operator with lots of experience if it is to be done well. The technique is performed as follows.

The laparoscope is inserted together with a fine instrument to enable the surgeon to grip the fallopian tube. An electric current then fuses the tissues into a solid mass, so closing off the tube completely. The procedure is then repeated for the other side. It is quick and almost totally safe. The only problems are that women who have had bowel operations before may not be suitable (because old scar tissue makes the procedure technically difficult to perform) and that fat women may also be difficult to laparoscope. From the woman's point of view though, it is simple, quick and safe and almost never involves more than one night in hospital.

About one third of women report that they are unaware that anything has been done; about a third have period-type pains but can carry on as normal; and the remaining third take a couple of days off to recover.

Other common sterilization procedures carried out under laparoscopic control involve the placing of tiny elastic bands or plastic clips on the fallopian tubes. These are quick and simple and mean only one night in hospital.

Some women consider the desirability of sterilization and give permission well in advance of the birth of their baby so that if a Caesarean section becomes necessary, they can be sterilized there and then. This should not, however, be a last-minute decision taken by a couple when they hear that a

Caesarean section might be necessary. Research shows that women who undergo sterilization immediately after the birth of a baby or after an abortion are more likely to regret it later than those who have made a more considered decision.

## Post-operative progress

Once a woman has been sterilized (other than by laparoscopy) she will be home again within three to five days and there are no changes in her menstrual cycle or her sexual functioning except, of course, that she cannot conceive. The egg she produces each month is reabsorbed by the body just as a man's body reabsorbs his sperms after a vasectomy. Some women are very upset by the thought that they can no longer conceive but most are happier than before because they no longer need to bother with contraception. Because of this, some couples' sex lives are greatly improved as a result of sterilization.

Unfortunately, sterilization is virtually irreversible. Many researchers are working on reversal and reversible procedures but the task is technically very difficult because the fallopian tubes are so tiny and the operation to sew up the cut ends involves operating under microscopes and using stitches little thicker than a human hair. Clearly such a delicate operation cannot readily become widespread. The placing of clips or elastic bands on the fallopian tubes damages a much smaller length of tube and so may improve the chances of reversal if the couple decide they want more children.

According to a major US survey carried out by the International Institute for the Study of Human Reproduction, a large majority of men and women who have been voluntarily sterilized are satisfied with the operation. A large majority also reported no change in their sexual activity or desire after the operation. However, it appears from UK studies that women who are sterilized immediately after a birth (or abortion) and those who have sexual or marital problems are more likely to be unhappy about having been sterilized and may even seek a reversal of the procedure. Younger women too seem to regret having been sterilized, a fact which is causing concern among gynaecologists because the age at which women are being sterilized (currently at about 32–36) is falling. This way well mean, on present evidence, that increasing numbers of women are going to want a reversal of the operation. A poor marriage is a bad reason for seeking sterilization, especially now that divorce is so common. As many as one in seven women regrets having been sterilized.

# STOMACH CANCER

**What is it?**
Cancer affecting the stomach is becoming less common. It affects twice as many men as women and usually occurs over the age of 40.

There are several signs and symptoms of stomach cancer, any one of which (or combination of many) may be present. Unfortunately, many people have no serious complaints until the cancer has spread. There may be upper abdominal pains, a loss of appetite, vomiting, weight loss or anaemia.

The diagnosis is usually easily made on a barium meal (see page 420) X-ray or on gastroscopy (see page 387) which provides the added advantage of enabling a biopsy to be taken to be sure the growth is malignant. Most tumours of the stomach are malignant. Ulcers of the stomach are usually benign. (See Peptic ulcer, page 278).

**Why operate?**
Surgery is essential once a stomach cancer has been diagnosed because it should be removed so that it does not invade other local organs. Surgery is also often advisable for gastric (stomach) ulcers that appear to be malignant. Really large stomach cancers may so obstruct the passage of food that a new channel has to be made to bypass the growth. This can prolong life for a few months, especially when combined with anti-cancer drugs and radiation therapy.

**How?**
Under a general anaesthetic an incision is made from the tip

of the breast bone to the navel, although some surgeons make the incision across the top of the abdomen. Most of the stomach usually has to be removed and nearby lymph nodes and other tissues are often taken away too. If the entire stomach is removed, the small intestine is connected directly to the oesophagus (gullet). The whole procedure takes about two to three hours.

### Post-operative progress

There is the usual post-operative pain as experienced after any major abdominal operation but the person can be up a day or two after. The wound heals within two weeks, after which bathing can be carried out as normal. After about two weeks in hospital the person can be back at work within two months.

As we have seen, many people come to doctors with their stomach cancers already in a rather advanced stage. This means that by the time the surgeon operates the growth is already large. Only about 10 per cent of men and 15 per cent of women are alive five years after the diagnosis is first made but for early stomach cancer the survival figures jump to 37 per cent and 43 per cent respectively. About a third of these are still alive at ten years.

Early surgery is definitely valuable and increases the person's outlook but it is not practical to screen everybody over the age of 40 for stomach cancer, so many will inevitably go undetected until too late.

Long-term complications can be a problem too, though many are relatively easily overcome. If the stomach has been removed, the person can only eat small meals, which have to be taken slowly. Vitamin $B_{12}$ has to be given by injection because the loss of intrinsic factor (a substance produced by the lining of the stomach which facilitates the absorption of this invaluable vitamin) means none of the vitamin is absorbed from food. Apart from these small physical problems there are the psychological ones. Quite naturally, anyone who is told he has stomach cancer is going to feel depressed about it. Until the actual operation there may be doubt as to whether the growth is malignant (unless a biopsy has been done using a gastroscope) so there is always hope that the operation will not be as serious as anticipated. However, even if one can come to terms with the malignancy, it is always difficult knowing that one's life expectancy is probably reduced.

# THYROID OPERATIONS

The thyroid gland is an 'H'-shaped organ that lies in front of the throat with the limbs of the 'H' on either side of the windpipe just above the top of the breastbone. Though a relatively small gland, it is very important because it controls the metabolism of the whole body. Utilization of food energy at a cellular level is controlled by the hormones produced by the thyroid gland and circulated around the blood stream.

Underactivity of the thyroid gland makes a person cold, sluggish, slow to react and think, and liable to put on weight. This can be remedied by giving thyroid tablets. Overactivity of the gland produces weight loss, nervousness, excessive sweating, trembling, a feeling of warmth, palpitation and sometimes a bulging of the eyes with a rim of white visible all around the iris.

A goitre is a swollen thyroid gland and can be caused by too little iodine in the diet (add iodine and the gland returns to its normal size), or by thyroiditis, an inflammation of the gland with fever (treated with steroid drugs). It may also become nodular for no apparent reason. The thyroid gland can also become enlarged because of a tumour but this is usually confined to the gland itself, so removal results in very good cure rates.

Thyroid diseases are usually diagnosed clinically but blood tests and radio-isotope scanning of the gland (see page 405) give more detailed information to the doctor and help him decide whether drugs or surgery are indicated.

Goitre caused by insufficient iodine is rare today as some table salt has iodine added to it. If the gland is overactive (producing a condition called thyrotoxicosis), drugs are usually used to suppress the production of thyroid hormone.

Radioactive iodine can also be given by mouth to be concentrated by the thyroid where it destroys some of the gland and cures the problem. Unfortunately, it is not always easy to gauge exactly how much of the isotope to give and too much thyroid tissue may be killed, leading to low thyroid activity which then has to be counteracted by giving thyroid tablets for the rest of the person's life.

### Why operate?
Surgery is needed when medical treatment has improved but not cured the trouble; when a scan of the gland shows a 'cold' area (of non-active thyroid gland); or when the gland is so large that it is pressing on the windpipe.

### How?
Under general anaesthesia an eight to ten centimetre long incision is made around the contour of the neck above the collarbone. This incision leaves so fine a scar that a year later it is almost impossible to see where the cut was made. At the operation the surgeon removes part, half, or all of the gland, depending upon the underlying trouble. If compression of the windpipe was the reason for the operation, then perhaps only the cross-piece of the 'H' that lies across the windpipe need go. If there is a benign tumour, only that part of the gland affected by the tumour is removed. Even with some cases of cancer, only half of the gland is removed, though more often the operation is more extensive.

Thyroid surgery is very delicate because so many important structures pass nearby and have to be preserved. This particularly applies to the parathyroid glands which control calcium metabolism in the body and to a nerve which supplies the muscles to the vocal cords.

### Post-operative progress
There is very little pain post-operatively and the wound heals quickly. There may be hoarseness for a few days but this is rarely troublesome. Because the area is so richly supplied with blood vessels, a drain is left in place for two to three days

so that there is no build-up of blood to form an internal bruise.

All the previous thyroid symptoms are cured by surgery. It is relatively easy to remove too much of the gland when operating for overactivity, so leaving the person with too little functioning tissue, but thyroid tablets can redress the balance easily. Needless to say, thyroid tablets are essential after removal of the whole of the thyroid gland.

Return to work is in order within two to three weeks of going home, which is usually about a week after the operation. Careful check-ups are done to monitor your thyroid state after the operation just to make sure that no new problems have been produced.

# TONSILLECTOMY

**What is it?**
The removal of the tonsils, often along with other glandular tissue nearby called the adenoids.

At the back of the throat there is a collection of lymphoid tissue. This tissue helps provide a defence against infection in the air we inhale and in food and the things we put in our mouths. It forms a ring which consists of two tonsils, the adenoids and nodules on the base of the tongue. When harmful bacteria are inhaled, healthy tonsils enlarge as they produce protective white blood cells. The tonsils are relatively small in the first year of life and increase in size as the child grows. They are usually at their largest between the ages of four and seven years and then get smaller during the next five years or so.

Tonsillitis is an infection of the tonsils that occurs when their natural resistance is overwhelmed by infection. It may be seen as part of a generalized infection of the throat but can occur in isolation too. Most cases of tonsillitis are caused by a viral infection for which there is no cure. Some, however, are caused by a bacterium called a streptococcus. Antibiotics are useful in preventing complications of streptococcal sore throats (rheumatic fever, nephritis and middle ear infection) and are widely and justifiably used in these circumstances. Unfortunately, it is very difficult to differentiate between viral and streptococcal sore throats unless a swab is taken and sent to a bacteriology (microbiology) laboratory, though children with a streptococcal infection are more likely to have a headache, tummy ache, vomiting and enlargement of the lymph nodes in the neck than are children with viral tonsillitis.

The size of the tonsils is not a reliable indication as to the type or severity of the condition. Some tonsils that meet in the middle of the throat are quite healthy.

If the tonsils become chronically infected, causing recurrent tonsillitis, bad breath, difficulty in swallowing and long-term swelling of the glands in the neck, then tonsillectomy should be considered. This is rarely necessary before the age of four years and is often avoidable after that. If the tonsils are still active in defending the body against infection, the child will get no benefit from tonsillectomy unless they are so large that they are making swallowing difficult. However, if they give rise to attacks of tonsillitis of such severity or frequency that they outweigh the disadvantages of an operation, then they should be removed.

Remember, before pushing your doctor to remove your child's tonsils, that doing so may not produce any decrease in the number of coughs, colds and sore throats the child will have; any decrease in the frequency of chest infections or laryngitis; nor any decrease in the number of middle ear infections, sinusitis or nasal allergy. Your child can still get sore throats after a tonsillectomy but he may well feel better, eat more and lose his bad breath. Having a tonsillectomy will mean that he will have to stay in hospital, possibly for no good reason, and be subjected to an anaesthetic and the dangers of an operation, however small.

### Why operate?

An operation is worthwhile if the tonsils cause frequent and severe attacks of tonsillitis; if the obstruction to eating or breathing is unpleasant or dangerous; or if the tonsils are small, fibrous and of no protective value to the child. A previous history of a quinsy is also an indication for surgery.

## How?

Both children and adults can have their tonsils removed. The vast majority of tonsillectomy procedures are carried out on children because upper respiratory infections affecting the tonsils are most common in childhood.

A general anaesthetic is used. The operation is performed through the mouth: there are no external incisions. The surgeon grasps the tonsil, dissects it off its bed on the back of the throat and places a wire snare around the stalk. Once this stalk is cut through, the tonsil is freed. Adenoid tissue is snipped off the back of the nasal cavity. The two procedures can be completed in half an hour.

## Post-operative progress

Most children (and especially adults) complain of a sore throat for up to a week but this is clearly not a serious or life-threatening problem. Immediately after the operation the person will have to lie on his side so that he cannot choke on any blood that might ooze from the removal sites. Do not be alarmed if you see a small amount of blood coming from your child's mouth post-operatively; this is normal and stops within a few hours.

Pain is the most unpleasant side-effect of the operation and it may be referred to the ears. Most children only want fluids and very soft foods such as ice cream for a day or two but surgeons differ on how soon they let a child eat normally again.

Bleeding can occur within an hour or so after surgery (in which case it will be noticed and treated at once) or later between the fifth and tenth days. If this occurs when the child is back home, tell your doctor at once so that he can stop it or telephone the hospital with a view to taking him back.

Many children return to normal life two weeks after the operation and they are usually perfectly well or fit for school within three weeks.

Pain in the throat at meal times, sometimes radiating to

the ears, may continue for up to ten days or so after the operation. It may be controlled by taking a suitable dose of a household painkiller twenty minutes before meals.

For details of children in hospital see page 74.

# TORN CARTILAGE

The knee is a complex and stable joint but is often the site of trouble, one of the commonest of which is a torn cartilage. Damage to the cartilage of the knee occurs when weight is placed on the joint while the body twists with the foot fixed. Because this collection of manoeuvres happens fairly frequently in sports, it is sportsmen who mostly suffer from torn cartilages. Cartilages can, however, be torn outside the sports field and are not only seen in sportsmen.

The cartilages that get torn are crescent-shaped buffers that lie between the ends of the thigh and lower leg bones. They are cleverly contoured to help the smooth working of the knee and act as shock absorbers in rather the same way as the intervertebral discs do in the spine. In each knee there are two cartilages, one on the inner and one on the outer side of the joint.

When a cartilage is torn, the piece that tears away becomes jammed in the joint on movement, causing it to 'lock'. This produces pain, swelling, an unwillingness to put weight on the leg and an inability to straighten the knee.

### Why operate?
An operation is not always necessary for such symptoms. Surgery is often needed though because most of these tears occur in young people who are active sportsmen and wage earners who are naturally loath to be off work or incapacitated for months. Also many sufferers complain that they are continually uneasy about the stability of the joint and that they would rather have an operation 'to be sure of a cure'.

## How?

Very recently, a team in the UK has started removing torn cartilages without actually opening up the knee joint at an operation. They do this using an operating arthroscope and are achieving excellent results, with their patients up and about the day after the operation and walking normally again within days. This operation down a telescope inserted into the knee is still not widely available though and most people have their cartilages removed at an open operation in which a ten centimetre long incision is made across the knee joint under general anaesthesia. The operation takes about half an hour and is very satisfactory. A compression bandage is applied together with a plaster backsplint and the person is in hospital for about ten days.

The day after the operation, exercises are started so as to strengthen the thigh muscles that help keep the knee stable. About two days after the operation the person is allowed to put weight on the affected leg but it takes four to six weeks before normal activities can be resumed.

Apart from the scar, which is unsightly, there are no after-effects and the knee seems to function perfectly well without its cartilages.

# TRANSPLANT SURGERY

To many people, the possibility of being able to replace diseased or damaged organs in an otherwise healthy person seems an ideal way out of many health problems. Science fiction writers have used their imaginations to further enhance this dream and is it only natural to hope that one day we will be able to replace body parts just as we can those of a car.

So far, excellent results have been obtained with transplanting corneas, skin and bone but other organs and tissues are proving more difficult for various reasons. The main cause for much of the failure to date has been the phenomenon known as rejection. When any 'foreign', that is 'non-self' material enters the body, defence machanisms come into play. These usually involve the production of white cells which produce antibodies to the foreign substance. Eventually, the body's defences overwhelm the foreign intruder and the transplanted tissue dies.

Given that most of the mechanical aspects of transplanting organs can be overcome with improved equipment and surgical technique, the main barrier to greater advances in transplantation surgery is that of rejection. In the early days, surgeons used large doses of radiation to dampen down the body's defence mechanisms. Unfortunately this proved impractical because those treated were left with no natural defences at all and died of any infection that came their way.

Drugs of the steroid group such as prednisone were then tried because they too suppressed rejection mechanisms and these, combined with radiation therapy, were used for some time but again with little success. Today's advances in transplantation are coming about because we now understand rejection phenomena better and can monitor suppressive drugs much more carefully than ever before. Newer substances such as anti-thymocyte globulin (ATG) are now being used in heart transplants particularly but it is too early yet to know if they will produce a dramatic improvement in rejection rates.

Apart from the corneas, bone and skin, only four other organs are being transplanted with any degree of regularity and success. These are bone marrow, kidneys, livers and hearts.

**BONE MARROW TRANSPLANTS** Children born with certain bone marrow disorders can be treated with some success using bone marrow grafts either from close relatives or from carefully matched outsiders. These provide the child with the lacking red and white blood cell-producing material. The marrow transplant is given via a vein but the cells find their way into the recipient's bone marrow quickly. Here they function as if they were his own marrow cells. In order to prevent rejection, the child is kept in a germ-free atmosphere during the time when his body's natural defence systems are unable to cope. This can be very wearing for the adults around, especially the parents, but does not seem to bother the children too much. Bone marrow transplants are not often done and have not caught the public's imagination in the same way that livers, kidneys and hearts have, even though individual cases have received considerable publicity.

**LIVER TRANSPLANTS** were first carried out in 1963 and since then over 300 have been performed, mostly in two centres, one in Denver and the other in London. Although some progress has been made on artificial liver machine design, these cannot maintain people for long periods as can kidney machines, so transplants are the only answer for those with certain kinds of liver failure. In many ways, selected people with proven inoperable cancer of the liver are the best candidates for liver transplantation because they are young and have a very poor outlook if nothing is done. The US centre in Denver believes that liver transplants should only be done on young people and sets an upper age limit of 45 years but the London group has had good results in people in their 50s.

Cancer of the liver and cirrhosis are the two main conditions that make the surgeons working in these centres consider transplantation, although only a small proportion of these people are suitable. The liver does not seem to suffer too badly from rejection by the body as does the kidney and the London team has found that fewer than ten per cent of their livers are rejected. Early transplants were not very successful but now that the donor livers are being obtained much sooner (with improved operative and transport techniques), many patients remain alive for some years after receiving their new livers. The longest survivor in the world lived for seven years and several people are now alive five years after the transplant. It is confidently predicted that very soon the overall and long-term results of liver transplantation will be better than kidney transplantation and that, money permitting, many more people with killer diseases of the liver will be saved.

**KIDNEY TRANSPLANTS** are by far the most numerous of all major organ transplants and many thousands have been performed since the first one was done in 1954. Every year, scores of thousands of people in the West face death as a result of kidney failure and some of these are kept alive by dialysis on artificial kidney machines. Such lucky people can lead an almost normal life while they wait for a kidney to become available. There are about 50 dialysis centres in the UK but home dialysis is now so successful that most long-term patients treat themselves on their home dialysis units.

However, the emphasis is firmly on transplantation because although dialysis tides the person over while awaiting a kidney, it is much more expensive than a transplant and tends to disrupt his life.

Renal transplantation is now no longer thought of as experimental. A successful graft returns the person to virtually normal health but unfortunately, only about half of all donor kidneys are capable of providing this. The best results come from using a closely matched kidney from a relative, when 80 per cent of recipients experience a five-year graft survival rate. Unfortunately, in the UK, relatives rarely offer kidneys, so donor kidneys (following death) are most often used.

If you are to have a renal transplant, you will be carefully examined *before* your operation with a view to any necessary treatment. Once you are admitted to a transplant programme, you will be checked to ensure that you have no infections anywhere, such as in your teeth, lungs or nose. You will have a barium meal and enema (see page 420) to rule out ulcers and diverticular disease and the state of your skeleton and bone metabolism will be examined. If you have high blood pressure, it will be treated. Then you have to wait for a suitably matched kidney to become available.

The operation itself is a relatively routine procedure today. The new kidney is placed in the pelvis and its arteries and veins connected to blood vessels there. The urinary outflow tube (ureter) is implanted into the bladder. The whole operation takes about two hours.

At the time of the operation, rejection-suppressing drugs are started and rejection episodes are treated by increasing the doses of these drugs temporarily, with or without other drugs and radiation.

Results are now fairly good. Over half of all transplanted

kidneys are still working well after one year and about a quarter at ten years. Closer tissue matching of donors and recipients results in improved survival of the kidney. Half of all the failures result from rejection and about one third of recipients die from something else despite a normal, functioning kidney. There is no doubt that results *can* be improved and that this will come about as tissue matching methods improve and as the handling of rejection phenomena improves. There is every hope that the three year functioning kidney transplant survival rate will soon reach 50 per cent.

Most big centres today run an integrated dialysis and transplant programme, with transplantation being potentially available to all those who are suitable. Some people will, because of their age or for immunological reasons, be unsuitable to be included in the transplant programme and will have to stay on long-term home dialysis. In such units the outlook for renal transplant patients is improving steadily. One centre reports, for example, that its success with renal transplants is now better than that achieved with cancer of the rectum and colon. As so many of those receiving kidneys are young and have work and family responsibilities, every effort to prolong their active lives is well worth while both in human and economic terms. Successful kidney transplantation offers a better way of life for an increasing proportion of those with otherwise untreatable kidney disease.

The most dramatic and emotive of all transplant procedures are **HEART TRANSPLANTS**. Ever since Professor Christian Barnard performed the first operation successfully in 1967 in Cape Town, the public has been understandably fascinated by the subject.

After the first flush of success in the late 60s, many centres attempted the operation and in 1968 more heart transplants were done than in any subsequent year. Overall, the results were very poor indeed and public and medical enthusiasm waned. The most recent group of heart transplants in the UK has been remarkably more successful than the early operations in the late 60s and 70s.

Although the subject dropped out of the headlines around the world, a research team at Stamford University in

California kept up their efforts and were able to so improve survival rates (to 65 per cent at one year and 50 per cent at five years) that others were encouraged to match them.

Ironically, this improvement has not come about as a result of some miracle drug or discovery but rather from increased skill in using existing drugs and in the selection and clinical management of the recipients. The very poor early results are now thought to have been caused almost entirely by the misuse of anti-rejection drugs. One new procedure *has* helped though. Today's heart transplant patient has regular biopsies of his heart muscle taken using a simple technique that does not involve re-opening the heart – indeed it is done under a local anaesthetic. This has meant that rejection can be picked up a critical day or two earlier than was previously possible and then combated with drugs. Also, dietary control and the use of drugs to prevent clogging up of the new heart's blood supply have meant that the new heart lives longer.

Everyone has an opinion on whether or not heart transplants should be done, though many people form their opinions on insufficient evidence. Now that we have come through the ethical arguments about removing a beating heart from a donor (an argument which could have threatened the whole transplant programme but which has now been resolved by improved ways of defining brain death), people are worried about the economic implications of spending so much money on any one patient at a time when the National Health Service needs money so desperately. This argument is in fact fallacious because each heart transplant only costs about £17,000 and most of this expenditure is on pre-operative investigations and post-operative care. When social security payments paid to the patient or his widow are also taken into account, it has been calculated that alternative forms of medical management would cost at least as much.

The other criticism people have is that the money spent on heart transplants should be chanelled into research to prevent heart disease in the rest of the population. This is also a fallacious argument because in practice the relatively small amount of money spent on heart transplants would *not* be rerouted to prevention.

Coronary artery surgery is expanding at a considerable rate and this, together with existing open heart operation programmes, could soon bring the total to 15–20,000 such operations each year in England and Wales alone. Given that so few people are suitable for heart transplants, they will only ever form a tiny fraction of this large number of heart operations. The two major centres in the UK currently performing this operation, for example, are transplanting fewer than twenty hearts a year between them.

# TRIGEMINAL NEURALGIA

### What is it?
An extremely painful condition of the face of unknown cause. The pains are mostly sharp, stabbing or shooting in character and occur in bouts lasting from a few seconds to 20 minutes. They are brought on by touching the face (as on blowing the nose or shaving) or by facial movements (such as talking and laughing).

The condition is seen most commonly in women between the ages of 50 and 70. The first attack typically lasts for a few weeks and may not return for months or years.

### Why operate?
Early attacks of the disease are treated with painkilling drugs but in really severe cases these may not prevent frequent and severe painful episodes. Anticonvulsant drugs produce some pain relief in about two thirds of sufferers but eventually some will need surgery.

### How?
The fifth cranial nerve is the one involved in this strange condition and it can be cut or injected to relieve the pain. If the injection (which produces a numb face over the area supplied by the nerve) works, the person can usually live

happily with the numbness but no pain. A more permanent job can be done at an operation on the nerve through a burr hole in the temple area. If the whole half-face has been numbed, you will have to wear glasses with a sidepiece to protect the now insensitive cornea of the eye from ulceration.

# TUBERCULOSIS

**What is it?**
A bacterial infection affecting any organ of the body but in the western world especially the lungs. Until 30 years ago pulmonary (lung) tuberculosis (TB) was a very serious disease killing millions of people worldwide every year and producing debilitating illness in millions of others. In the West, as in the rest of the world, the greatest single reason for the decline in the level of the disease has been the tremendous improvement in sanitation, public health, living conditions and nutrition. TB thrives in countries where all these are poor. TB was well on the way to being eradicated by these improvements alone in the western world when chemical agents which actually kill TB bacteria were introduced just before the Second World War.

Today in the West, TB is an uncommon disease. It is, however, still common in several third world countries.

Medical treatment with good food, rest and drugs cures the vast majority of TB cases today but if these should fail, diseased lung segments can be removed.

TB can affect other parts of the body but such infections are rarely seen today in the West.

**How?**
Under general anaesthesia, a long incision is made in the chest and the diseased part of the lung removed or abscesses drained. Sometimes, the affected part of the lung cannot be removed because the TB has involved the pleura (chest lining) or other vital structures in the chest. Collapse therapy (thoracoplasty) may be used in these cases. This involves the removal of part of a series of ribs to collapse the underlying

lung. It is rarely done. There are two other ways that the lung can be collapsed and so rested: air can be introduced into the affected side of the chest or a certain nerve crushed. This increases the likelihood that medication and other non-surgical methods of treatment will have a beneficial effect but such collapse therapies are now rarely used.

Lung resection (in which part or all of a lobe of the lung is removed) is never done until at least six months after starting drug therapy and then only when the disease is unstable; the scars on the lung are considerable; or where medical treatment has failed to control the disease. Only very rarely does the whole lung have to be removed. Lung resection, once very common, is now a rare operation.

# ULCERATIVE COLITIS

**What is it?**
An inflammatory disease of the colon (large bowel) usually affecting adults between the ages of 20 and 40. No one knows what causes it but bacterial, allergic and emotional factors are thought to be involved though not all in each case. It seems to be more common in fussy, meticulous people and an acute attack is often brought on by an emotional crisis.

This distressing condition is characterized by bloody diarrhoea which occurs in bouts with free periods between. The diarrhoea also contains pus and slime (mucus). The attacks of diarrhoea are sometimes accompanied by a high fever and unpleasant abdominal cramps. Less severe attacks involve milder cramps, a slight fever and a loss of appetite. If the attack gets worse (though many do not) nausea and vomiting set in, the cramps become severe, the diarrhoea voluminous and the person can die from severe fluid loss.

In between bouts the person returns to normal.

The diagnosis is made from the clinical history, by looking into the colon using a sigmoidoscope (see page 406) or colonoscope (see page 386), and by taking barium enema X-rays (see page 420) which produce characteristic pictures in this disease, and by a biopsy.

**Why operate?**
About a seventh of patients with ulcerative colitis have one attack and then completely recover but more often the story is one of repeated attacks. A limited number of drugs are used for ulcerative colitis but the failure of medical treatment (see below) means that an operation will be necessary.

Surgery is also necessary if there is severe bleeding or a complication such as perforation with peritonitis, obstruction, peri-anal abscess, or cancer. Cancer develops in about ten per cent of people who have had the disease for more than fifteen years.

**How?**
Medical treatment is always tried first unless there is an acute complication which demands urgent surgical intervention.

Bed rest, a low residue diet and blood transfusions, if necessary, often get the person feeling a lot better. Drugs can be given for the pain, the diarrhoea and the cramps.

For those who do not do well on this regime, steroid drugs are given in the form of an enema. The person lies slightly head-down on a bed and retains the enema for as long as possible. Prednisone can also be given by mouth or by suppository and can produce long remissions. Some doctors claim good results with a particular type of sulphonamide but the results of studies with this drug are conflicting. Those people in whom it does produce a reduction or total relief of symptoms should take the drug for life.

When an operation *is* necessary, the whole of the colon and the rectum are now removed (a proctocolectomy) and the intestinal contents discharged at the surface of the abdominal wall by bringing the end of the small bowel there to form an ileostomy (see also page 224). This is major surgery but is safe and effective if anaemia and dehydration are corrected before the operation. The dose of steroids the person is on has to be increased to cover the stress of the operation.

It is often very difficult for a surgeon to know when to

operate because it is tempting to leave the person alone while
he is well in between attacks but equally it is dangerous to
wait until he has an attack because he may then be too ill for
the operation. In a severe attack the usual procedure is to
try steroids for a week or so and to proceed to an emergency
operation if this produces no result. It has been shown that
conservative surgery (removing only part of the affected
colon) is ineffective because the disease recurs elsewhere
later on.

## Post-operative progress

The person is out of bed within three days of the operation
but he will be somewhat restricted because he will still have
an intravenous drip. A nasogastric tube (see page 403) will be
in place to rest the intestine by removing gastric secretions
and the intravenous drip containing nutrients will keep him
going until he starts eating normally after five or six days.

Many surgeons keep ulcerative colitis patients in hospital
for several weeks post-operatively so that they will get well
again and learn how to live with their ileostomy. The idea of
having an ileostomy revolts most people but the majority are
a lot happier after they have met other people who have one
and see how little it has changed their lives. Follow-up
studies show that more than 90 per cent of people with
ileostomies are quite happy with them and can live with only
the most minor of dietary restrictions. Many of them swim,
dance and play sports, women marry and have children
normally and there are no life assurance problems. There are
now ileostomy clubs with branches around the country and
many other countries have them too. For the address of the
Ileostomy Association of Great Britain, see page 428.

At first the output from an ileostomy is very fluid because
the colon usually does the job of re-absorbing water from the
food residue so that our bodies do not lose it all. As time goes
by, the small intestine seems to become more water-
absorbing and the output from the ileostomy is less liquid. It
never becomes like normal motions though, unlike the
output from a colostomy (see page 147). Today's ileostomy

patient has the advantage of disposable plastic bags with air-tight, odour-controlling seals. Many hospitals have a stoma specialist who will be a great help and reassurance to you both in hospital and after you leave.

# UNDESCENDED TESTIS

The testes, the male sex glands, usually hang in the scrotum where they produce sperms and some male sex hormones.

While a baby is in the womb his testes move down from inside the abdomen to come to lie in the scrotum. If for some reason this descent is interrupted, the testes may not be down at birth but may appear some time later. It is important for both testes to be down in the scrotum, particularly after the age of five or six years, because an undescended testis is less able to produce sperms (so making the man infertile) and rarely becomes cancerous later in life.

However, if your son's testis cannot be felt, do not worry. The vast majority of such testes are 'retractile' – they pop back up into the canal above the scrotum at the slightest stimulus. A doctor may be able to push the testis gently down into the scrotum but it often pops back up again at once. So long as it will come down it does not need any other treatment.

It is now thought wise to bring an undescended testis down into the scrotum at about the age of five or six years. Under general anaesthesia an incision is made in the groin and the spermatic cord freed of fibrous tissue, so allowing the testis to be brought down. The surgeon then tethers the bottom of the testis to the scrotum with a stitch or two.

There are no post-operative complications and the boy usually ends up with normal sperm production, especially if the operation is done before the age of six years. If the condition affects both sides, many surgeons will do both operations at the same time.

# URINARY STONES

## What are they?

Stones are produced in the urinary system as a result of infection in the urine or because the urine contains an excess of a particular organic salt which crystallizes out in the form of stones. The stones produced vary in size from tiny gravel to large 'staghorn' calculi which fill up a major part of the kidney.

No one knows why the majority of kidney stones develop but certain disorders of the body systems that control the salts in urine can produce stones. Parathyroid disorders and gout, for example, by releasing excessive levels of salts into the urine, favour the formation of urinary stones.

Most of us have produced small stones in our urinary systems but have passed them without even knowing we have had them. Many quite big stones do not produce symptoms for some time but then suddenly start giving pain which is the main symptom of kidney stones. As long as they sit in the kidneys they are usually 'silent' but as soon as they start going down the ureter (the fine muscular tube that takes urine from the kidney to the bladder) the trouble begins – and it can be very alarming indeed because the pain is so severe.

As well as pain, there may be tenderness over the kidney on that side, fever, shivering, pain on passing water, blood in the urine and eventually the person can become so ill that hospital admission becomes essential. As the ureters strain to squeeze the stone along, the doctor gives painkilling drugs and waits to see if the stone will pass spontaneously. It is always better not to intervene surgically if possible, though on rare occasions the pain may be so severe and atypical that a person with a stone will have an exploratory abdominal operation (laparotomy, see page 242), because the surgeon cannot take the chance that it might be another even more serious condition.

The vast majority of people who have urinary stones pass

them after a few days. Once they are through the ureter, the narrowest part of the journey is over and they then come out easily. However, stones over about one centimetre in diameter will probably never pass and may become lodged in the urinary system. Some become impacted in the kidney itself, others in the ureters and some in the bladder. If a stone blocks a ureter, urine builds up behind it, stagnates and can become infected, with serious consequences. Such stones need operating on.

Bladder stones are less common than kidney and ureteric stones and occur mostly in older men with stagnant urine caused by an enlarged prostate gland (see page 289). The signs are frequent, painful urination, often with blood. The stones can be seen on X-rays or down a cystoscope (see page 163). The diagnosis is usually made from the clinical picture and from finding blood in the urine. However, an emergency intravenous urogram (see page 423) may be done to visualize the stones and to check kidney function. This also helps the surgeon to see exactly where the stone is stuck so that he can plan the best operation to perform, if one becomes necssary.

### Why operate?
Operations are necessary to remove stones that are too big to pass; to remove stones that are not being passed, even though they are quite small; to remove stones that are causing a blockage of the urine flow; and, of course, to remove stones which are damaging the kidney itself.

### How?
If a stone is caught at the lower end of the ureter (quite a common place for this to occur), a surgeon can remove it using an operating cystoscope. Under a general anaesthetic the cystoscope is passed (see page 163) and a special catheter with a loop at its tip inserted into the bottom end of the ureter. It is then possible to pull the stone down into the bladder from which it is removed via the cystoscope. It is also possible to stretch the lower end of the ureter so that the stone can pass more easily. There are several gadgets that can be

tried before an open operation on the ureter has to be contemplated.

Only about ten per cent of all urinary stones need operating on but when they do, the operation is usually a major one. An incision is made in the abdomen or over the kidney, depending upon the site of the stone. The kidney or ureter is then opened and the stone removed.

Kidney stones are more difficult to remove than stones in the ureters and there may be a drain left coming out of the wound so as to keep the kidney free from urine and blood while it heals. Very large stones, especially if they have been present silently for years, may have so damaged a kidney that it will have to be removed.

Bladder stones can often be removed via a cystoscope and large ones can be crushed and the pieces washed out using an operating cystoscope. Very large stones that cannot be crushed have to be removed at an open operation on the bladder. The operation is straightforward, takes less than an hour, can be performed under local or spinal anaesthetic if the person is very old and frail, and is not too traumatic, even in the elderly. It usually means a stay in hospital of two weeks.

### Post-operative progress

With either location of the stones, the person is out of bed within a day or two and home after fourteen days. Stones frequently recur but if they do your surgeon will do special blood tests to rule out overactivity of the parathyroid glands. This can itself be cured by operating on the parathyroids.

# UTERUS OPERATIONS

(See also Cervix operations; Fibroids; Hysterectomy.) The most commonly performed operation on the uterus is its removal (hysterectomy, see page 219) and uterine cancer is one of the reasons for its removal. Fibroids are probably the commonest reason that hysterectomies are done but the operations for these are described elsewhere (see page 182).

Cancer of the uterus is less common than cancer of the cervix but has recently been catching up. It is a condition of the older woman, having its maximum incidence in the 50–60 year age group. If the cancer is confined only to the lining of the uterus, 65 per cent of the women operated on will be alive five years later. As the growth spreads to involve more of the uterus or even other organs, the outlook gets worse.

It is usual to irradiate the uterine cavity by inserting caesium (a radioactive isotope) for 24 hours. This has a direct effect on the lining cells and prevents them being spilt at hysterectomy a few weeks later. Often there is no tumour left when the hysterectomy specimen is examined.

# VARICOCELE

## What is it?
A condition in which there are varicose veins around the spermatic cord just above the testis (usually on the left). Although the condition is not serious it can cause a pulling sensation. It is the cause of infertility in about 30 per cent of infertile men. Normally fertile men can have varicoceles though, and the mechanisms by which sterility is produced are unknown. There are several theories, most of which are backed up by the finding that curing a varicocele results in an improvement in or a return to a normal sperm count in 80 per cent of men. Most men who have the operation become fertile as a result and half of their partners will be pregnant within a year of the operation.

## Why operate?
To cure infertility or reduce discomfort.

## How?
The operation is simple and involves tying off the left spermatic vein through a small incision in the groin.

# VARICOSE VEINS

**What are they?**
Swollen, twisted veins in the lower half of the body, usually the legs. It used to be thought that haemorrhoids (piles) were a sort of varicose vein but there are new ideas on this today. Some women suffer from varicose veins around the genitals in pregnancy but the vast majority of varicose veins are of the legs and are found predominantly in women.

Swollen, twisted veins can be seen in the legs of many people. The main thing that bothers their owners is that they look unpleasant, but they can also cause swelling, pain and inflammation, and may even actually ulcerate and bleed. In short, they are a nuisance at best and potentially fatal at worst. They are rare in developing countries, but are appearing in the towns even of these countries as the rural people become urbanized. In the UK, between 10 and 17 per cent of adults have varicose veins and a study of multi-nationals in Switzerland found an incidence of 29 per cent. Between the two of them, haemorrhoids and varicose veins cause three million lost work days a year in Britain alone.

Rather like haemorrhoids, varicose veins have been attributed to many causes. The oldest theory is probably that man has not yet adapted to being an upright animal, walking only on his hind legs. At first sight there seems to be some sense in this. Blood from the legs has a long way to go to get back to the heart and it is uphill. But nature gave us two systems to overcome this problem. Every time we walk, the muscles at the back of the leg below the knee contract and squeeze the blood up the deep veins of the calf until most of it reaches the groin. This mechanism is called the 'soleal pump' after the big calf muscle – the soleus. Blood flows upwards towards the heart in the long veins just beneath the skin, where it is trapped in sections by valves allowing blood to pass upwards but not downwards. In this way, blood from the legs is pumped up into the large collecting vein in the abdomen – the inferior vena cava – from where it travels to the heart. As long as this pump mechanism does not fail, the one-way valves keep the blood from flowing back down under gravity and all is well. Because the head of pressure is quite considerable, if the valves fail the columns of blood in the veins cause their walls to bulge and even to burst. The deforming of the vein walls renders the valves even more ineffective and a vicious circle sets in.

To maintain that Man as an animal has failed to adapt to his upright posture in this regard is clearly untenable, especially as millions of people, notably those in the developing countries eating unrefined diets, rarely get varicose veins yet have exactly the same anatomy as we do. It must be something else. Perhaps we in the West are of inferior stock, with a second-class set of leg veins that we pass on to our children. This too is an unlikely hypothesis because the very people who never get varicose veins soon do so if they live in our society. American blacks and whites have the same incidence.

For years, long periods of standing were thought to be the cause, but this is unlikely be true. Prolonged standing undoubtedly makes existing varicose veins worse, but as far as we know does not initiate them. In fact, many rural peoples are on their feet for very long periods indeed and yet have less than one hundredth the varicose vein problem that we have in the West. Similarly with pregnancy: the number of babies born per woman in developing countries is much higher than in the West, so if pregnancy were a cause they would have a lot more trouble – not less. None of these widely held theories in fact explains why it is that varicose veins are so common in the West and so uncommon in peoples who eat unrefined foods. Recent research is providing some answers though. People who eat highly refined foods pass small, hard, sticky stools and do so with great difficulty. The straining involved raises the blood pressure in the veins of the legs and could well weaken the valves in them, so leading to varicose veins over many years.

The treatment of varicose veins to date is less than spectacular. Early cases get some benefit from elastic stockings, which simply compress the superficial veins of the leg and do the valves' job of holding back the blood. But elastic stockings are not popular (except with older people) because to be of any use they have to be thick and so look unpleasant. Injecting veins with a solution that causes the local formation of tough fibrous tissue is a widely used technique but does not always produce a permanent cure. Surgery provides the only long-term cure, and it is usually combined with tying off the veins in the groin where all the leg veins congregate before entering the abdominal veins. Even surgery has its drawbacks and second operations are not uncommon.

The answer must surely lie in prevention. People on unrefined diets do not get varicose veins nearly as much as we do in the West, as we have seen, so it is well worth learning from them. On high-fibre foods there is no straining to pass stools and therefore there are no surges of pressure down the leg veins.

But primitive rural people also have another protective factor – they squat when passing stools. This squatting position may help to shut off the leg veins at the groin so that no pressure can be transmitted down to them. Our modern western style of lavatory ensures that as we strain to pass our hard, small stools, all the pressure goes straight down the veins to damage or deform them.

## Why operate?
Surgery is necessary if the varicosities cannot be cured any other way and if the pooling of blood in the legs is considerable. If this occurs and is allowed to continue for months or years, varicose ulcers may form. These can bleed profusely or become infected and can take a long time to heal, so a varicose vein operation is well worth doing to cure small ulcers and prevent new ones forming.

## How?
There are five ways of treating varicose veins, three of which are operative.

ELASTIC SUPPORT STOCKINGS are used as a first line of attack in early cases and can actually prevent young women from having to have an operation at all. The strength of the supporting stockings forces blood from the superficial sets of veins in the leg to the deep ones. This may be all that is needed to cure troublesome symptoms and put off or even prevent an operation.

**INJECTION TREATMENT** involves the injection of irritant solutions into the varicose veins. It is suitable for a person with many varicose veins or for treating the remaining veins left after a stripping procedure (see below).

For many years surgeons have injected varicose veins with limited success. An irritating solution was injected into the vein in the hope that it would block it off and relieve the trouble. However, this often failed to work so a variation of the method is now being used. This seems to give even better results. In this, the fluid is injected at several points along the vein where it is thought that the superficial leg veins enter the deep ones. The whole leg is kept bandaged for six weeks so that the walls of the veins are kept together and they grow across actually to close off the cavity. This is called compression sclerotherapy and produces early results that are as good as those produced by surgery though the long-term results are not as good. The procedure is done as an out-patient and you are asked to walk three miles a day for a while.

**SURGERY.** For severe varicose veins many surgeons advise stripping the long veins in the legs. This procedure is especially used when there is a lot of pooling of blood in the legs with a backward flow of blood.

Under general anaesthesia an incision is made in the groin of the leg to be treated and the varicose vein is displayed and divided. One of the main veins of the leg is then exposed by a small incision just below the knee or at the ankle and a flexible vein stripper passed up inside the vein from the bottom to emerge at the top. It is tied to the open end of the vein, the whole leg is bandaged firmly and the stripper (complete with its surrounding vein) pulled out from beneath the bandage. Small tributaries may be tied off at other places in the leg too. In a second type of operation surgeons concentrate more on dealing with the vein at the groin and then use very small cuts to deal with the individual veins in the leg.

The person is encouraged to get up and walk about on the leg after the operation as this reduces the risk of a deep vein thrombosis forming (see page 56). You will be in hospital for only a few days and normal bathing can be resumed in about two weeks.

Crêpe bandages are worn for three to four weeks or even longer if the swelling has not subsided. It can take two months for the leg to feel normal again. After this time, the surgeon inspects the leg and injects any residual veins, if necessary.

Varicose veins can recur, even after a stripping operation because new veins open up from the deep to the superficial system.

The third type of operation is one to divide these perforating veins and may be used for people who have had varicose ulcers.

Results are good for the stripping procedure and the leg scars are hardly visible within a few months.

As varicose veins are so common, some centres are now operating on a day-case basis so that more people can be treated.

Even in places that favour this approach, careful pre-operative screening is essential to ensure success. One recent survey found that only one per cent of day-care patients had to be re-admitted. About one quarter of the patients they treated in this way had minor complications but they were all easily treatable by their general practitioners, community nurses or both. There is little doubt that when it comes to operations such as those for varicose veins, day-case or five-day wards could be the answer to reducing the long waiting lists that exist for such common conditions. Having said this though, it will always tend to be the younger, fitter patient with a good home background that will be most suitable for such day care. Many varicose vein sufferers will, however, not fall into this category and will need full hospital admission.

Results of surgery and injection methods have recently been compared in a large trial that followed 249 patients for five years after their treatment. By three years, 14 per cent of those treated surgically and 22 per cent of those treated by injections needed further treatment or support stockings. The probability of having to have no further treatment is greatly increased in those treated surgically and the improved outcome after surgery was especially marked in people over 45.

# VASECTOMY

**What is it?**
An operation in which the sperm carrying duct (vas deferens) is cut and tied off on each side as a means of permanent sterilization in a man.

**Why operate?**
Increasing numbers of men are concerned that their wives should not have to bear the burden of long-term contraception and find the sheath cumbersome or unsatisfactory in other ways. For such men a vasectomy is a very good operation. Like the female forms of sterilization though, it must be considered to be irreversible and so deserves very careful consideration by both partners before action is taken.

**How?**
A vasectomy is a simple and quick operation, usually performed as an out-patient. There is no special preparation necessary but a little shaving either side of the top of the scrotum is often suggested.

After thoroughly cleaning and disinfecting the area around the scrotum, the surgeon injects a small amount of local anaesthetic into the areas where he will make his incisions. These incisions are small (about 1 centimetre long) and are made about 5 centimetres above the testes where the root of the scrotum is joined to the lower abdomen. The vas is very superficial and easily found. It looks like a thick piece of yellowish string. The surgeon ties the vas in two places and cuts out a piece about a centimetre long. Any bleeding is stopped and the wound closed with two small stitches. The procedure is then repeated for the other vas. Both sides together only take about 20 minutes and the man can go straight home but has to wear a scrotal support (rather like a jock strap) and avoid lifting and strenuous exercise for ten days. It is probably sensible to have a day off work following a vasectomy but after this everything should be back to normal.

In order to understand why a vasectomy works we need to look at the male anatomy in some detail. Sperms are produced in the testes and stored in the epididymes next to the testes. The sperms stay here for several weeks then travel from this storage area up the vas deferens on each side before being ejaculated. Sperms themselves form only a small part of what a man ejaculates: the rest is fluid added by various glands along the way. However, the sperms are the part that can make a woman pregnant and are thus most important when it comes to sterilization.

In a vasectomy, the cutting of the transport tube from testes to penis means sperms are trapped in the testes and the man becomes sterile. A man who has had a vasectomy still produces sperms as usual but they cannot get out. They dissolve and are re-absorbed by the body. However, unlike women, who become sterile as soon as the fallopian tubes are cut (because no eggs can get past the block) a vasectomized man can be fertile for weeks or months simply because he has some sperms 'in store' in his reproductive tract.

## Post-operative progress

Complications after the operation are very few indeed. Any pain there may be can be controlled with simple painkillers and bruising will soon disappear but little else ever happens.

As with any kind of sterilization procedure, the most crucial question is – does it prevent pregnancies? As we have seen, the answer is not as simple as in the case of women. Because a man can remain fertile for so long after the operation, two or more sperm counts are carried out between eight and sixteen weeks after the operation. The man supplies a specimen of semen which is examined microscopically for sperm activity. In this four-month period, the man (or his partner) has to use an alternative method of contraception. Once the hospital has given the go-ahead, these other methods can be abandoned and the man can be sure he is not fertile.

Most men are concerned about their sexual potency and those who undergo vasectomy are no exception! One of the commonest questions men ask is – 'Will it affect my sex life?' Unfortunately the answer is not all that simple. Many surveys have been done on the subject but they seem to show the same thing – that men whose sex lives were satisfactory before the operation rarely have problems but those who had difficulties before may have problems after. There is nothing physically damaging to a man's sex organs about a vasectomy: a simple tube that carries sperms is cut and none of the erection-producing mechanisms is touched. So if a man becomes impotent after a vasectomy it must be for psychological reasons and not physical ones.

When it comes to reversal, things are not so good although in the best centres success rates of 50 per cent are claimed. Numerous studies have been and are being done to try to devise a truly reversible vasectomy. Some researchers have even worked on a small, magnetically operated tap that the man could switch 'on' and 'off' by placing a magnet over the tiny equipment in his vas deferens. Sewing the small bore vas tubes back together again is very difficult technically and anyway a proportion of men whose 'plumbing' is put back to normal again still do not produce fertile sperms. It is thought that this is because they have produced antibodies to their own sperms.

A vasectomy is a very safe and effective sterilization procedure but should only be carried out in men with normal sexual histories and currently satisfactory sex lives and must be considered permanent. Very rarely a large bruise can occur in the scrotum and some men complain of pain at the vasectomy site – vasectomy is not totally without complications.

# WARTS

### What are they?

Warts are viral skin lesions with many appearances. They tend to disappear in time whether they are treated or not.

Although warts occur mostly in children, adults too are frequently affected. They may be solitary or multiple and most people have or have had a wart at some time in their lives. Common plane warts are flat, brownish masses which vary in size from 2 millimetres to 2·5 centimetres across. When a wart like this grows on the sole it is called a plantar wart or verruca. This becomes deeply embedded in the sole and can be very painful. Such plane warts are also found on the face, neck and hands.

Warts can occur anywhere on the body and are caught by person-to-person contact or are transferred from place to place on the body by the person himself.

### Why operate?

As over 80 per cent of warts disappear whetever you do to them, the value of treatment is difficult to judge. Simple remedies can be bought over the chemist's counter but some warts are resistant and need further treatment. Various caustic agents can be used to burn the wart chemically and in cases that do not respond to this treatment surgery may be necessary.

### How?

Only the most serious of warts need any form of real surgery and even then they are easily removed using small incisions. More often, liquid nitrogen is used to burn them off or alternatively electrosurgery can be used. If many warts are to be treated by this latter (cautery) method, a general anaesthetic will be used but otherwise warts are treated without anaesthetic or at most under a local anaesthetic.

# Part III
# Procedures and Investigations
# (in alphabetical order)

# PROCEDURES AND INVESTIGATIONS

There are literally hundreds of investigations and clinical procedures that can be carried out on a surgical patient but many of them are rarely performed. Some have mainly research value, even though they do provide useful information which can alter the course or outcome of your treatment.

The following section of the book covers most of the tests that are likely to be done on the average surgical patient in a general hospital. One or two of the more unusual tests have been included for interest.

In practice, most people have very few investigations performed although more may be done in teaching hospitals. This is because doctors in training have to learn and because such hospitals are also research-orientated and may be doing studies to compare and contrast the value of one treatment against another in various clinical situations. However, no test or investigation should ever be done without your informed consent and it is up to you to ensure that a doctor or nurse tells you what is going on. Just as with any procedure in hospital you may not by law have anything done to you without your informed consent. Most people are quite content to undergo tests and investigative procedures without question, but if you feel that your test needs further explanation, do say so.

The following list covers most of the commonly performed procedures and investigations.

| | |
|---|---|
| Amniocentesis | Bone marrow puncture |
| Aspiration | Catheterization |
| Audiometry | Cervical cytology |
| Auriscopy | Culdoscopy |
| Auscultation | Electrocardiography (ECG) |
| Biopsy | Electroconvulsive therapy (ECT) |
| Blood pressure | Electroencephalography (EEG) |
| Blood samples | Endometrial Biopsy |
| Blood tests | Endoscopy |

Enemas
Epidural analgesia
Hysterosalpingogram
Hysteroscopy
Intravenous drips
Laparoscopy
Lumbar puncture
Nasogastric tube
Ophthalmoscopy

Radio-isotope tests
Rectal examination
Tubal insufflation
Ultrasound
Urine testing
Vaginal examination
X-rays
X-ray computed tomography

# AMNIOCENTESIS

The removal of a small amount of amniotic fluid from around a baby while it is still in the womb.

A baby is contained in a bag (the amnion) of fluid (liquor) inside the mother's uterus. The fluid comes from the placenta and the membranes around the baby and circulates through the baby's lungs and kidneys. The baby also swallows the liquid and then passes it out as urine. A fetus under 14 weeks of age has too little amniotic fluid for the doctor to be able to get to it but after this time the volume increases considerably until there is so much that the baby can literally swim around in it.

Having an amniocentesis is much like having an injection. The doctor takes an ordinary syringe with an ordinary blood-taking sized needle and inserts it in the midline between the navel and the pubic hair line. The skin is sterilized first to ensure that no bacteria are introduced into the baby's world. A local anaesthetic may be used. Although it is not essential, many doctors prefer to scan the abdomen with an ultrasound machine so as to localize exactly the greatest area of amniotic fluid and so be able to insert the needle into that and not into the baby. This is especially important in early pregnancy, when there is little fluid, and in mothers with rhesus negative blood in whom any bleeding in the baby (caused by the needle) could provoke rhesus disease.

Amniocentesis does not hurt much and there is no leakage

of amniotic fluid as the needle hole is so small. There is a small (one per cent) risk of the mother miscarrying if the procedure is carried out early in pregnancy but the later it is done, the less the risk. The main danger is that the placenta may be punctured. This is unlikely to occur if the doctor has ascertained by ultrasound the position of the placenta before inserting the needle.

There are many ways in which a sample of amniotic fluid can help doctors help mothers. Perhaps one of the best publicized is that of fetal abnormality detection. Many pointers can make a mother or a doctor suspect that a fetus may be abnormal. If it is likely to be, the parents may wish to have the pregnancy terminated. Ideally an abnormal fetus should be aborted as early as possible, so the earlier the amniotic fluid sample can be obtained, the better. This is difficult before 14 weeks, as we have seen, but the sample needs to be taken as soon as possible after this.

Amniocentesis can help doctors diagnose an abnormality in several ways. The fluid extracted contains cells that have been shed from the body of the fetus. As each body cell contains a replica of all the genetic material of the body, doctors can tell from one cell if the fetus has a major chromosomal abnormality such as mongolism (Down's syndrome). This can be useful if the mother has already produced such a baby, or in older mothers, because it is known that women over the age of 35 are more likely to produce Down's babies than are younger women.

It is possible to tell the sex of the fetus from the cell studies, and this is a pleasant bonus to most mothers, but there are certain conditions such as haemophilia in which this information is really helpful. Haemophilia is known as a 'sex-linked' disease because it is only seen in males. Females act as carriers but do not suffer from the disease. If there is a family history of a sex-linked genetic disease, it helps to know the sex of the fetus. Cells from the amniotic fluid can be examined to tell the sex of the fetus. A male fetus will have a 50–50 chance of suffering from such a disease. The parents are asked to decide before the amniocentesis whether they want the fetus aborted if it is a male, on the understanding that it would have a 50–50 chance of suffering from the disease if they do not.

Disorders such as spina bifida and anencephaly can also be detected early by measuring the level of a substance called alpha-fetoprotein in the amniotic fluid.

The maturity of the fetus can be very important when the mother is uncertain of her dates or when a planned premature delivery is being considered. Newborn babies weighing less than 2500g are at risk because immature lung function may lead to the respiratory distress syndrome, and it is therefore vital to ensure that babies are not delivered too early unless absolutely necessary. Both the cells and the amino acids in the amniotic fluid can help in this respect. The larger the number of greasy skin cells (shed by the fetus in increasing numbers as pregnancy progresses), the more mature the fetus. Sophisticated measurements of naturally-occurring substances (lecithin and sphingomyelin) reflect the maturity of the fetal lung.

The rhesus positive fetus of a rhesus negative mother who has rising levels of rhesus antibodies during her pregnancy is in danger of becoming severely ill even before birth. Amniocentesis enables the amount of bilirubin in the amniotic fluid to be measured, giving doctors a guide as to whether to induce the labour early.

Amniocentesis is one of several techniques that enable doctors to predict the birth of damaged or severely ill babies. Parents may wish to avoid such births. It is, however, relatively expensive in that highly trained staff are needed to carry out the test and to analyse and interpret the changes in the fluid. At present amniocentesis is only justifiable when there are medical reasons for suspicion about the outcome of the pregnancy.

If you have had an amniocentesis to rule out a certain condition (such as Down's syndrome) and the answer proves to be negative, it does not necessarily mean that there is nothing else wrong with the baby. Many parents are shocked when they have a baby with an abnormality after having a 'normal' result from an amniocentesis but it is important to remember that the sample of fluid the doctors remove is not – and cannot be – tested for every abnormality.

# ASPIRATION

The removal of fluid from a body cavity or organ. All the body's cavities contain tiny amounts of lubricating fluid. For example, joints are lubricated by synovial fluid produced by their linings and the abdominal cavity's contents are lubricated by fluid so that they can slide easily over one another as we and they move. The amount of fluid in any one place is very small but in disease these fluids can become more plentiful and actually produce trouble. A collection of fluid in a body cavity is called an effusion and when it occurs in certain situations it is given a specific name. For example, excess fluid in the abdominal (peritoneal) cavity is called ascites (dropsy).

As the cavities concerned normally contain only small amounts of fluid, an effusion can be very unpleasant for the patient because it distends the walls of the cavity and puts the contained and surrounding structures under pressure. Aspiration or removal of the fluid can relieve symptoms quickly and dramatically, especially if a joint is involved. Not only does this help the patient directly, but also indirectly because the doctor can analyse the fluid removed and perhaps find a clue to its cause. Although the simple removal of an effusion may actually be curative in itself, in most cases it is only a temporary measure, leaving the underlying condition still to be treated. Once a cause has been found, however, specific treatment may lead to a successful cure.

Aspiration is technically very simple. A local anaesthetic is injected into the skin over the effusion to be aspirated, using a fine needle to minimize discomfort. Once the anaesthetic has taken effect, a larger bore needle is passed through the skin and into the fluid. The plunger on the attached syringe is withdrawn and the fluid taken off. The amount that comes off varies according to the cavity and the size of the effusion but can range from a few cubic centimetres from the knee joint to several litres from the chest. The needle used has a special two-way valve so that when the syringe is removed to expel the fluid from it, air does not rush into the cavity being aspirated. With this and the usual sterile precautions taken with invasive procedures on the body, aspiration is quite safe and usually painless.

The most frequently aspirated cavities are those surrounding the lungs (pleural cavities), the heart (pericardial cavity) and the abdominal organs (peritoneal cavity) but cavities such as those produced by tuberculosis (TB) can also be aspirated. Where there is known disease, the doctor may well take the opportunity of injecting through the aspirating needle drugs that will act locally to control or eliminate the disease.

Aspiration is being increasingly used to obtain cells from inside tumours so that treatment can be planned before the tumour is removed. There is no doubt that this procedure can be valuable to the surgeon. About 95 per cent of tumour aspirations produce a satisfactory specimen for pathological examination. The accuracy of this procedure varies with the type of tumour. In breast lumps, pathologists can now detect malignancy, when it is present, in over 90 per cent of specimens and the 'hit' rate for lung tumours is even higher. There is debate in medical circles as to how important or valuable it is to have aspiration specimens to examine before an operation is performed, but from the patient's point of view it is certainly helpful to have some idea of the likely outcome so as to be able to discuss the subject with the surgeon before the operation is done.

# AUDIOMETRY

A test of hearing using an electronic instrument called an audiometer. A trained operator, by manipulating the controls on the apparatus, chooses a tone (a sound of a particular frequency) which is fed into the patient's ear by means of headphones. The whole procedure is carried out in a soundproof booth or room to cut out extraneous noises. By operating another control the volume is increased until the patient signals that he can just hear the tone. The volume and frequency readings are then recorded and the test repeated over a whole range of frequencies and volume levels. A graph (audiogram) can then be drawn of exactly what the person can hear under very carefully controlled conditions and this helps the doctor to determine the proper treatment for that patient.

Needless to say, audiometry is completely painless. The only problem is that it takes quite a long time and the subject has to keep concentrating to be sure to report the tones as soon as they appear.

Children often need to have their hearing tested and there are several ways that this can be done. 'Free field' audiometry is that in which the child turns to the source of the sound and is suitable for children from about nine months of age. Older children can be tested with the adult type of audiometer but may be asked to perform a manoeuvre (such as moving a ball from one box to another) each time a sound is heard.

## AURISCOPY (OTOSCOPY)

The use of an auriscope (otoscope) to examine the outer parts of the hearing system.

The human ear consists of three main sections. The outermost part on the side of the head is called the *pinna*. This leads sound down a blind tube (the auditory or ear canal) to the eardrum. This canal and the eardrum can be visualized and examined with an auriscope. From the eardrum inwards is the *middle ear* – consisting of three small interlinked bones – and lastly there is the nervous mechanism for transforming sound and balance sensations into nervous impulses interpretable by the brain. This innermost part is called the *inner ear*.

An auriscope is a mains or battery operated hand-held instrument which simply shines a light down a funnel-shaped tube (speculum) inserted into the outer ear. It contains a tiny magnifying lens so that the deep parts of the ear can be seen more easily when illuminated. The speculum comes in different sizes to fit different sized ears and the doctor uses the biggest one he can so that he can get as good a view as possible.

In a clean ear, no preparation is necessary. The doctor simply inserts the auriscope gently (after warming if it is cold) and pulls the outer ear upwards and backwards so as to allow the instrument to pass easily. If the ear is full of wax, the auriscope can be left in place and delicate instruments or swabs passed down its nozzle to clean out the wax before proceeding with the examination of the ear. Wax can also be cleaned out with the aid of a wax-softening oil used for a day or two before the examination.

Although a good doctor will note everything he sees as the auriscope passes down the ear canal, the main centre of interest is usually the eardrum. This thin layer of skin walls off the delicate middle ear from the outside world and undergoes characteristic changes in certain ear diseases. Children are especially prone to ear infections because they have a relatively short and horizontal eustachian tube (joining the back of the nose to the middle ear). In affected children the eardrum is first dull, then red, and finally bulging or even ruptured with pus flowing out of it. This is called otitis media and needs medical attention.

One final word. Never try to poke things into ears yourself. You can easily damage the lining of the canal and cause infection or, even worse, pierce the eardrum. If you are worried about your ears or your hearing, see your doctor.

# AUSCULTATION

Literally another word for listening. Auscultation can be a useful aid to doctors in making a diagnosis. A doctor will look at you, take a clinical history, feel and do all kinds of sophisticated tests but still one of the most valuable things he can do is to listen to parts of your body. This is why a stethoscope is so useful to a doctor.

When doctors first started listening to parts of their patients in the early nineteenth century, they were labelled as quacks by their contemporaries but today doctors rely a great deal on stethoscopes and their electronic successors for instant help in diagnosis. At first the heart and lungs (the most obviously 'noisy' parts of the body) were the only things to be listened to with a stethoscope but today this has extended to listening to bowel sounds; abnormal blood flows in arteries and in glands such as the thyroid.

Most of us will have experienced a doctor listening to our heart and lungs but what he is listening for and what can he hear? The sound of air entering and leaving the lungs has a characteristic quality in health and disease. This is why a doctor will ask you to say '99' – because saying it generates a deep note which he can interpret at different places over the lungs. Any deviations from the normal are readily understood by a doctor who, by listening alone, can often foretell the results of X-rays and other tests very accurately. Because X-rays are so sophisticated today and can give such accurate information about what is happening in the lungs, some doctors feel that even the best auscultation is a dying art. This is a shame if it is true because we should not expect to X-ray everybody for the slightest chest complaint and a good doctor with a stethoscope can often be just as helpful without the patient having to undergo the inconvenience and potential danger (however small) of repeated chest X-rays. A doctor with a stethoscope can diagnose chest conditions such as asthma, bronchitis, lung abscess, tuberculosis (TB), fluid on the lung, broken ribs, heart failure, pneumonia and many others simply by spending a minute listening. It would be difficult to find a machine that could do that in a minute!

Now to the heart. At each beat of the heart (of which there are about 70 per minute in a healthy person) there are two major sounds to be heard. The first sound is produced by the closing of the valves between the upper and lower chambers and the second by the snapping shut of the valves in the large outflow vessels to the lungs and the body. Even in health the quality of these sounds varies but in diseases of the heart and especially diseases that affect the valves, these sounds are greatly modified. If a valve has been damaged, blood flows past in rough eddy currents rather than smoothly as normal. These abnormal blood flows produce characteristic sounds (murmurs) which can tell a doctor exactly what is going on. Not every murmur implies heart disease, especially in children, but the murmurs associated with serious heart disease are quite distinct and very valuable in diagnosis. We marvel today at clever machines but there is still little to beat the skilled ear of the physician. We have mentioned the two main heart sounds but a trained ear can detect up to six sounds during each heart beat. When you remember that each beat lasts under one second, that is quite an achievement! Today there are electronic listening devices that record on paper exactly what is happening in the heart. (These are not like an ECG that records *electrical* potentials coming from the heart.) But as for the chest, the stethoscope still reigns supreme because all but the rarest of conditions are readily detectable by a competent doctor without recourse to expensive equipment. Lastly, it is worth remembering that the fetal heart can also be heard in the pregnant mother's abdomen from about the 24th week of pregnancy. This is usually done using a special ear trumpet. This can, in the later stages of pregnancy and labour, be a useful guide as to the condition of the fetus and may indicate that immediate action must be taken by the attendant staff if the fetus becomes distressed.

Lastly, let us consider some of the other things a doctor may listen to with his stethoscope. Most often he will be using it to listen to the pulse of the blood coming through in the brachial artery as he lets the pressure off the blood pressure cuff around your upper arm. (See page 363). As the blood flow restarts, characteristic sounds are heard which cease as the flow becomes continuous. Many abnormally large blood flows can also be detected with a stethoscope. These can occur over a very active thyroid gland in the neck or even over diseased bones. Even tumours can produce strange sounds because their blood circulation is abnormal. Similarly, any abnormal narrowing of a blood vessel causes typical noises because of the disturbed flow of blood at that point. Lastly, the bowel, that greatly underestimated organ, works away unseen and (mostly) unheard! Intestinal obstruction and several other conditions can be detected using a stethoscope, so do not be surprised if your doctor seems to be listening to some very odd places – there are many things to listen for.

# BIOPSY

A method of obtaining a tiny piece of tissue from the body – usually without an operation.

When part of the body is diseased it is often helpful to know exactly what is going on at a cellular level. This can only really be achieved by obtaining some tissue and examining it in a laboratory. In other words, however good a doctor may be and however good his interpretation of X-rays and laboratory tests, he may still be unable to diagnose with certainty exactly what is happening. This is especially true for several kinds of tumour. The findings are not simply of academic interest but can often suggest the best sort of treatment for a particular case.

The advantage of a biopsy is that it is a minor and minimally invasive technique, seldom requiring a general anaesthetic. The technique is as follows. After the skin has been cleaned and rendered sterile with antiseptic, a local anaesthetic is injected using a fine bore needle to minimize the pain. The method of biopsy then varies according to the organ being studied. If it is the skin, a tiny piece is cut out and the incised area closed with a stitch. If it is a bone, a large-bore needle is used and if it is a kidney a special 'punch biopsy' needle is used. This latter is struck firmly as it hits the kidney so that it penetrates the body of the organ, leaving a cross section of it within the cavity of the needle. The needle is then removed and the tissue examined microscopically. Similar needle biopsy techniques can be used for examining lung, liver, muscle and bone marrow.

The small bowel can be biopsied using a special capsule which is swallowed while attached to a fine bore tube. Once the capsule is in the stomach, you will be able to eat and drink normally as the tube and attached capsule pass through the stomach into the small bowel. The end of the tube open to the air is attached firmly to the face by sticking plaster, so there is no possibility of it being 'lost' into the bowel. Before the biopsy is taken, the position of the capsule is checked by taking an X-ray just in case it is still in the stomach and has not passed on into the small bowel beyond.

When the doctor is sure it is in the right place he will apply suction to the open end of the fine tube with a syringe which draws a piece of bowel wall into the capsule and operates a tiny knife to cut off the small sample obtained. The tube is then pulled up and the capsule containing the sample comes with it.

One of the commonest biopsies performed today is a breast biopsy. This may be done by aspiration (see also page 355) or excision (see below). Breast lumps are extremely common and although four out of five are not malignant, surgeons are always careful to make the most accurate diagnosis possible before they operate. This is greatly helped by obtaining some cells from the lump – a procedure which can be done as an out-patient. The most widely used out-patient method is that in which a special needle is used to suck up cells from the lump. This is called an aspiration biopsy.

An aspiration biopsy is simple and only takes two minutes. The skin over the lump is disinfected and a local anaesthetic given. The doctor steadies the lump with one hand and inserts a special needle (which is very fine). The needle is then moved backwards and forwards in the lump while suction is maintained via a syringe. This needle aspiration technique produces a satisfactory specimen in over 90 per cent of women.

The attraction of the technique is that the woman knows before she goes into the operating theatre whether or not she has a tumour and therefore whether or not she will have her breast removed.

In some hospitals an excision biopsy will be done instead of an aspiration biopsy. This procedure is usually carried out in an operating theatre. The surgeon removes a small piece of the breast lump and sends it to a pathologist for an immediate opinion as to whether or not it is cancerous. Because the pathologist fast-freezes the tissue so that he can cut it in fine sections to look at it, this procedure is called a 'frozen section'. Once the results of the frozen section are back with the surgeon in the operating theatre (this only takes minutes and the woman remains anaesthetized) he can decide what to do next. If the lump turns out to be a cancer he will remove the lump alone or the lump and the breast, depending on many factors (see page 121 for more discussion of this). If the lump is not cancerous he will simply remove it and the operation is over very quickly.

## BLOOD PRESSURE

Perhaps one of the most frequently performed 'tests' carried out whether you are going to have an operation or not is having your blood pressure taken. There are lots of books that go into the causes and remedies for high blood pressure. Here we will look at how the blood pressure is measured.

Blood flows around the body in elastic walled tubes called arteries. These vessels do not simply carry blood around as would a rigid drainpipe – they actually reflect the heart's pumping action and control the flow of the blood inside their cavities by the tightening and relaxation of the muscles in their walls. Of course the most direct way of measuring the pressure of the blood would be to insert a pressure measuring device into an artery. Unfortunately this is not practical on a day-to-day basis but has been done in research situations (and was indeed done in animals and man by the pioneers of blood pressure measurement). What these laboratory-based techniques have taught us though is that the commonly used method of measuring blood pressure is very accurate if performed correctly.

The blood pressure cuff known to us all works on the following principle. If you have liquid flowing down an elastic tube, by applying pressure you can stop the flow altogether. If the pressure is removed slowly, the point at which the fluid flows again is the pressure of the fluid in the tube.

To measure the blood pressure a cuff is placed around the upper arm. The width of this cuff is important and there are large and medium-sized adult ones and small ones for children. The cuff is inflated with air by squeezing a hand-held rubber bulb until the pulse at the wrist can no longer be felt. The cuff is connected to a mercury column that registers the pressure of the air in millimetres (mm) of mercury. Mercury is used simply because its column is not very high at blood pressure levels. If water were used the apparatus would need to be several feet high! Some more modern instruments no longer use mercury columns but read off directly on dials or even on electronic digital displays. But however the result is presented the underlying principle is the same. The gradual release of the cuff pressure produces an audible pulse, heard by listening with a stethoscope over the artery below the obstructing cuff. The pulse is caused by the return of the blood flow. The doctor notes the level of the mercury when the pulse is heard and in a normal person this is about 120mm and is called the SYSTOLIC PRESSURE. This reflects the maximum pressure produced in each heart beat, as measured in an artery in the arm.

Once he has recorded this result, the doctor listens for the beats of the pulse to disappear as the cuff pressure is further reduced. The normal value of this is about 80 mm of mercury and is called the DIASTOLIC PRESSURE. This second point is the pressure at which the blood is able to flow freely through the artery even in the 'relaxed' phase of the heart beat when it is not being forced through in pulses. 'Diastolic' is the name given to the relaxation phase of the heart and diastolic blood pressure reflects this; 'systolic' is the name given to the active, contracting phase of the heart beat and the systolic pressure reflects this.

The relative importance of systolic and diastolic blood pressures has been argued for decades by doctors but today it is widely held that the diastolic pressure (the lower one) is the more important because it is less easily influenced by superimposed conditions (such as exercise or anxiety). Diastolic blood pressure is also more directly related to the elasticity of the arterial wall and it is this that we know to be of importance in many arterial diseases (especially those that affect the heart).

The taking of the blood pressure is an important part of any clinical examination but has to be done well to be of any value. Blood pressure varies in normal, healthy people with emotion, pain, exercise, meals, tobacco, alcohol, temperature and bladder overfilling, and it even changes during the day. Because of this, it is essential to be relaxed, not to have eaten or smoked for at least 20 minutes and preferably to have rested for a few minutes before your blood pressure is taken. Do not run into the surgery; make sure you have had time to sit and relax before the reading is taken; do not roll up your sleeve into a constricting band; and sit yourself comfortably with the 'blood pressure' arm level at the level of your heart. If all these rules are adhered to, blood pressure readings are accurate and reproducible and thus of use to the doctor and patient alike. If the first blood pressure reading is high your doctor will ask you to return for another measurement before he starts any investigations or treatment. As many as half of all patients who have raised blood pressure the first time it is taken have a normal pressure on the next reading. If you are taking any tablets for blood pressure, tell the doctor. When it comes to having surgery, you will be perfectly safe, provided your blood pressure is well-controlled but your surgeon and anaesthetist should be told what tablets you are on well before the operation.

Should you be one of the many thousands who suffer from longstanding blood pressure problems you may want to take your own blood pressure at home to save you making repeated trips to your doctor or specialist. Several surveys have been done on this subject and they show that most people take their blood pressure very accurately and happily. Most of those studied have found that they were reassured by being able to take their own blood pressure and some have taught themselves to relax and so lower their blood pressure. Some hospitals provide a do-it-yourself blood pressure machine and others start you off on one and then suggest you buy your own. Ask your doctor if he minds you altering your anti-hypertensive drug dose according to the blood pressure you get when you do the readings yourself. Taking your own readings will certainly help you remember to take your tablets and should enable you to control the condition better than would otherwise be possible by infrequent blood pressure-taking visits to hospital. This sort of relationship has existed for years between diabetics and their doctors and is being taken a step further as machines are becoming available to enable the diabetic to measure his own blood sugar at home. The home measurement technique is popular with patients and saves a lot of doctor time too.

Although doctors have traditionally been reluctant to put day-to-day responsibility into the hands of their patients, the tide is turning and increasing numbers are encouraging their patients to take a greater responsibility for their own health. There are very strong arguments for the person with high blood pressure to be allowed to look after himself much more than he currently does.

Equipment for the home measurement of blood pressure is widely available in the US and it is not difficult to buy in the UK.

# BLOOD SAMPLES

As medicine has progressed in recent years, more and more emphasis is placed on the results of blood tests. This means that many people coming into contact with a doctor end up having a blood test done.

Venepuncture, as the taking of blood is properly called, is simple, safe and without side-effects in good hands. Today, many hospitals have technicians who do all the blood letting. Very simply, a cuff is applied to the upper arm in order to obstruct the flow of blood in the veins and make them stand out more prominently. The skin is then cleaned with an antiseptic or simple alcohol and when this has dried the needle is inserted at a low angle (almost parallel to the skin surface) into a superficial vein. As soon as the tip of the needle is in the vein the syringe plunger is pulled back to draw blood into the syringe. In people with very small or poorly visible veins the venepuncturist may ask you to 'pump' your hand a few times to encourage further blood flow and so make the veins more prominent before inserting the needle. The veins are also more prominent when you are warm.

The volume of blood removed is usually small (a few cubic centimetres) but as tests become more numerous, larger volumes of blood are being withdrawn. Having said this though, as anyone who has been a blood donor will know, we can easily lose a lot more blood than is ever likely to be required for diagnostic purposes. You can easily lose a pint of blood without suffering ill effects.

Once the blood has been withdrawn the cuff on the upper arm is released, the needle quickly but gently removed and the puncture area pressed on through a swab or adhesive dressing for a minute or two. The hole in the vein soon closes and after the average venepuncture no bruising should occur. Ideally, a new site should be used for future venepunctures because repeated blood taking from exactly the same place can damage the vein wall and make it go hard. This is, however, the counsel of perfection because many people only have one 'good vein' which, if many tests are necessary, gets well used. There is no danger in this but in time it may become so hard that it will cease to be a useful vein for venepuncture purposes and another site will have to be found.

If only a tiny amount of blood is needed for a test, it can be obtained from a pin prick on an ear or fingertip.

In some conditions, arterial blood may have to be taken. This is usually obtained from the femoral artery in the groin where it runs very near the skin. This is a more serious procedure than venepuncture; is more difficult technically because an artery is firm and more likely to 'escape' the needle tip than a fat, thin-walled vein; and lastly, can be painful for the patient. Arterial blood sampling is not commonly done, nor should it be, except for special tests.

In babies, veins are often almost impossible to find on the

limbs so paediatricians use the veins on the scalp or the large veins in the neck (jugulars). Neither seems to cause the baby distress. For details of blood tests and what they measure, see below.

# BLOOD TESTS

There are well over 300 blood tests that can be carried out in most large hospitals and there are scores of other laboratory tests that can be done in addition to these. It is probably fair to say that more tests are being done now than ever before in the history of medicine and that many of them are unnecessary. In the USA medico-legal considerations now demand that certain tests are done routinely, even if there is no clear indication for them, so that the physician or surgeon cannot be sued for negligence. This situation has not yet spread to the rest of the world but the signs are that it might do so and today many millions of blood and other simple tests are performed quite unnecessarily as 'routine' procedures.

If you are a 'normal' surgical patient the chances are that apart from your specific surgical condition, you will be in good health. If this is so, then you will have very few blood tests indeed. There is some sense in using a hospital admission as an excuse to screen people for all kinds of diseases but most surgeons do not think this advisable or cost-effective. Uncommonly, a new case of diabetes or hypertension will be detected (though not by blood tests) and this new knowledge will influence the way in which the surgeon considers the person as an operative risk. The anaesthetist will certainly be glad to know of any such condition. Most often though, all the tests are normal.

Probably the commonest of all blood tests performed on surgical patients is a HAEMOGLOBIN estimation and an examination of some of the many other constituents of the blood. This enables the surgeon to find out how well you could tolerate blood loss and is essential for major procedures in which blood may have to be given. A raised white blood cell count points to an infection in the body. Your blood group is ascertained unless it is already known. No major surgical procedure will be undertaken unless the surgeon knows your blood group.

All the other blood tests of importance to surgical patients are biochemical with the exception of clotting tests. With the increasing use of heparin and other anticoagulant drugs as a preventive against thrombosis (see page 56) many more surgical patients need tests done to monitor blood clotting.

Here are just a few of the more commonly performed blood tests.

**ACID PHOSPHATASE** is an enzyme normally present in the blood in tiny amounts. Men with cancer of the prostate may have greater amounts of it in their blood. The estimation of this enzyme can be useful diagnostically but can also help by monitoring the effectiveness of treatment. It can be raised after a rectal examination, so blood should be taken first.

**ALKALINE PHOSPHATASE** is an enzyme normally present in small amounts in bone, kidney, liver and other tissues and also in tiny amounts in the blood. It is raised in some specific conditions such as hepatitis, glandular fever, some bone diseases, pregnancy and cirrhosis of the liver. It can be very high in children.

**ALBUMIN** is the main blood protein. A lower level than normal suggests kidney or liver damage. It also falls in longstanding infections and with malnutrition.

**AMYLASE** is an enzyme in the blood produced by inflammation of the pancreas. It can also be found under similar circumstances in the urine.

**AUSTRALIA ANTIGEN** is a protein found in the blood as part of the body's response to acute serum hepatitis.

**BILIRUBIN** is a blood pigment which becomes increased in amount in liver disease and in certain anaemias.

**CHOLESTEROL** is a naturally-occurring fatty substance essential for life. There has been considerable debate as to the importance of the cholesterol level in the blood but medical opinion now doubts whether it is as important as was previously thought. High serum cholesterol levels are found not only in heart disease (for which cholesterol has become best known) but in underactive thyroid states, diabetes, inflammation of the pancreas and in certain kidney diseases.

**CREATININE** is a nitrogenous compound formed by muscles. It is usually present in small amounts in the blood but levels are increased in certain kidney diseases and with kidney failure.

**ELECTROLYTES** (sodium, potassium, chloride and bicarbonate) are essential ions in the blood that ebb and flow between the tissues and the blood stream, bathing cells and providing the right environment for them. These chemical substances can become unbalanced in various diseases and also if a patient is not drinking after an abdominal operation or is having intravenous fluids to replace lost body fluids.

**GLUCOSE** is a sugar produced by the breakdown of carbohydrates in the intestine. It is the body's main fuel and can be stored in the liver in another form (glycogen). Single blood glucose estimations are helpful but not nearly as valuable as repeated ones, especially after a glucose load has been given by mouth. A higher than normal level of glucose suggests diabetes. In the glucose tolerance test, blood samples are taken at regular intervals to confirm or rule out the diagnosis of diabetes. The disease is usually characterized by the presence of glucose in the urine too.

**LDH (LACTIC DEHYDROGENASE)** is an enzyme found in many tissues but present in increased amounts after tissue injury. This test is usually used after a possible heart attack because damaged heart muscle releases the enzyme into the blood in the days immediately following the attack.

A **PBI (PROTEIN-BOUND IODINE)** estimation is a measurement of the amount of thyroxine, produced by the thyroid gland, bound to blood proteins. Low and high levels of thyroid activity produce correspondingly low and high levels of protein bound iodine. There are other more accurate and useful tests of thyroid function today, including the measurement of thyroxine and its precursors in the blood.

**SGOT (SERUM GLUTAMIC OXALOACETIC TRANSAMINASE)** is an enzyme normally present in the heart and liver especially which also circulates in the blood in very small concentrations. Its level rises in the blood after a heart attack (rather like LDH) and also with inflammation of the heart (rheumatic fever), liver damage, muscular dystrophy, glandular fever and after taking aspirin and cortisone. A raised level therefore has to be interpreted with caution unless there is an obvious cause for it.

UREA (blood urea nitrogen, BUN) is a by-product of protein metabolism, put out of the body by the kidneys in the urine. Poorly functioning kidneys do not remove enough urea from the blood and levels rise. The urea level also rises after massive haemorrhage, with severe infections, with untreated diabetes and with certain cancers. The blood urea level is low in some liver diseases, malnutrition and pregnancy.

# BONE MARROW PUNCTURE

Red blood cells and certain types of white blood cells are produced in the bone marrow and in certain uncommon conditions doctors will need to compare what is happening in the bone marrow with the circulating blood picture. Often in a large hospital this procedure is carried out by a specialist in blood disease – a haematologist.

Some centres give a pre-medication just as before an operation but this is not always necessary as the area is fully infiltrated with local anaesthetic. The skin is cleaned over the breastbone (sternum) and a local anaesthetic put into the area. A special needle is then inserted firmly into the breastbone itself. This can produce a feeling of pressure as it goes in, but if it is painful, do say so. The central stillette of the needle is then removed, a syringe attached and suction applied. This can be distressing but if you are expecting it, it is not too unpleasant.

A very few drops of bone marrow are removed and placed in a watch glass by the bedside. Smears are made on to glass slides and the remainder taken away for further examination. The needle is withdrawn and the puncture site dressed with an adhesive dressing. There are no side-effects.

# CATHETERIZATION

The insertion of a tube into a body cavity. When the tube is threaded through a blood vessel into the heart the procedure is called cardiac catheterization but to most people the term means the insertion of a rubber or plastic tube into the bladder via the urinary passage (urethra).

Bladder catheterization is done in any condition in which the spontaneous passage of urine is difficult or impossible. It is sometimes carried out in the last stages of labour to reduce bladder size and enable the baby to come out more easily. Many women find this unpleasant and some suffer urinary infections afterwards as a result. Perhaps fewer women would really *need* to be catheterized if the conditions surrounding birth enabled them to be up and about more, so encouraging them to pass urine spontaneously. Another way of avoiding catheterization during labour is to ask for a bedpan regularly. Old men with enlarged prostates (see page 289) and people with paralysis may have catheters either permanently or temporarily in place.

A catheter is basically a simple flexible tube up to about 30 centimetres long. If it is to remain in place it will have a balloon just behind the tip. This balloon can be inflated, once the catheter has been pushed into the bladder, by injecting water through a special one-way valve at the end that remains outside the body. Once the balloon is inflated, the catheter stays in place and permits long-term drainage of the bladder.

Putting a catheter in is a simple, pain-free procedure. In women the urethra is only just over three centimetres long and the catheter slips in easily, usually without the need for any local anaesthetic jelly. In men though the urethra runs the whole length of the penis, down through the prostate gland and up into the bladder. Because the catheter has further to go, most doctors use a local anaesthetic jelly. This jelly is squeezed into the opening at the end of the penis and a clip placed around the penis so that it does not all ooze out again. After about five minutes the anaesthetic will have acted and the catheter can be gently inserted. There are many different widths of catheter and a good doctor will choose just the right width for the patient in each case.

Occasionally the catheterization may be difficult because of a stricture (narrowing) or a very large prostate and then a general anaesthetic will be given so that special instruments can be used.

As soon as the catheter is in place the urine flows out of the open end. Once the bladder has been drained a plastic bag is connected to collect future urine. If the catheter is being inserted to remain in the bladder long-term a spigot or plug is put in the free end. The spigot can then be removed periodically by the patient to empty his own bladder. In some cases, especially in the elderly or the paralysed, the catheter's open end may be connected to a polythene bag strapped to the person. This collects the urine for future inspection or analysis and is of particular value in patients with kidney failure because their doctors need to be able to determine accurately the quantity and quality of the urine passed in order to ascertain their kidney function.

Suprapubic catheters are often used after repair operations for prolapse as they allow spontaneous voiding of urine but can remain *in situ* to check and drain any residual urine.

There is only one potential problem with urinary catheters and this is infection, although many people complain of some slight soreness for a few hours after their removal. A scrupulous aseptic technique must be used whenever anything is put into the bladder because a urine infection can go on to affect the kidneys and kidney infections are potentially harmful, even with today's good antibiotics. A doctor inserting a catheter will often put on a mask, wash his hands well, use sterile surgical gloves and, today, a disposable plastic catheter. With these precautions a person who has a catheter should not get a urine infection and the procedure of catheterization should be completely safe and trouble-free.

# CERVICAL CYTOLOGY (CYTOTEST)

Cancer of the cervix is the second most common cancer in women and most usually occurs between the ages of 30 and 50. It is almost always curable in its earliest stages and is worth diagnosing early. Unfortunately, in the early stages it usually produces no symptoms and so needs to be actively looked for.

The way in which it is diagnosed is by a Papanicolau (Pap) smear test. This involves the insertion of a vaginal speculum (see page 414) and then the gentle scraping, aspiration (sucking) or swabbing of the mouth of the cervix to obtain some of its surface cells. This should not be confused with a scraping of the lining of the womb, as in a D and C (see page 166) as the womb is not entered during a smear test. A smear of cells is then made on a glass slide and sent to a trained pathologist who specializes in this type of work (a cytologist). A skilled cytologist can tell whether the cells are cancerous or even pre-cancerous and so advise the gynaecologist whether or not to proceed with a local cutting away of the involved tissue. The amount of tissue removed is very small (usually smaller than your little finger nail). This clearly does *not* mean removing the whole womb, as is required for cancer of the uterus itself but medical opinion varies as to how this so-called 'cancer-in-situ' should be handled, once diagnosed.

Because the smear has to be sent away to a cytologist, you will not be given the result of the test for some days – or even a couple of weeks. If the result comes back negative you may be asked to return for another routine smear at a later date. If it is positive, do not worry – the smear often picks up other things that are nothing to do with cancer but which nevertheless need treating. Even if it is positive for cancer there is no cause for concern because the operation is simple (you will only be in hospital for a day or two), cures the condition in almost every case and has no effects on your sex life or your ability to have children.

The test is simple and painless and has no after-effects.

If it hurts, tell the doctor because it might mean you have an ulcer on the cervix which he could treat. Any woman about to undergo a Pap test should not douche before the test as this could wash away the very cells the doctor is trying to obtain. Ideally, all women between the ages of 30 and 50 should have a Pap test done every five years (and every year if they are on the Pill).

The screening of women for cervical cancer is a complex subject. The number of women having cervical smears is going up but the growth in numbers is coming from women who are not at any great risk of developing cervical cancer (ie young women). Women usually have a cervical smear either because they have no choice (it is done as part of the routine in certain clinics) because they have chosen to have a check-up in case there might be something wrong or because they have gynaecological symptoms. Of all cervical smears done, about half are repeat smears and nearly a third are done in response to a woman complaining of symptoms. Studies suggest that increasing numbers of smears are being done to diagnose something specific rather than as a preventive or screening measure. Experts are now questioning the validity of spending so much public money on routine smear taking in women under 35, unless they have symptoms suggestive of cervical disease.

# CULDOSCOPY

A technique in which an instrument is passed through the top end of the vagina into the pelvic cavity so that a doctor can examine the external surfaces of the pelvic organs. It is a test most usually employed in the investigation of infertility.

As long ago as the 1940s culdoscopy was widely used in the investigation of gynaecological conditions but today it is only used on any scale in the investigation of infertility and even then is not commonly used in Europe. Many doctors have a poor opinion of culdoscopy because they remember the relatively unsophisticated instruments of 20 or 30 years ago but today's instrument with its high-powered light source is a very different thing and the results can be most helpful.

Many women who are infertile have fibrous bands of tissue in their pelvic cavities, bands which have formed as the result of a previous infection – usually gonorrhoea. These bands which deform, or even completely block off the fallopian tubes (so causing infertility), can be seen and even divided at culdoscopy.

Another condition, endometriosis, in which patches of tissue exactly like that lining the uterus are found in the pelvic cavity, also causes infertility. Culdoscopy enables these patches to be seen and treated locally. Endometriosis is a treatable cause of infertility and so is well worth diagnosing.

Culdoscopy involves the passing of a telescope with its light source through the top end of the vagina into the abdominal cavity. With proper organization in a special clinic the whole procedure need only take 15 minutes.

If you are to have this procedure carried out under local anaesthetic, as is common in the US, you will be given a painkilling tablet to take before you arrive at the hospital and you will also have to have given yourself an enema the night before to clear out the bowel. You will be asked to eat nothing after midnight and to have no breakfast. You will be given a tranquillizer to take about an hour before the procedure and you should go along with a friend or relative. Women undergoing this procedure used to be shaved but this is no longer done. Once on the table, the doctor will place you face down with your bottom in the air and your legs apart. He will arrange the table so that you are as comfortable as possible and you will have a nurse with you at the head end of the table all the time.

The surgeon makes a tiny incision in the roof of the vagina and inserts a thin telescope into the abdominal cavity. In expert hands the whole examination, including photography if necessary, takes only five to ten minutes. Once the procedure is complete, the table is levelled and carbon dioxide gas is pumped into the abdomen through the telescope's outer tube to displace the air that has been sucked in during the procedure. Carbon dioxide is used because it is absorbed more readily than air. The equipment is then removed and, if necessary, a tiny stitch used to close the vaginal hole, though usually nothing is required. You will be asked to lie down for an hour afterwards to make sure you are all right and you should not take any strenuous exercise for the next 24 hours. If you get any problems at all once you are home, telephone the clinic.

In the UK and Europe culdoscopy is not very popular with specialists because most consider a general anaesthetic desirable and feel that laparoscopy is a more valuable procedure, given that a general anaesthetic is needed anyway.

Culdoscopy is valuable though in diagnosing endometriosis which is responsible for nearly 40 per cent of female infertility, according to many studies, and is treatable. A further 20 per cent of women have some pelvic inflammation and this is very well seen on culdoscopy. Adhesions after old surgery are found in about 16 per cent of infertile women and culdoscopy gives a good view of these.

# ELECTROCARDIOGRAPHY
## (ECG or EKG)

Heart disease is now the greatest single killer in the West and has attained epidemic proportions. Many people who are to have operations that are nothing at all to do with their hearts will have an ECG performed pre-operatively, so for this reason the procedure is included here.

An ECG machine is simply an apparatus that measures the electrical currents created by the heart's muscle at several different places on the body and displays the result on paper or on a TV-type screen. Every time the heart contracts, minute electrical impulses are produced by its muscle. These are detectable all over the body but the commonest kind of ECG machines use 3 leads or electrodes to pick up these impulses from the body and 9 further leads to monitor the heart area itself. Each of these gives a different perspective on the heart electrically speaking and so enables the person interpreting the ECG to tell what is going on in various parts of the heart at the same time.

At any one time a person having an ECG will only have four or five electrodes strapped to him. These are placed at both wrists and ankles – with or without the addition of a single chest electrode if one is to be used. By combining these readings though, 12 electrically different 'pictures' of the heart are possible – each one showing a separate perspective. So it is that an expert can, by looking at various combinations of leads from an ECG, get a complete picture of what is happening in the heart. This is why such a seemingly simple test is so valuable.

An ECG is painless, quick, and has no side-effects. A small amount of jelly is smeared on to the ankles and wrists (because the skin is a poor electrical conductor and would not otherwise give a good reading) and the four limb electrodes are strapped on. These are then connected to the ECG machine which can be mains or battery powered. Six of the possible 12 combinations of leads are recorded simply by the operator flicking a switch. At no time does any electricity enter the subject being examined.

A small suction pad – the chest lead – is then applied to the chest wall in six different positions (again some conducting jelly is smeared on the skin first) and once this is done, the ECG is finished. The whole procedure can be completed in ten minutes although it will take longer if the doctor wants to see the results of exercise on your ECG.

An ECG is valuable because so much information can be obtained from a good trace and because the trace, if obtained on paper, can be kept as a record to compare with future ones.

Just as with many other 'expert' pieces of gadgetry, the ECG readout looks like something from space until it is explained. Tracings from all parts of the body have certain common characteristics though. The first wave in any heartbeat, which is usually upright but may be inverted, is called a P wave and is caused by contraction of the atria or collecting chambers of the heart. The next wave is a small downward deflection called the Q wave which is followed by a big, upright one called an R wave. This is followed by a further downward deflection – the S wave. The whole QRS wave complex represents the contraction of the ventricles – the real pumping parts of the heart muscle. The intervals between and nature of these waves varies according to the disease present. If the heart is damaged or its internal conducting system is faulty, changes occur in the intervals between these waves and notably between the P and the R waves.

So from an ECG doctors can tell (i) the rate of the heartbeat; (ii) the rhythm with which the heart is beating; (iii) the nature of any abnormal rhythms; and (iv) the timing of all the key events in one heart cycle (which is less than one second long). From these pieces of information they will be able to diagnose literally scores of conditions affecting the heart.

If someone is severely ill either post-operatively or after a heart attack, he may be wired up to a cardiac monitor. This is basically an ECG machine that takes its electrical information from the patient (often only via a single adhesive chest lead) and displays it on a TV-type screen rather than on paper. This is done when prolonged monitoring of the ECG is needed and when miles of recording paper would be a positive nuisance! The design of such equipment varies enormously but is mainly contrived to display the ECG trace for immediate surveillance. Other refinements include the possibility of recording any interesting abnormalities as they occur; recording events and the heart's behaviour immediately prior to these events; and sounding alarms if the heartbeat steps outside pre-set limits. Unfortunately, such equipment, whilst of some help to doctors, can be distressing to patients who, apart from the constant feeling of being watched over electronically, are only too aware that something adverse is happening as alarms go off and staff come running. Such equipment is valuable in certain clearly defined situations but its value and indeed the value of intensive monitoring of post-heart attack patients is under scrutiny in many centres, partly in the light of evidence from the UK that certain patients under such scrutiny do not necessarily fare any better than those looked after at home.

None of this takes anything away from the simple ECG itself though which is an invaluable tool in skilled hands and enables a doctor to make crucial decisions about the state of the heart before, during and after an operation. If there is any hint of heart disease or if you have had a heart attack, the anaesthetist may well stick a single adhesive electrode on your chest before the operation so as to be able to keep a watchful eye on your ECG throughout.

# ELECTROCONVULSIVE THERAPY (ECT)

The application of an electric shock to the brain. The electrical current produces a fit, rather like that of grand mal epilepsy and this is how it first came to be used. In 1934 Dr von Beduna of Budapest made the observation that epilepsy was very uncommon in schizophrenics. He then deduced (for no good reason that we know of today) that these two conditions must therefore be virtually incompatible. This led him to suggest that epileptic fits might be used to cure schizophrenia. It soon became clear that schizophrenics did not benefit in the way he had hoped but it was found that depressives did improve.

Fits were first induced using the injection of very painful chemicals into muscles but in 1937 the Italians Cerletti and Bini passed an electric current through the brain and this is the basis of modern ECT.

Because the passage of a current through the brain causes a violent contraction of all the body's muscles, the person receiving ECT must be anaesthetized and paralysed by a drug. Because the body's muscles are paralysed, no violent contractions occur and the previously encountered dangers of dislocations and fractures of bones (especially in the spine) are now not seen. Clearly, if the body's muscles are all paralysed, the person cannot breathe, so the anaesthetist has to inflate the patient's lungs artificially for the very short duration of the procedure.

Once the electric shock has been given, by applying electrodes to the head in the region of one or both temples, the person is allowed to wake up and is usually conscious again within ten to fifteen minutes. Some people feel restless or emotional for a while but often fall asleep and wake an hour or two later to resume daily life. There may be a slight headache, loss of memory or confusion but in most people these disappear quickly.

There are some disadvantages though, as opponents of ECT are quick to point out. Some people, especially the elderly, suffer some permanent memory loss. Opponents of ECT are also concerned that it might be being used against the will of the patient compulsorily detained in mental hospital. There is no evidence that this occurs on any scale.

Some people – and even some experts – had until recently questioned whether ECT actually worked at all, or whether it might only have a placebo effect. Studies have now been carried out in the UK and elsewhere which show without doubt that patients given dummy ECT (an anaesthetic and the muscle paralysing drug yet no shock) fare less well than those given ECT. Also, one very good study from Edinburgh found that whilst patients did not positively enjoy ECT, most believed it had helped them and found it less frightening or unpleasant than going to the dentist. Other research found that when matched groups of depressives were examined using tests of memory and other high level brain functions, there was no difference between those who had and those who had not received ECT. What some of the patients studied did find unpleasant was hearing other patients being treated but this should be easily preventable in a unit run by thoughtful people.

ECT is mainly used in the treatment of depression and related disorders. It is also valuable in manic states, in certain types of schizophrenia and in some hypochondriacs. Most psychiatrists advise a course of six to eight treatments.

After 40 years of the medical use of ECT, only lately have

any useful studies been carried out. Until as recently as 1974 only a tiny amount of money had been spent on ECT research and even today we do not know how it works. There are many theories but the physical convulsion that occurs is certainly not an essential element.

Although the controversy over ECT is likely to continue for some time, thousands of people will continue to have it simply because for many it is the best treatment available. Opponents make much of the unknown factors involved, the loss of memory that can occur and the 'big brother' image of patients in mental hospitals being treated against their wills but all of these criticisms can be levelled against the use of many of the psycho-active drugs which are used with gay abandon by millions of people.

ECT is not a panacea for mental illness, nor is it the bogey it has been made out to be. Further research may help explain how and why it works and then perhaps we will be able to come to terms with this controversial therapy.

# ELECTROENCEPHOLOGRAPHY (EEG)

The EEG is a piece of equipment which measures electrical impulses arising from the brain. Every moment of our lives our brain cells are 'firing off' as we sense things in the world around us and as our bodies perform voluntary and involuntary activities. Somehow, and no one knows how, this seemingly dissociated mass of independently-firing nerve cells produces patterns of nerve activity recordable as brain waves.

Of course, the most logical way of recording the brain's electrical activity would be to insert fine electrodes into the organ itself but this is clearly not suitable for clinical use. Luckily most of the waves get through the bone of the skull and can be recorded on the scalp. An EEG machine then simply measures differences in electrical current over the scalp at many places.

There are four main types of brain wave, alpha, beta, theta and delta, and each is dominant under various conditions. Certain wave types are more plentiful when we are at rest, others as we awake, others as we dream and yet others when we are active. EEG studies of sleeping people have greatly furthered our understanding of the nature of sleep and dreams, for example.

Unfortunately, even the very best EEG machines are crude (in modern terms of scientific expectations) in what they can tell us about the brain. Only a fraction of the whole brain's mass can be examined using an EEG and more recent inventions such as computerized tomography (see page 424) have added a new dimension to understanding diseases inside the skull. An EEG is, for example, not helpful in diagnosing mental and emotional disorders but can be extremely useful in epilepsy.

Having an EEG done is painless and completely without danger. It does, however, take about an hour to do and you will be asked to keep your eyes closed for long periods. First, the technician measures your head to ensure that he can place the many electrodes accurately. These electrodes are stuck on to the scalp and each electrode lead is then plugged into the EEG machine. Tracings are made of the brain waves on large sheets of paper that display all the leads at once. The technician will ask you to perform certain manoeuvres as he records the brain waves for later interpretation by a doctor who specializes in reading EEGs.

Electroencephalography is still a relatively new technique but the future must hold promise of better, more useful machines as computers help to improve the value of the readings just as they have improved X-rays in computerized tomography.

Having an EEG is painless and needs no special preparation. Your doctor may take you off certain sorts of drugs if you are on them. Wash your hair the night before the test but do not put on any grease.

# ENDOMETRIAL BIOPSY

A test in which a sample of the lining of the womb (the endometrium) is taken and examined under a microscope.

An endometrial biopsy is usually done as part of the investigation of infertility and can be done at any time from the time you think you have ovulated until the day your period starts. The type of tissue seen in the pathology laboratory tells the doctor whether ovulation has taken place. The main cases of infertility in women are disorders of ovulation and an endometrial biopsy and special blood tests can help decide whether ovulation has in fact occurred.

An endometrial biopsy essentially involves the same technique as does a D and C (dilatation and curettage – see page 166), and can be performed without a general anaesthetic and as an out-patient. Some doctors use local anaesthetic around the cervix to numb it and most give some painkilling tablets beforehand. With you lying flat on your back and with your legs up in stirrups the doctor gently stretches the cervix with dilators which increase in size until the cervix is wide enough to take a tiny scraper (curette). He then scrapes this gently around the inside of the womb and removes some tissue. An alternative method involves using a thin (about the thickness of a piece of spaghetti) plastic catheter (a Vabra catheter) to suck out the uterine lining for examination. This is much narrower than the curette's blade, is not nearly so uncomfortable and is less likely to damage the cervix. Most women, especially if they have not had children, find the stretching of the cervix very unpleasant, which is why some kind of painkiller, tranquillizer or local anaesthetic is advisable. Many women say that if gynaecologists had had the procedure themselves, they would probably find another way around it. Some gynaecologists have now done this and rely much more on blood progesterone levels or use the Vabra catheter to obtain the same information. However, the endometrial biopsy still has a place in showing the doctor the quality of ovulation and how ready the endometrium is for the implantation of an egg. In some clinics the procedure is always carried out under a general anaesthetic. Ironically, this investigation for infertility sometimes results in a pregnancy, though no one knows why. For this reason some experts advise that no other investigations be performed for three months following the taking of an endometrial biopsy so as to give the couple a chance to conceive before proceeding further.

# ENDOSCOPY

Doctors are understandably keen to be able to see at first hand what is going on in any particular organ. X-rays can tell them a lot, especially when methods involving contrast media (radio-opaque substances) are used, and radio-isotope studies can tell a lot about the functioning of various organs. But in many cases the best thing a doctor can do is actually to see for himself what is going on and so come to a better decision on how to treat the patient and his problem. There are basically two ways he can do this. He can open up the patient at an operation (laparotomy, see page 242) and look directly, or he can use instruments that save the patient an operation yet allow him to see inside.

Instruments have therefore been designed to look into almost every nook and cranny of the human body and today we can look, without an operation, into much of the digestive system, the bronchial tree, the pleural cavity, the pelvic organs, the urinary passages, all the orifices of the head and even the arteries. Such 'looking in' is known as *endoscopy* and the instruments involved are called endoscopes. Many of these pieces of sophisticated engineering not only make it possible for the doctor to see inside the body but also enable samples of tissue to be taken and even permit minor surgery to be performed.

**FIBRE-OPTIC ENDOSCOPES** These have revolutionized endoscopy because they are flexible, give a good, clear view of the subject and enable quite sophisticated combinations of air, blowing, suction and minor operations to be carried out under excellent illumination.

The principle behind all fibre-optic instruments is much the same. They consist of a bundle of hair-like glass fibres, each of which is coated with a substance of lower refractive index so that all the light passing down the fibre is reflected internally. This phenomenon of total internal reflection allows a powerful beam of light to be transmitted from a light source outside the body so as to give intense illumination with no heat. The image at the distant end of the instrument is transmitted undistorted to a magnifying system and thence to the eye. The tip of the instrument can be guided from outside the body, thus enabling to steer it into exactly the right position. Most modern endoscopes, especially those used for examining the digestive tract, are of the fibre-optic kind, although a fibre-optic light source can also be used for a rigid instrument such as a sigmoidoscope.

**PROCTOSCOPY.** Perhaps the simplest of all endoscopes is the proctoscope. It is a short, rigid, tubular, steel instrument that enables a doctor to look at the back passage (anus). It is simply a tube with a light attached (see page 406 for more details).

A **SIGMOIDOSCOPE** allows a surgeon to see even further into the bowel and is described on page

A **COLONOSCOPE** is a good example of how fibre-optics have changed endoscopes. It is a flexible bundle of 30,000 glass fibres down which a cold light is sent so that the operator, by looking down an eyepiece at the end, can see everything as the tip of the instrument advances. The examination is usually performed under sedation but you should tell the doctor if there is any pain at all. The success of the examination depends on very good bowel preparation for 36 hours beforehand. This is usually achieved by limiting the intake of high-residue foods and by taking laxatives or having an enema done. Sometimes an X-ray technique is used to show the doctor exactly where the tip of the instrument is along the length of the bowel.

Colonoscopy is usually done to clarify a dubious X-ray finding in the large bowel and can be valuable in people who show no abnormality on X-ray or sigmoidoscopy yet still have rectal bleeding or diarrhoea. Colonoscopy can find the cause of rectal bleeding in about half of those complaining of this symptom. It is also a useful instrument for keeping an eye on inflammatory conditions of the bowel to assess the value of treatment, although many surgeons use a sigmoidoscope for this. Polyps can be removed with a special attachment to the colonoscope and since some polyps become malignant, this is a valuable thing to be able to do without having to operate on the patient.

Colonoscopy is time-consuming (it may take up to an hour) and is very expensive, mainly because the instrument only lasts for a few hundred examinations and because the training of a doctor to use it is expensive. It is, however, a very safe way of seeing almost all the large bowel and could greatly help prevent some of the 8,000 deaths a year that occur in England and Wales from cancer of this organ.

A **GASTROSCOPE** is a flexible, fibre-optic instrument which is passed through the mouth into the stomach. You will be asked to fast overnight before this examination and will be given a sedative or tranquillizer an hour beforehand. Some hospitals also ask you to suck a local anaesthetic lozenge about half an hour before the examination.

The procedure is simple and is not an operation – simply an examination. You will be asked to lie on your side and may be blindfolded. The blindfold is really only cosmetic so that you do not have to watch what is happening but you can leave it off if it bothers you. The doctor then inserts the gastroscope into the back of your mouth and pushes it gently down the gullet into the stomach. The duodenum, stomach and gullet can then be fully examined. Once the procedure is over you should not eat or drink anything for three hours if you have had a local anaesthetic spray or lozenge because you could unwittingly damage your throat. Some doctors will ask you to stay in hospital overnight but this is by no means always the case. Most European countries and Japan do not use a sedative at all and studies have been done to find out whether sedation is necessary. Gastroscopy is poorly tolerated without sedation by women, patients under forty and those with a special type of heartburn. Heavy drinkers tolerate gastroscopy badly regardless of sedation. Having said this though, many people are perfectly happy to swallow a gastroscope without sedation and one study found that 61 per cent of patients prefered it to a barium meal (see page 420).

**BRONCHOSCOPY** – looking down into the lungs using an instrument inserted down the throat – is now usually carried out using flexible, fibre-optic equipment, like so many other endoscopic procedures. Bronchoscopy can be performed under local anaesthetic in an emergency (for example to remove an inhaled foreign body) but is often done under a general anaesthetic. The procedure is carried out in the ward or in an operating theatre but, either way, it is not an operation in the true sense of the word, but an investigation. If the instrument is passed through the nose (as is usual) some minor bleeding may occur afterwards and some people have difficulty in speaking for a while. Most often though, a sore throat for a few hours is all that the person complains of. This is a small price to pay for the considerably increased accuracy of diagnosis that bronchoscopy allows, particularly of a tumour of the lung – the biggest single cancer problem in the western world.

**ARTHROSCOPY** is a procedure in which an endoscope is inserted into a joint so that a doctor can diagnose and treat disease there. The knee joint is especially suited to this procedure because lots of things go wrong with it and because an operation does not always provide the answers. Also, most knee problems affect young people who are valuable to society and their families and cannot afford weeks off work after an open knee operation.

Under full operating theatre conditions and under a general anaesthetic, the patient has the arthroscope inserted into the knee joint through a tiny swab incision. Once again fibre-optics have revolutionized the procedure and enable the operator to get a very clear look at all the structures in the joint; to take samples of tissue, if necessary; to take photographs for record and teaching purposes; and even to remove cartilages that are damaged. After the examination, the wound is closed with one stitch and a crêpe bandage applied firmly. As soon as you have recovered from the anaesthetic you can walk and you will usually be allowed home the same day. No particular precautions are necessary after the investigation and you can go about your daily life normally.

A **LAPAROSCOPE** is a special form of endoscope for looking inside the abdominal cavity (see laparoscopy, page 389). The laparoscope is mainly used by obstetricians and gynaecologists to diagnose and treat pelvic disease in women and to sterilize them. Increasingly though it is being used as a diagnostic tool by other doctors, notably physicians in the assessment of liver disease, abdominal malignancy, in diagnosing lumps in the abdomen, for trying to find a cause for fluid in the abdomen and for assessing large spleens.

**CYSTOSCOPY** is a commonly performed endoscopic manoeuvre (see page 163) for which rigid instruments (as opposed to flexible, fibre-optic ones) are still popularly used. These instruments are, however, becoming increasingly sophisticated and use fibre-optic light sources to increase illumination, allow photography and enhance the use of the instrument as an operative tool. Today, most men who have their prostates removed have the operation performed down an operating cystoscope (resectoscope) as it is much safer than the open abdominal operation. For more details on prostatectomy, see page

There is no doubt that as technology advances, even more ingenious pieces of equipment will be invented to look into every corner of the human body. This, together with improved diagnostic methods (ultrasound and computerized tomography), should mean that fewer open operations with all their attendant dangers and hospital stays will be necessary.

# ENEMAS

Whenever the large bowel is to be examined (at colonoscopy or a barium enema X-ray, for example) it will have to be cleaned out very effectively so that the procedure can be of maximum value. In the past, enemas were used for many disease conditions and were thought actually to be curative in their own right. Today, enemas are performed in hospital to empty the bowel before investigative procedures and in the constipated person in whom other methods of bowel emptying have not worked. A sensible diet rich in dietary fibre (roughage) will mean that you will never become so constipated that an enema is necessary, but even if you eat a healthy, non-constipating diet like this, you will still need an enema to prepare your bowel for certain tests or surgery.

Basically, an enema involves filling the lower bowel with a fluid which, when passed, carries with it the contents of the bowel. A variety of solutions can be used from soap and water to castor oil and today, disposable plastic enema packs are widely used. The technique is always the same, no matter what the fluid.

The patient is placed on his left side with a towel and a polythene sheet under the buttocks. A wide bore tube is attached to a funnel (or a plastic bag of fluid) and the tube lubricated and inserted into the back passage. A pint or two of fluid is then allowed to flow into the bowel and the patient asked to keep it in until he wants to open his bowels. Once the stools have been passed with the fluid the person can go about things as normal. If the enema contains medication for ulcerative colitis, for example, you will be asked to lie flat (often with the foot of the bed raised) and to retain the enema for some time. If this is the reason you have enemas, you will be given disposable bags of medicated enemas to perform the procedure at home on your own.

Should the retained stools be very hard the nurse may have to soften them by putting olive oil in the rectum, where it is retained for 20 minutes. A normal enema then usually removes the retained matter.

Occasionally, in old people, the hard masses of stool still do not come away and have to be removed by hand. This can normally be done under normal ward conditions but may need a general anaesthetic. Using as many fingers as he can the doctor (or nurse) removes the hard faeces and may end up by giving an enema to clear out the remainder. If you find the procedure unpleasant or painful, tell the person doing it.

# EPIDURAL ANALGESIA

A procedure, used for abdominal and lower limb operations as well as in labour, which involves the injection of local anaesthetic into the surroundings of the spinal cord so as to deaden pain. In the UK, epidural analgesia is used very much more often for pain relief in labour than for any other purpose.

Labour is a painful process for many women and today's women are understandably loath to accept pain if they think it can be alleviated safely. There are several well tried and tested ways of relieving pain in labour but all have their disadvantages. Psychoprophylaxis is fine provided you can stick to it when it comes to the crunch (some can: others cannot); 'gas and air' is good but is not suitable in labours that go on for many hours; and injected drugs are effective but may end up affecting the baby adversely, especially when it comes to initiating breast feeding.

Epidural analgesia is by no means without its problems but it does have two major advantages. Firstly, you feel no pain, yet are awake, do not feel sick (as can occur with pethidine and similar drugs) and are able to enjoy the birth of your baby and share this pleasure with your husband. Second, if forceps are needed to help the baby out, or an episiotomy be called for with its inevitable stitches, no further anaesthetic is necessary. You can even have a Caesarean section under the epidural, if necessary.

Although epidurals have been available for over 40 years it is only in the last decade that they have become really popular and widely used. Some hospitals in the UK use this method in over half of their labours and the figure is even higher in some hospitals in the United States.

Epidurals are particularly useful in premature labours in which the baby's head might be soft, as a more controlled delivery with forceps is possible using this method. This is important because a soft skull offers less protection against internal brain damage if it 'pops out' of the vagina in an uncontrolled way. Very long labours in which the mother gets distressed and exhausted are helped greatly by an epidural which is also safer than repeated injections of painkillers which can depress the baby's breathing. Women with high blood pressure in pregnancy also benefit from an epidural because, by its very nature, it tends to lower the blood pressure.

The technique is basically simple and in experienced hands is safe and quick. Quite simply, local anaesthetic is placed around the spinal cord in the lower back at the area where the nerves to the uterus, vagina and bladder come off. The procedure is usually carried out by an anaesthetist with special training in the technique and starts off with a tiny injection of local anaesthetic into a previously sterilized area of skin on the back. When this area of skin is deadened by the local anaesthetic the doctor inserts a needle into the epidural space surrounding the spinal cord. In order to make this easier the doctor will have asked you to lie on your left side with your knees tucked up as far as they will go.

When he knows he is in the right place he threads a fine polythene catheter (tube) down the hollow needle so that its tip lies in the epidural space. The hollow needle is then removed leaving the catheter protruding through the skin. He tethers this to the skin of the back with sticking plaster and connects the other end to a drip bottle full of the local anaesthetic or to a bacterial filter into which injections can be made when necessary. Ten millilitres of a special anaesthetic are usually injected as a starter and this lasts a long time. Because nerves to muscles are more difficult to deaden than nerves carrying sensation, a woman with an epidural will often be able to move her legs (albeit with difficulty) yet feel no pain at all.

After about two hours the epidural will need topping up but this is a completely pain-free procedure. In good hands epidurals are very satisfactory as a method of pain relief but they depend on the woman telling her attendant as soon as she feels the beneficial effects beginning to wear off.

There are very few medical reasons why a woman should *not* have an epidural and it is now a widely accepted and popular method of pain control. However, it is not without its problems. Most of these, to be fair, arise when the procedure is performed by inexperienced people or because of poor technique rather than as a result of any intrinsic dangers of the method itself. Having said this though, some women find that an epidural simply does not work for them. This is usually because the catheter is in the wrong place or because it is not being topped up often enough.

Low blood pressure can be a real problem. Because the blood vessels of the legs are dilated (enlarged) by the effects of the epidural, more blood than normal is pooled there and the woman's blood pressure falls. This is especially likely to be a problem if she is lying on her back because the baby's weight compresses the veins that carry the blood back to the heart – so lowering the blood pressure further. This problem can be overcome by lying on one side but this can be uncomfortable after a while. Because of this potential fall in blood pressure many hospitals put up an intravenous drip so that if the blood pressure falls too low (and so endangers the blood supply to the baby) they can quickly 'fill up' the blood circulation with special fluids.

But probably the greatest single disadvantage of epidurals is that they tend to reduce the urge to push and this means that the mother cannot play such a big part in actually pushing the baby out. This in turn means that obstetric forceps are used very often in epidural births and this entails an episiotomy (see page 178) with all its subsequent discomfort. Forceps are used to deliver first babies more often than subsequent ones but in many centres epidural analgesia leads to the use of forceps as a routine, even though they may not strictly be necessary. As far as the mother is concerned at the time, she does not feel anything from the forceps, of course, because of the epidural. The stitching up of the episiotomy is also pain-free without injections.

Over a few hours the feeling comes back to the legs and there are usually no after-effects at all. If the doctor has accidentally entered the fluid surrounding the spinal cord as he was inserting the needle (a so-called 'dural tap') a headache may be a problem and this can last for several days. This should be a rare occurrence though. Some surveys have shown that babies delivered to epidural mothers are more likely to become jaundiced but this is usually only transitory and is not serious.

# HYSTEROSALPINGOGRAM (HSG)

An X-ray procedure which gives special information about the inside of the uterus and fallopian tubes. It is carried out in an X-ray department but is done as an out-patient procedure. It is usually done as part of the investigation of infertility.

In women who have trouble conceiving there is often a blockage in one or both fallopian tubes as they lead from the ovaries to the uterus. Such a blockage can be responsible for infertility and may be treatable so it is useful to know how and where the tube is blocked. If the tubes are open (as they are in a healthy woman) then other causes for the infertility will be sought. There is little point in stimulating a woman's ovaries to ovulate using 'fertility drugs' if when she does so her eggs cannot get to the sperms to be fertilized. Because of this, tests to find out about the state of the fallopian tubes are usually an early part of the investigation of any infertile woman.

Some women who have had an infection involving their fallopian tubes want to know whether or not it has affected their tubes adversely and so try to get an HSG done to find out. This is not often possible on the National Health Service but could be arranged privately.

Once on the X-ray table with your legs up in stirrups you may be given a local anaesthetic injection around the cervix to reduce the pain as a special nozzle is inserted into the cervical canal. It is this stretching that is painful and if it is too much you should tell the doctor. With the nozzle in the cervical canal, a radio-opaque substance is injected into the uterus and X-rays taken as the fluid passes up the tubes and out into the abdominal cavity. You may experience painful cramps like severe period pains when the fluid is injected but if you tell the doctor he can allow the cramps to go before proceeding further.

The whole process is usually shown on a TV screen as well as being recorded permanently on X-ray film. If the radio-opaque fluid cannot go along the tube the doctor will wait for a while in case the tube is in spasm. If the spasm goes and the tubes are then clear, all is well. Even with this fairly sophisticated test, false negatives and positives can occur, and this has made many experts unwilling to accept HSG results alone as final. One study, for example, found that 'HSG was completely inaccurate in 19 per cent' of women.

A recent German study found that the results of laparoscopy (see page 398) and HSG concurred in 76 per cent of the women they examined and that in the remaining 24 per cent the so-called 'normal' findings on HSG had to be reviewed after laparoscopy and vice versa. HSG therefore has not been overtaken by laparoscopy. The two tests should be used as complementary to each other.

As with tubal insufflation (in which gas is pumped through the fallopian tubes), some women seem to have their tubes cleared by this procedure and conceive after the test. Why this should happen is not known but whether the fluid pressure actually breaks down small blockages and debris or whether the tiny dose of X-rays stimulates the ovaries, the result is an unexpected but welcome pregnancy in a small percentage of women. Some doctors think that the stretching of the cervix may be what enables a pregnancy to occur because some women get pregnant after having an endometrial biopsy (see page 384) and in this test nothing is done to their tubes. Whatever the reason, some doctors will suggest that you keep on trying to conceive for a clear three months after either of these tests before embarking on further infertility tests, whatever the test result, simply because each test may be curative in itself.

Many women find this test very unpleasant, so doctors give a tranquillizer and painkiller to be taken before the test. About 20 per cent of infertile women have blocked tubes though, so it is worth going through with it if you really want to get to the root of the problem. The test is normally done in the first half of the menstrual cycle.

# HYSTEROSCOPY

A technique in which a fine telescope is inserted into the uterus through the cervical canal. Looking inside the uterus is very difficult technically because it is difficult to get enough light; because the cervix is so tight that the telescope has to be very small in diameter; and because it is very hard to distend the uterus so that its walls are parted sufficiently to allow their inspection. With the development of fibre-optic instruments (see page 385) which allow a powerful, cold light source to illuminate even the darkest holes, hysteroscopy has now become a reality.

It is used to examine the inside of the uterus for abnormalities and also in the search for a cause for infertility.

The instrument is inserted into the uterus via the cervix under either general or local anaesthetic. Because stretching the cervix is so painful, many doctors prefer to use general anaesthesia. The cervix is stretched, the telescope inserted and the uterine cavity filled with fluid or carbon dioxide gas. The doctor can then see the whole of the lining of the uterus, the openings of the fallopian tubes and any abnormalities of shape and structure of the uterus. This method often gives far more accurate results than does a hysterosalpingogram (HSG, see page 394), because with an HSG, small filling defects with the radio-opaque fluid are often difficult to interpret and small areas of trouble can escape detection altogether. Hysteroscopy followed by laparoscopy is probably more valuable than a hysterosalpingogram alone and is now replacing it in some centres.

# INTRAVENOUS DRIPS

Now that intravenous fluids can be produced in ways that ensure they are free from bacterial contamination, more and more people are being given them in hospitals. There are basically two kinds of fluid that are given. The first, blood (or plasma), is used to replace that lost in serious accidents, after or during an operation or in certain conditions in which there is profuse internal bleeding such as occurs with bleeding peptic ulcers. The second group of fluids is specially constituted to replace body fluid and certain specific chemicals in the body if they become depleted after, for example, prolonged diarrhoea or vomiting. More uncommonly, a person who cannot eat is kept alive by intravenous feeding. Sometimes a person who it is thought might need blood will be started on a drip of a plain fluid (glucose saline is commonly used), while blood is being matched and made ready for him.

Intravenous infusions (as drips are properly called) are simple procedures today, mainly because plastic and polythene have made it possible for everything to be pre-sterilized and disposable. This starts with the cannula or needle that goes into the vein. The insertion of this is simple. Preparations are made exactly as for venepuncture (see page 366) and then a special cannula is put into the vein. If only clear fluids are to be given through the drip, a small bore needle will be used. In fact there is a very small and unobtrusive type of cannula called a 'butterfly' which is so fine that it slips into the vein painlessly and can remain strapped in place for days if necessary. If blood or intravenous feeds are to be given, a larger needle will be required. This may be inserted after a local anaesthetic has been put in the skin over the vein but as today's cannulae are so well designed and sharp (because they are used once and discarded) this is not often necessary. If you would rather have a local anaesthetic – ask the doctor. Once the cannula is in the vein, it is strapped in position with adhesive tape. Tell the doctor if you know that you are allergic to any particular kind of adhesive dressing – as some people are. Some hospitals and clinics have switched entirely to non-allergic adhesive dressings to overcome this problem. If you are ill enough to need a drip, then you will not want a skin reaction to the adhesive dressing to add to your problems. Finally, the arm is securely bandaged and the tube from the drip pack hanging by the bedside tethered so that you cannot pull the whole thing over when you move about in bed.

Changing the bags (they used to be bottles) of fluid is easy today and because they are centrally produced in scrupulously sterile plants, there is no danger of infection from such packs. If you do have a drip up and you are well enough to be able to watch it is worth keeping an eye on the level in the bottle or bag to ensure that it does not run out without the nursing staff noticing. If it were to do so it would not be dangerous but could mean that the cannula in the vein might clot up and so have to be replaced – at some possible discomfort to you.

If you are severely ill and are being given lots of intravenous fluid it is possible that you will have to have a urinary catheter in place (see page 372) to collect your urine. Urine will be drained off into a bag or bottle under the bed so that the doctors can keep an eye on your fluid balance. Clearly there must be a careful balance between fluids put in and urine coming out or you could retain fluid.

If your drip stops flowing (you will be able to tell by looking at the drops in the chamber beneath the bag), do tell someone. Also, be sure to tell a nurse or doctor if there is any pain or if your arm swells up. If this occurs the drip will have to be taken down and another vein used but most often a stopped drip that has not caused swelling can be restarted without a new venepuncture. Sometimes a small clot lodges at the tip of the cannula in the vein but this can be dislodged with some saline injected into the tube.

In the uncommon event that the doctor cannot find a vein into which to put a drip, he may well expose a small section of a vein, often at the elbow, groin or ankle, so as to be able to give the life-saving fluids. Do not be alarmed by this, it is only a slightly more serious form of a normal drip procedure.

# LAPAROSCOPY

A technique which enables a surgeon to examine many of the contents of the abdomen and pelvis and even to perform simple operations, without opening the abdomen.

The concept of laparoscopy is at last 40 years old and is

very simple. A tube with a light on the end is inserted through the skin of the abdominal wall and enables the operator to see inside the abdominal cavity.

There are many occasions on which a surgeon (and especially a gynaecologist) wants to look inside the abdomen to help him sort out a difficult diagnosis. X-rays, computerized tomography (see page 424), and ultrasonic scanning (see page 410) can all help but even with these aids there are still occasions when it is necessary to have a look at what is actually happening inside the abdomen in order to make a definitive diagnosis. Until the invention of the laparoscope, it was necessary to perform a major 'look and see' operation known as a laparotomy (see page 242). Today though in spite of the widespread use of the laparoscope by gynaecologists, it has not caught on in a big way with general surgeons, mainly because their problems in terms of diagnosis and management are different. There are signs that this is changing as the instrument becomes more refined.

Basically a laparoscope is a steel, tubular instrument with a light at one end and an eyepiece at the other. Early models had ordinary small light bulbs as their source of illumination and the level of light produced was rather poor. Today, with the introduction of fibre-optics, very powerful illumination can be obtained and it is this more than anything else that has really made laparoscopy a useful and safe diagnostic and operative technique. The most recent instruments enable the surgeon to operate down them rather than through a separate entry and this has created even greater possibilities for the future.

Laparoscopy is carried out for three main groups of conditions. First are the undiagnosable problems in women with pelvic pain for which no cause can be found. The laparoscope can help rule out macroscopic diagnoses such as adhesions (from previous abdominal surgery or pelvic infection) and a condition called endometriosis (which is usually treatable once a doctor knows what he is treating). The second group of people who can benefit from laparoscopy are infertile women. The view of the female sex organs through a laparoscope is extremely good and it is possible to see whether the ovaries are producing eggs properly, for example. It is also easy to examine the state of the fallopian tubes – a common seat of infertility-producing conditions and easy to check that the fallopian tubes are not blocked off by disease (and so producing infertility) by having an assistant insert some dye into the uterus and watching through the laparoscope for it to emerge from the ends of the fallopian tubes inside the abdominal cavity. Previously this would have meant having X-rays.

The last group of women who can benefit from laparoscopy are those who want to be sterilized. The laparoscope enables a gynaecologist to burn, cut or clip the fallopian tubes quickly and easily. One recent method involves the placing of tiny elastic bands around the fallopian tubes. This is a quick and simple way of sterilizing a woman which involves only one night in hospital.

Most surgeons perform a laparoscopy under general anaesthesia. This is almost essential because the technique involves inserting two litres of carbon dioxide gas into the abdominal cavity. This gas forces the diaphragm upwards and makes breathing difficult so a general anaesthetic combined with a mechanical means of controlling the patient's breathing is essential. The technique is as follows. Under general anaesthetic a tiny nick is made in the skin just below the navel. A fine needle is then inserted into the abdominal cavity and carbon dioxide gas pumped in. This gas helps separate the abdominal organs, enables a good view to be obtained and creates an unnatural 'cavity' around organs so that the surgeon can see and operate more easily. Once the two litres of gas have been pumped in, the fine needle is withdrawn and a wide one inserted into the same half inch long incision in the skin. The laparoscope is then inserted down the tube. For certain procedures another, smaller incision (about two millimetres long) is needed – especially when elastic bands are being used for sterilization. This nick in the skin is also in the midline and below the original laparoscope one. Once the laparoscopy is over, the gas is removed as completely as possible and the procedure is complete. A single skin clip or suture is used to close the wound.

Because laparoscopy is a quick and simple procedure it is also very safe. There is only a tiny risk of complications. A survey in the UK of more than 50,000 laparoscopies carried out all over the country during one year found that only 0.8 per thousand women had any anaesthetic complications; 2.5 per thousand had bleeding from the abdominal wall wound; and 1.8 per thousand suffered internal damage as a side-effect of the laparoscopy. These are very small numbers of complications for such a useful procedure and it has to be borne in mind that many of these women would probably have been subjected to a more major operative procedure had they not had a laparoscopy. The major advantage of laparoscopy is in fact its speed. It reduces the amount of time the patient spends under general anaesthesia which is bound to make it safer for her. One night in hospital is usual.

There are very few side-effects but some women complain of shoulder tip pain post-operatively. This is caused by trapped carbon dioxide gas irritating the under surface of the diaphragm which in turn causes referred pain to the shoulder tip. It disappears very quickly.

## LUMBAR PUNCTURE

Several diseases of the nervous system, and meningitis in particular, produce specific changes in the fluid that surrounds the brain and spinal cord – the cerebrospinal fluid. The whole of the brain and spinal cord 'floats' in a bath of this special nutrient fluid which is contained by the skull and spinal bones. Normally the fluid (CSF) is clear and colourless. In disease though its protein, glucose, chloride, cell content and pressure can all be changed in varying degrees. A knowledge of these changes helps greatly in the diagnosis of certain diseases and it is essential in meningitis to find out which organism is responsible for this dangerous infection. Only when a doctor knows the organism involved can he hope to treat meningitis effectively and since by definition the organism affects the nervous system, the only place it can be obtained for culture is from the fluid around the nervous system. If there were any other way of arriving at the same diagnostic end point, doctors would use it and not resort to a lumbar puncture because, although it is safe in good hands, it is still an intrusion into the body that is not undertaken lightly.

As with so many of the tests described in this section of the book, a lumbar puncture is something people fear, yet it is simple, quickly carried out and, in good hands, completely safe.

First, the person is turned on his left side on the bed and asked to draw his knees up to his chest. This is done so as to bend the spine in such a way as to open up the gaps between the vertebrae and thus make it easier for the doctor to insert the lumbar puncture needle. The skin is then scrupulously cleaned with an antiseptic and the area covered with sterile towels. The doctor feels for the gaps between two adjacent lumbar vertebrae (at the base of the back) and inserts local anaesthetic into the skin with a fine needle. While this is taking effect he checks that his equipment is ready. He then inserts a needle (about twice the bore of an ordinary blood-taking needle) through the anaesthetized skin and into the fluid surrounding the spinal cord. Some of the fluid is collected for analysis. He then measures its pressure using a very simple glass tube and after possibly asking an assistant to press both sides of the patient's neck to see the effect this has on the pressure in the tube – he will be finished. He withdraws the lumbar puncture needle, covers the area with an adhesive dressing and asks the patient to lie flat.

If you ever have a lumbar puncture this last piece of advice should be well heeded because if you try to sit up within 24 hours of a lumbar puncture, you will probably experience a very unpleasant headache. This should be the only side-effect of a lumbar puncture and is completely avoidable if you lie flat or even with the foot of the bed raised for the next day. Having a lumbar puncture is very similar to having epidural analgesia (see page 391); the difference is only technical in that the needle does not go so far in with an epidural as with a lumbar puncture. Also with an epidural no fluid is removed nor are any measurements taken.

# NASOGASTRIC TUBE

Many people who go into hospital have to have a nasogastric tube passed down the nose and into the stomach. Perhaps the commonest reason for doing this is to allow the constantly-produced acid secretions of the stomach to be sucked out when the bowel is not working properly – as often occurs after abdominal operations. A nasogastric (Ryle's) tube can also be inserted to investigate the secretions produced by the stomach or to wash out the stomach after an overdose of drugs or poisons. The tube may be passed during an operation but often it needs to be in place beforehand.

Most people find having a nasogastric tube passed unpleasant, but in good hands the whole procedure is soon over and once the tube is down it is not too bad. First, the doctor or nurse will ask you to sit up and then will look at your nose to see which nostril looks wider. The tube is lubricated and pushed gently into the nose while you breathe in and out through your mouth. As the tube goes down further you will asked to swallow. Sometimes a few sips of water help at this stage. Although many people choke (gag) on the tube as it goes down, it usually goes into the stomach quickly and easily. If it proves difficult, the whole thing can be repeated using a narrower tube. You may feel you would like to pass the tube yourself – some people feel better doing it themselves.

Once the tube is in place the doctor or nurse will blow some air down it from a syringe while listening for bubbling noises over the stomach area of the abdomen with a stethoscope. This confirms that the open end is in gastric juice. The gastric contents are sucked up and tested, if necessary, and the free end of the tube is stuck to the face with sticky tape. Its end may be shut off with a plastic spigot or joined up to a bag. Sometimes the tube becomes blocked and the staff may have to inject a syringe-full of saline solution or air down it to clear it. Taking the tube out is easy. It is simply pulled out while you swallow several times.

# OPHTHALMOSCOPY

An ophthalmoscope is a battery or mains operated hand instrument which enables a doctor to look into the eye and diagnose disease there.

Clearly, any condition or disorder of the eye visible to the patient himself when looking in a mirror is not going to present much of a visualization problem for a doctor. However, several conditions affecting the eye do not manifest themselves so easily and have to be diagnosed with the aid of this simple but effective instrument.

Unlike an auriscope (see page 357) which is actually put into the ear, the ophthalmoscope never touches the eye but is brought up close to it as the doctor looks through a magnifying lens into the illuminated eye. The illumination is produced by a tiny bulb which is part of the instrument and it is this that enables the back of the eye (the retina) and all the other internal structures to be so clearly seen.

The retina can be seen with an instrument in front of the eye because by looking through the pupil (the dark centre section of the eye) most of the back of the eye can be visualized and even photographed. As well as giving information about the retina, an ophthalmoscope also enables a doctor to examine the lens of the eye and to look for cataracts in it.

But although specialists in ophthalmic or neurological disease may look into the eye with all kinds of diagnoses in mind the physician or surgeon working in a hospital looks into the eye very often, yet is not specifically looking for eye disease. This apparent contradiction can easily be explained. The retina is the most readily visualized part of the body that displays its arteries and veins for all to see. This means that by looking in the eye the doctor has a window on the entire blood vessel system. So useful is this that the effects of diseases that affect blood vessels (diabetes and high blood pressure are two good examples) can be minutely observed in life. Since both of these diseases are characterized by specific changes in blood vessels all over the body, by being able to see what goes on in one small section of the body so clearly, doctors can better understand the total picture. Of course, the blood pressure machine (see page 363) tells one how high the blood pressure is – but what it does not tell a doctor is the effect that *that* level of hypertension is having on a particular person and we are all very individual in this respect. Similarly with diabetes. It is all very well knowing how many units of insulin a person is taking but it does not give doctors any clue to the total disease picture as it affects all the organs of the body. Ophthalmoscopy enables the doctor to do this and so provides a valuable tool in everyday practice – after all diabetes and hypertension, to mention but two such easily-diagnosed conditions, affect millions of people in the western world today.

An ophthalmic surgeon will, of course, be mainly concerned with actual eye disease or malfunction when he looks in your eye. If you have had a head injury, doctors can find out about the pressure of the fluid around the brain by looking in the eye too.

So, if a doctor looks in your eye with an ophthalmoscope, do not be surprised or wonder if he has got the right patient – he may be looking for something that is nothing to do with your vision at all.

## RADIO-ISOTOPE TESTS

Nuclear medicine (the use of radioactively tagged compounds in diagnostic and curative medicine) is of increasing value as the number of isotopes available increases. Medically used radio-isotopes are man-made variations on normal chemical elements such that the body's tissues recognize them as normal chemicals but in fact they have been altered (often by bombardment in a nuclear reactor) so as to make them emit radiation which can be detected with special equipment.

A small dose of a radioactively 'labelled' substance is given by mouth, inhalation or intravenously and the radiation this fixed dose emits is measured extremely accurately. Detector machines scan the body and this scanning produces a picture of the organ or tissue by which the isotope was absorbed.

Radio-isotopes have the advantage of being actively taken up by a particular tissue or organ and so can give a doctor a very good idea of the functioning of that organ. This can only rarely be achieved by any other method. X-rays and most other image-producing methods yield only anatomical pictures of tissues and organs and say little about how they are functioning. Specific radio-isotopes tend to be taken up by certain body tissues. This means that an organ or system can be demonstrated clearly yet the rest of the body remains virtually free from the radio-isotope. Within an organ there may be areas where the isotope has been taken up in large quantities. These areas are called 'hot spots' and usually mirror an increased blood flow to the area. Places where no isotope is taken up may indicate growths of various kinds.

Isotopes have therapeutic uses too. Certain thyroid diseases and some types of leukaemia and other blood diseases respond well to therapeutic doses of isotopes. You will be told whether your isotope is for an investigation or treatment.

Lastly, you need have no fear about the dangers of radio-isotope studies. The doses are extremely small and the fall-off of the radiation is very fast. The isotopes do not remain in the body for long or cause any harm.

# RECTAL EXAMINATION

Two common conditions occurring predominantly in middle-aged men are easily diagnosed by rectal examination: an enlarged prostate (see page 289) gland and a rectal cancer. Because both are amenable to treatment (but only if caught early in the case of rectal cancer), a rectal examination is an important part of the physical examination of any man over middle age and is commonly performed by surgeons. A vaginal examination is probably of more value for examining the pelvis in women but if a specific rectal disorder is suspected, then a rectal examination is done too.

Quite simply the person to be examined is asked to lie on his left side with his knees drawn up to his chest. The doctor puts on a glove and inserts a well-lubricated finger into the anus (back passage). Apart from the embarrassment most people feel when having a rectal examination and the slight discomfort of unfamiliarity, it can hardly be said to be painful and is over very quickly. There are no after-effects.

Bleeding from the rectum is a very common problem in the West – mainly because so many people have piles (see page 200). However, bleeding is also a sign of rectal cancer – a very unpleasant disease that has to be caught early if treatment is to be successful. A rectal examination is well worth doing, even in someone with definite piles, because the bleeding could be coming from two sources.

In children, if a rectal examination has to be performed, the doctor will use a well-lubricated little finger which should not cause much distress to the child.

A rectal examination is often followed by **PROCTOSCOPY** if there are any suspicious findings. A proctoscope is a short, wide, tubular steel instrument that can be inserted into the anus. The patient lies in the same position as for a rectal examination and the doctor inserts the well-lubricated proctoscope gently. The 'open' end is filled in by a blunt but rounded end piece which is removed once the instrument is in position. The proctoscope may have its own light source or can have a light shone down it from outside. It is only a few inches long and so does not cause great discomfort. The great advantage with a proctoscope is that it can reveal internal haemorrhoids and trouble in the anal canal. It can also allow access for the treatment of some conditions.

This examination is often followed by a sigmoidoscopy which allows inspection of the rectum.

A **SIGMOIDOSCOPE** is a long tube, made of steel, with a light at the end. It enables the doctor to look much deeper into the large bowel after inserting the instrument into the back passage. Both this instrument and the fibre-optic colonoscope call for very careful cleaning of the bowel before the procedures are done, as there will otherwise be too much stool in the way for the doctor to be able to see the walls of the bowel. Methods of preparation vary but often an enema will be given about an hour before the procedure. If you are having it done as an out-patient, you will be given a disposable enema and instructed how to use it. If the examination is to be carried out in the afternoon, you should have a light breakfast but no lunch.

Having said this, many surgeons do not like to prepare the bowel for sigmoidoscopy at all. Scrupulous bowel preparation is, however, always necessary for a colonoscopy.

Sigmoidoscopy is usually carried out with the person lying on his left side and his knees pulled up to his chest. Some surgeons use other positions. No general anaesthetic is necessary but if you feel pain at any time, do tell the doctor. The instrument is lubricated and then passed gently into the back passage after the doctor has first done a rectal examination with his finger. Once inside a little way you will hear the doctor pumping air into the bowel with a hand-held bladder pump. Do not be alarmed at this: it is simply to force air into the bowel so as to push the walls open and allow the instrument to go through easily. The whole manoeuvre only takes half an hour at the most, even if the doctor decides to take a little sample of bowel tissue for subsequent microscopic analysis.

Any inflammation (such as occurs in ulcerative colitis – which affects the bottom end of the colon in most people with the disease) or tumour can be seen, and if necessary a sample of tissue can be taken. Special long-handled biopsy forceps enable the surgeon to excise a tiny piece of the tissue for laboratory examination and thus to make a more accurate diagnosis.

# TUBAL INSUFFLATION (RUBIN TEST)

This is the oldest of the tests used to find out whether the fallopian tubes are open or blocked by past infection, and was first described by Dr I. Rubin in 1947.

After ovulation problems, damage to or blockage of the fallopian tubes is the next most common cause of infertility. In fact about 20 per cent of all infertile women are thought to have abnormalities of their tubes. The fallopian tubes run from the ovaries to the uterus and normally carry an egg down to the uterus each month. Fertilization of the egg by a sperm takes place in the tubes and any malfunction or blockage of the tubes can prevent this happening and leads to infertility. The commonest cause of blocked tubes by far is adhesions caused by infection, usually gonorrhoea or a perforated appendix. The tubal insufflation test was designed to assess the fallopian tubes' ability to convey an egg to the uterus and in effect tells the doctor whether the tubes are open or closed.

Just before ovulation is thought to be due, the woman goes to the clinic as an out-patient or is admitted for the investigation to be done under anaesthetic. She is positioned with her legs in stirrups and an instrument with a nozzle is inserted into the cervical canal. Carbon dioxide gas is blown down this tube under pressure, and the pressure carefully watched. The gas escapes from the open ends of the fallopian tubes, if indeed they are open. The doctor listens with a stethoscope over the lower part of the abdomen to hear if gas is escaping and then asks the woman to sit up. As she does so the gas rises to the top of her abdominal cavity (under the diaphragm) and causes pain to be felt in the shoulder. This in itself is diagnostic that the tubes are not blocked because if they were, the gas could not have got there. The gas is absorbed harmlessly by the body and leaves no after-effects but the Rubin test is uncomfortable and does not produce reliable results. It is very difficult to tell whether a tube is really blocked or is simply in spasm; the doctor can never know whether one or both tubes has let the gas through, and it can produce both false negative and false positive results.

In its favour, it is easy and quick to perform, is not too uncomfortable and can sometimes even clear small blockages in the tubes. Because of these advantages it has not been entirely abandoned but most experts would rather rely on other methods. The best known of these and the most widely available is a hysterosalpingogram (see page 394).

# ULTRASOUND

A procedure in which very high (inaudible) sound frequencies are used to visualize structures inside the body.

The principle behind ultrasound diagnostic techniques is exactly the same as that used in the echo sounder on a ship. In a marine echo sounder sound frequencies are beamed to the ocean floor, bounce back up and are collected by the instrument again. The time taken for this cycle is noted and the depth of the water under the boat calculated with great accuracy.

In medical ultrasound the same principle applies. After first wetting the patient's skin with oily fluid, a probe is rubbed gently over the skin surface. The probe emits high frequency sound waves and picks them up fractions of a second later. The images are fed into an electronic system which converts the sound wave reflections from the organs under the probe at any one moment into a TV picture, where it is 'frozen' for examination by the operator. The pictures on the TV screen can be photographed or printed out automatically to provide a permanent copy of the information to store in the patient's medical file.

Ultrasonography is still in its early days in the medical diagnostic world but is fast improving in usefulness. It is relatively cheap, may be portable and is used by a radiologist or radiographer with extra training. CT (computerized tomography) scanning (see page 424), its main rival, can offer none of these advantages although at its best and in certain conditions it produces better information.

Although the value of CT scanning has yet to be proven outside its use as a diagnostic tool in the brain and its value in planning the treatment of certain cancers, ultrasound is becoming more and more useful every year. It has a proven place in obstetrics and other areas of medicine are finding just how valuable it can be.

From the patient's point of view it is simple, quick and harmless, and of course has none of the disadvantages associated with X-rays.

In obstetrics, ultrasound has enabled doctors to be able to tell the age of the fetus very accurately (to within eight days) and can display several abnormalities likely to cause miscarriage. It is also useful for diagnosing multiple births (for example, twins). The fetal heart can be seen from seven and a half weeks onwards and certain congenital abnormalities of the fetus such as spina bifida can often be picked up early too. It is frequently used to locate the pool of amniotic fluid so that the doctor can be sure of avoiding both baby and placenta when performing an amniocentesis. Sometimes there is doubt as to whether a woman's intra-uterine contraceptive device is inside the uterus or has perforated into the abdominal cavity. Ultrasound will tell the doctor quickly and easily not only whether the IUD is there at all but whether it is in fact in the uterus.

The liver, gall-bladder and pancreas can all be visualized with ultrasound but at the moment, except in the very best hands, X-rays offer more information. Ultrasonic studies of the heart give valuable information without the problems associated with radio-opaque fluid techniques. The diagnosis of breast lumps was one area in which it was hoped ultrasound would be a great help but as yet this hope has not been fulfilled and other methods are currently more reliable. Advances in the technology of ultrasound could alter this within a very few years.

Ultrasound *can* give indications as to the functioning of the organs it shows on the screen – but usually only shows their anatomy. Often, the altered anatomy enables the doctor to deduce information about the workings of the organ but in most cases the use of radio-isotopes is far more accurate. Today, ultrasound is often used in conjunction with radio-isotope studies. X-rays are associated with a small potential danger, so whenever possible doctors use ultrasound instead, if they are happy that the quality of the information is as good. Pricing will be a major factor in favour of ultrasound as the newer machines become even more sophisticated. X-ray plates are photographic film which depends for its existence on silver – a metal of increasing price and rarity. With the photographic print-out from an ultrasound machine costing only a twentieth of that of a single X-ray film, this could become an important advantage of the technique in the next decade.

There is now some debate as to the superiority of the various new methods of 'imaging', as CT scanning and ultrasound are called, and there is no doubt that each has advantages over the other in certain ways. Ultrasound equipment is only one tenth as expensive to buy as computerized tomography equipment and costs about a tenth as much to run. This could change as ultrasound machines become more sophisticated and have computers built into them. The training of people to do ultrasound investigations takes much longer than for CT scanning and the quality of the information produced by the ultrasound machine depends very much more on the ability of the operator than does CT scanning. It takes a skilled eye to be able to interpret ultrasound pictures but any doctor can interpret (and therefore get clinical help from) CT scanner pictures because they look just like textbook pictures.

Because CT scanning uses radiation it is not suitable for use in obstetrics and it is here that ultrasound has a clear advantage, especially now that 'real-time' machines, as they are called, can display movements and not simply still pictures. It has no known disadvantage to mother or fetus. At the other end of the scale, ultrasound has almost no place in diagnosing conditions inside the head and CT scanning is extremely valuable here. CT scanning is also very valuable in diagnosing chest disease and bone problems – ultrasound is no help in these fields.

As the years go by and ultrasound is developed still further, it will undoubtedly prove to be an even more useful tool than it is today but better equipment usually costs more and this may mean that new generations of machines will be less widely available than the current cheaper ones.

## URINE TESTING

Most people who go to hospital as in- or out-patients will have a urine test at some time. Many valuable things can be learned from examining the urine but the most important part of the test starts with the patient himself – the clean collection of a sample. If the urine is being collected for chemical analysis, it really does not matter whether you collect it under sterile conditions but if the doctor tells you that he is looking for infection of the kidneys or bladder, any bacterial contamination during collection could jeopardize the accuracy of the result and your treatment could be delayed. If you are having your urine 'cultured' for bacteria, it should be delivered to the laboratory where this is to be performed within less than one hour of your passing the specimen. In the meantime, do not refrigerate the specimen or put it in the sun on a window sill.

The best way to collect uncontaminated urine is by the mid-stream method. The practical details differ in men and women but in general the idea is to pass a little urine first and discard it. This removes any cellular debris from the urinary passage. The subsequent specimen should now be clean and represent a true bladder specimen.

In hospital, the procedure is carried out as follows:

IN WOMEN, the vulva is swabbed with warm, sterile saline, wiping from front to back and never bringing the same swab back to the front of the vulva again, once used. Once this is complete, the woman is asked to pass urine and a middle-of-the-stream sample collected. This is then transferred to a sterile bottle and sent to the bacteriology laboratory.

IN MEN, the foreskin is pulled back and the glans cleaned with sterile saline. The man then passes urine and a middle-of-the-stream specimen is collected.

If you are asked to collect a middle-of-the-stream specimen at home it is not difficult to do. Simply let a little urine go first and then pass some more directly *into the sterile pot provided* by the doctor or hospital. Never pass water into another container first before transferring it to the real urine bottle or contamination will occur.

Many other things can be detected in the urine apart from bacteria. The pH (acidity or alkalinity) of urine can give a clue to several conditions and even the colour of the urine can help in certain diagnoses. The specific gravity changes in some conditions, so this is checked. Acetone (which smells like nail varnish remover) can be present in diabetes and certain other conditions and the presence of protein suggests infection, kidney malfunction, heart failure or certain toxic conditions, for example. Bile breakdown products can tell a lot about obstruction of the bile ducts and the presence of pus cells indicates infection. Sugar is always tested for in case the person has unrecognized diabetes, and blood is looked for too just in case there is microscopic blood loss, insufficient to produce red urine.

Urine testing in good hands is an invaluable tool in the investigation of a variety of diseases. Most often the results are entirely normal but occasionally further tests will be required to follow up the urine test findings.

# VAGINAL EXAMINATION

A clinical examination in which the doctor looks at, feels and possibly takes samples of fluid or cells from the vagina and mouth of the womb. It also enables him to feel the other organs that lie in the pelvis, such as the ovaries.

It is usually done to sort out gynaecological signs and symptoms such as excessive or too little menstrual bleeding, painful intercourse, vaginal discharge and in the assessment of pregnancy and labour. It is also the only non-operative way to assess the position and condition of the uterus and ovaries.

Any gynaecological or obstetric examination begins with

the doctor first inspecting and feeling your tummy. Once this is complete he will ask you to lie on your back or side (usually the left) while he examines your vulva (external vaginal area). He will look at the outside first, separating the lips (labia) with his fingers. At this stage, he will be able to see any abnormal hair distribution, clitoral enlargement, varicose veins of the vulva, swellings, sores, discharges or inflammation before going on to feel for any abnormalities.

Although a manual examination of the vagina reveals a lot of information quickly and painlessly, the doctor will often first want to see the inside of the vagina and also to see the cervix (mouth of the womb) so that a smear can be done to rule out cervical cancer and so that the hormone state of the cervix and vagina can be assessed. At the same time he may take a swab to be tested for gonorrhoea or other organisms causing infection and discharge.

This look inside is easily done by the doctor inserting a special instrument into the vagina. A speculum, as it is called, is a smooth, polished instrument which is sterilized and warmed, sometimes lubricated and then gently inserted in its closed position into the vagina. Once inside, it is opened so that the blades push the deepest parts of the vaginal walls aside and allow a view of these and the cervix at the end of the vagina. In this position the doctor can take a smear of the cervix to look for cancer or infection and can also look for other abnormalities.

Once these preliminaries have been completed, the doctor removes the speculum and puts on a rubber or plastic glove. Next he inserts his forefinger into the vaginal opening a little way and feels the labia in turn between finger and thumb to detect any swelling of the Bartholin's glands that lie each side of the vagina in the fat of the labia. The finger is then passed higher up the vagina. Some doctors find they get a more accurate impression of what is going on if they use two fingers but if this is uncomfortable for the woman he can still feel most abnormalities using one only. Once his fingers are inside the vagina, he places his hand on the woman's lower tummy just above the pubic hair and by pushing down into the abdomen with one hand and up from the vagina with the two fingers of the other hand he can feel the uterus or womb between his two hands. This enables him to judge its size, position and consistency and to feel for swellings and lumps.

Once he has felt the uterus he moves his fingers to each side to feel the fallopian tubes and ovaries. Any cysts or other swellings can often be felt quite readily like this.

All this sounds complicated but a good doctor skilled in vaginal examinations can tell a lot about a woman's reproductive organs within a minute or so. If you get any actual pain when the doctor is examining you, tell him because it might be caused by a condition called endometriosis (which frequently causes infertility) and can be cured.

There is nothing particularly pleasant about having a vaginal examination but there is nothing to be feared either. The most unpleasant part for many women is the coldness of the lubricating jelly or the instrument the doctor uses. Most women think of their vagina as very personal and private and find it difficult to relax while a doctor feels inside and inserts an instrument into it. Hard though it may seem to believe, it is something that you soon get used to and many who need repeated vaginal examinations find that after a while they get so used to them that they think no more of them than having a blood sample taken. If you find it difficult to relax, look the doctor in the face, press your bottom into the bed, open your legs as wide as possible and breathe deeply all the time. Doctors can tell a lot from a good vaginal examination but everything is based on informed guesswork – after all, he cannot see your tubes and ovaries. Because of this he may well have to suggest other tests to clarify things he finds on examining you.

Lastly, many women fear that the doctor might harm a baby in the uterus – a view which was further encouraged when doctors used to advise abstention from intercourse during pregnancy. However, it is worth pointing out that vaginal examinations done during pregnancy are perfectly safe.

# X-RAYS

Until 1895 when Wilhelm Roentgen, a German physicist, discovered X-rays it was impossible to see inside the human body. Today X-rays are an essential tool in the hands of doctors – a tool which helps them make a diagnosis and allows them to assess the results of treatment.

Although many people imagine that X-rays are only used to find broken bones, this is far from the case. Today, hundreds of different conditions can be diagnosed using X-rays, and for some of them X-rays are the best diagnostic method. Some of the more specialized X-ray techniques use radio-opaque substances which, when injected into the body, show up a particular part or system so clearly on the X-ray that it is almost like having a photograph in front of you to look at. Over the last ten years a remarkable new extension to radiology has been developed. This is called computerized tomography (see page 424).

X-rays work by casting a shadow on to a photographic film and show up tissues in the body according to their density. A 'gun' shoots a tiny dose of X-rays at the part of the body under examination after an X-ray-sensitive (photographic) film has been put behind the part. Some X-rays go straight through (where there is little tissue to interrupt them) and others are blocked by more solid tissues. Thus bones (very dense structures) let very few X-rays through and show up as white areas on the film behind and the lungs (very 'open' in texture and full of air) show up dark. All other tissues show up in varying degrees according to their density.

Once the X-ray film has been exposed, it, just like a film in a camera, has to be processed. After processing, the film is coded for future reference and is then ready to be interpreted by an expert. A radiographer is the person who actually takes the X-ray and the doctor who interprets the film is called a radiologist. Both are highly qualified professionals but the doctor obviously has a medical degree and specializes in performing X-ray investigations and interpreting X-rays.

Today's X-rays are safe. In the past there was concern about leakage from the equipment that produced the X-rays. Modern machines in hospitals today are much safer and all the staff who work in X-ray departments are checked at regular intervals for the dose of X-rays being received.

Sometimes you will see the doctor watching a TV screen when he is X-raying you. This allows him to use only very tiny doses of X-rays and through the TV set receive a perfect picture boosted in intensity by the electronics it contains. This is just one way in which modern technology is reducing the amount of radiation a person receives during radiological examinations. Today, unless you are having very large numbers of X-rays, there is no cause for alarm at all. Having said this though, it is sensible to tell the X-ray staff if you think you might be pregnant because X-rays could harm the unborn baby, though this is unlikely unless you are having lots of X-rays. Remember especially to think of this when taking your children to be X-rayed as you may get a dose of X-rays as you hold the child. If you are still within the childbearing age group, only have an X-ray in the first ten days of your cycle (the ten days after the start of your period) to be sure you have not just conceived. Most X-ray departments ask you to fill in a form asking whether you might be pregnant and the 'point' in your menstrual cycle that you are at.

Having an X-ray is no longer a dangerous or unpleasant affair. The machine makes buzzing noises but these are not alarming once you know what to expect. If you follow the radiographer's instructions you will be surprised how quickly and simply the whole procedure is over. If at any time you are worried or want to know what is happening, ask the radiographer or a doctor to explain. If you get any pain or strange sensations, tell someone: it may help them to help you.

Let us look now at some of the common X-ray procedures to see what is involved.

## Chest X-ray

Probably the most commonly performed X-ray and just about the simplest. No preparation is necessary. You simply stand with your back to the X-ray machine and with your chest flat against an X-ray film. You will be asked to take a long breath in and hold it at which time the X-ray will be taken. Sometimes you will be asked to stand sideways so that a picture can be taken at right angles to the first one.

## X-raying blood vessels (Angiography)

X-rays can now be used to show the blood supply of almost any area of the body. Most of these examinations are carried out under local anaesthesia with you awake and co-operative but others will be done under general anaesthesia, partly because they might be painful and partly because they can take a relatively long time which could be unpleasant for the person having it done.

CARDIAC ANGIOGRAPHY involves the positioning of a fine plastic tube in the heart. The tube is inserted into a vein in the arm or leg and then fed up into the heart under guidance from a TV-intensified image of the whole procedure. As veins end up in the right side of the heart this procedure is fine for looking at this part of the organ. If the doctor needs to know about the left side of the heart, the procedure is the same but the plastic tube is threaded up inside an artery and not a vein.

Once the catheter is in place, a radio-opaque substance is injected and films (still or movie) taken as the heart pumps the substance out into the blood stream. The picture obtained shows exactly what is happening inside the heart and movie films are particularly valuable when it comes to examining the heart's function as a pump. The substance is dispersed harmlessly within the body.

ARTERIOGRAPHY can be carried out under local or general anaesthesia. Two main methods are used. In the first, a radio-opaque substance is injected into the artery the doctor wants to examine. This is a good method for arteries in the limbs, the neck and even the aorta.

The second method is used when the radiologist needs to examine a distant arterial blood supply that cannot be directly approached by inserting a needle. A needle is inserted into an artery that leads to the area under examination. A fine flexible tube is threaded into the artery under X-ray control until the tip is in place near the area to be examined. The radio-opaque substance is then injected and still or movie pictures taken as it spreads through the area supplied by that artery. If you are not anaesthetized you may well feel a burning sensation as the substance is injected. Tell the radiologist if it is too unpleasant.

Veins can be X-rayed too. Usually the leg is the site of most interest because of deep vein thrombosis or varicose veins. A radio-opaque substance is injected into a superficial vein in the foot or can be injected into a bone in the foot or ankle under general anaesthesia. As it is injected into the veins, you will notice a burning sensation. If this becomes too unpleasant, tell the radiologist.

## Lymphangiography

This is an X-ray technique for demonstrating lymphatic channels. It can be used as a means of diagnosing diseases of the lymph system (Hodgkin's disease, for example). A small amount of blue-violet dye is injected into the toe webs on both sides of the body about five minutes before the procedure is to start. The lymphatic vessels then show up as fine blue-coloured streaks as they collect the dye particles. This enables the doctor to find the otherwise invisible lymphatic channels. Once the channels are visible he injects a radio-opaque substance and takes several X-rays as it travels up the leg to be dispersed in the body. The examination takes a long time and you will have to lie very still or the needles will fall out.

Your skin may go blue for the following 24–48 hours after the procedure but this is harmless and goes quickly. Also, your urine may go green or blue.

## X-rays of the bowel

By far the commonest type of X-ray done on the bowel involves swallowing a pleasant-tasting fluid, a barium compound: the 'barium meal'. Be sure not to eat or drink anything for at least eight hours before the examination but apart from that you do not have to do anything else at all.

The barium is given to you and you will be asked to swallow some as the doctor screens you in various positions on an X-ray table. Until recently you would have had to swallow a large volume of barium but today very small volumes (about a cupful) are used. This change has come about because many radiologists now use a new technique which does not rely on a large amount of barium being present in the stomach to show up any problems there may be. This new 'double contrast' method involves being given a powder or tablets to swallow immediately before the procedure. These produce gas in the stomach so that when a small amount of barium is swallowed there is a good spread of the barium all over the stomach lining. The gas shows up as dark areas and the barium as white and this enables the radiologist to see very fine details compared with the old method of filling the stomach with barium. At one stage you may be tipped 'head down' but you will not fall off the table and you are never completely upside down, only tilted so that the barium sulphate can coat the lining of the gullet and stomach just as milk coats a glass and renders it opaque. This produces excellent X-rays and all kinds of disorders can be diagnosed or declared absent within a few minutes. As most of the procedure is done under TV control, the doctor may let you watch, which can be fun and interesting – after all it is your stomach they are talking about. Some radiologists like to give a drug to encourage the stomach to empty slowly so that they can see how the duodenum and first part of the intestine shows up, so do not be alarmed if they suggest an injection. The whole procedure takes about 15–20 minutes.

If it is necessary to have pictures of the parts of the bowel that lead on from the stomach, the barium is allowed to pass onwards a little and is then re-X-rayed. If you are to have this examination (called a 'follow through', because they are following the barium through the bowel with their X-rays) you may be given a drug by mouth to help the stomach empty a bit quicker. The alternative is a lot of sitting around for three or four hours as the stomach empties naturally and passes the contents into the bowel.

If you are normally constipated, take a laxative after the

X-rays because the barium tends to have a further constipating effect.

The large bowel (colon) can be seen simply by taking a plain X-ray of the abdomen but this is rarely good enough for making a definite diagnosis of the conditions affecting it. A barium enema is therefore most often used. You will be asked to take some kind of laxative the night before and to open your bowels on the morning of the X-ray. In some hospitals you will be given an enema or even have your bowel washed out. The test is simple and not too disturbing although some people do not like the idea of it very much. A tube is passed into the back passage and barium is allowed to flow in under gravity while the doctor watches on a TV screen. Several films are taken of the key areas. The barium is then let out either through the tube or by your going to the lavatory. Sometimes it is necessary to pump some air in through the tube so that another type of X-ray can be done using the barium left coating the bowel lining. This can be uncomfortable but should not be painful. It does mean that you could spend the next few hours passing wind. The X-ray procedure itself takes about 45 minutes.

### X-rays of the gall-bladder

Sometimes a plain X-ray of the abdomen will show up gall-stones in the gall-bladder or in the ducts that carry bile to the intestine. However, most often a special X-ray called a cholecystogram will have to be done to be sure. Twelve hours before this test you will be given some tablets or powder which you should take with lots of water (about a pint). These contain a contrast medium which when eaten and digested passes through the liver and is put out in the bile.

You will be asked to take a non-fatty, easily digested meal the evening before the test and after that to eat nothing. You will also have to refrain from smoking until after the test has been completed. Because gas in the bowel can render the X-ray difficult to interpret, don't eat any wholemeal bread, crispbreads, fruit, vegetables or pasta for at least twelve hours before the X-ray.

X-rays of the liver area then show the bile system outlined

by the contrast substances and stones can readily be seen as dark areas within the white contrast substance. If the doctor needs to see if the gall-bladder is able to contract, you will be given a fatty meal or a commercial preparation, both of which make the gall-bladder contract in normal people. This squeezes bile and therefore the contrast substance from the gall-bladder into the ducts that take bile to the bowel, so showing up any stones that might be lodged in the ducts. There is also a method of X-raying the bile ducts which involves an injection of a radio-opaque substance into a vein but this is not as commonly used as the tablet method. Preparation for this involves having a fat-free meal on the evening before the X-ray and one slice of very thickly buttered bread and a cup of tea with milk on the morning of the test. The examination can take up to three hours.

## X-rays of the urinary system

IVU. By far the commonest X-ray of the urinary system is an IVU (intravenous urogram – it used to be called an intravenous pyleogram – IVP). You will be asked to ensure that your bowels have been opened for the two days prior to the X-ray so that no stools in the bowel lie in front of the kidneys. You will be asked to drink only one pint of fluid in the 24 hours leading up to the test and nothing at all in the six hours before the X-ray so that you will be relatively dehydrated.

A control film is taken and then you will be asked if you have a history of allergy – asthma, hay fever, drug sensitivities, food reactions and so on. If you have, a small test dose of the material to be injected may be given to see that you do not react to it.

In normal circumstances the radio-opaque substance is injected fairly quickly into a vein in the arm. If you feel strange at all, tell the doctor and he may give you a drug to counteract the effects. Usually, there are no side-effects, and X-rays are taken at intervals up to about an hour. Sometimes films have to be taken for much longer in order to 'see' the kidneys. Sometimes the kidneys will not show up on an intravenous urogram and you may have to have another sort of X-ray in which fine tubes are passed from inside the bladder up to the kidneys. This examination is usually done under general anaesthesia and involves injecting a radio-opaque substance through the tubes and then taking X-rays.

**MICTURATING CYSTOGRAM.** Sometimes a doctor will need to see how well the bladder is working. A micturating cystogram is an X-ray which involves passing a tube into the bladder up the urinary passage. The doctor then fills the bladder with a special fluid. This may be uncomfortable but say if it is too bad. Once the tube has been removed, more films will be taken whilst you are passing urine and again with the bladder empty. This whole procedure takes fifteen to twenty minutes.

# X-RAY COMPUTED TOMOGRAPHY (CT SCANNING, COMPUTERIZED TOMOGRAPHY)

Until this revolutionary way of producing X-ray pictures was introduced in 1972, the technique for producing X-ray pictures had hardly changed since Roentgen produced his first X-ray in 1895.

Research by a British company has produced a machine which overcomes the two main disadvantages of ordinary X-ray pictures. These disadvantages are: 1. the superimposition of three-dimensional information on to a single plane (photographic plate) makes diagnosis and interpretation difficult; and 2. only tissues and organs that have large differences in X-ray absorption relative to their surroundings will give good enough contrast for the human eye to distinguish them from their neighbouring structures.

CT scanning does away with the conventional concept of firing one burst of X-rays at the part to be examined and recording the results on a photographic plate. Instead, while you lie on a couch the machine emits a narrow fan of X-rays which passes through slices of the body, each about one centimetre thick or thereabouts, to be picked up by crystal detectors on the other side of the body. The picture is 'produced' as a result of a computer processing the readings of the emergent X-rays and is displayed on a TV-type screen built into the equipment. Prints are available of these TV pictures so that permanent records can be kept. The result is a picture that is like a three-dimensional anatomy book, with everything clearly visible rather as on a colour photograph.

From the patient's point of view CT scanning is simple and painless. Although the actual time the machine takes to 'write' one slice through the body is in the order of seconds, the doctors will usually look at many such sectional pictures, so the whole examination takes minutes. The amount of X-rays delivered to the patient is very small because the detectors are so sensitive. A photographic film used in normal radiography is only about one per cent efficient – the other 99 per cent of the radiated energy is lost. The crystal detectors of a CT scanner may well capture 95 per cent of the X-rays used and can in addition with the help of a computer distinguish far smaller differences in density contrast than can the human eye.

CT scanners are still in their early days, even though there are already 'fourth generation' models on the market. Having said this though it is difficult to see how much better they could become, except perhaps that they could be made more cheaply. The greatest disadvantage of CT scanning is its cost. Not only are the machines expensive but the staff and running costs are extremely high. This does not concern the person being X-rayed too much, especially if he is being saved from other, perhaps unpleasant, investigations by being CT scanned. Until CT scanning, 50 years old X-ray methods involving the injection of air or contrast medium into the brain could be unpleasant and were sometimes dangerous. For patients like these, CT scanning is a miraculous improvement. However, the value of these scanners outside the interpretation and diagnosis of brain conditions is far from certain. Whole body scanners can now look at slices of any part of the body but other diagnostic methods are often cheaper and can give just as good information for doctors to act upon.

For some investigations you may be asked to swallow

some special tablets; you may have to have an injection into a vein; or even an enema. These are all done to increase the contrast of the particular organ under study – but none of these procedures is painful or unpleasant and simply helps the doctors get a better picture than they otherwise might.

CT scanning is undoubtedly here to stay but because other cheaper diagnostic tools are fast becoming more useful and sophisticated (see ultrasound, page 410) and because it does not tell the doctor much about an organ's functioning (see radio-isotope, page 405) its role is likely to remain fairly limited, though valuable in special areas, such as the brain.

Remember that CT scanning is used to help in diagnosis and in planning treatment. It is not in any way a form of treatment.

# Some self-help organizations of interest to surgical patients

Action for the Disabled Association
26 Barker Walk
Mount Ephraim Road
Streatham, London SW16          Tel. 01-677-1276

Association for Improvements in the Maternity Services
(AIMS)
10 Stonecliff View
Leeds LS12 5BE                  Tel. 0532-634580

Association for Spina Bifida and Hydrocephalus
Tavistock House North
Tavistock Square
London WC1H 9HJ                 Tel. 01-388-1382

Back Pain Association
31/33 Park Road
Teddington
Middlesex TW11 0AB              Tel. 01-977-5474

British Kidney Patient Association
Bordon
Hants                           Tel. 04203-2021

British Pregnancy Advisory Service
Austy Manor
Wootton Wawen
Solihull
W.Midlands B95 6DA              Tel. 05642-3225

British Rheumatism and Arthritis Association
6 Grosvenor Crescent
London SW1X 7ER                    Tel. 01-235-0902

Cancer Aftercare and Rehabilitation Society
Lodge Cottage
Church Lane
Timsbury
Bath BA3 1LF                       Tel. 0761-70731

Cancer Information Association
Gloucester Green
Oxford OX1 1EA                     Tel. 0865-46654

Cardiac Spare Parts Club
9 High Street,
Harrold
Bedford MK43 7DQ

Colostomy Welfare Group
38-39 Eccleston Square
London SW1V 1PB                    Tel. 01-828-5175

Committee on Sexual Problems of the Disabled
c/o Radar
25 Mortimer Street
London W1A 8AB                     Tel. 01-637-5400

Compassionate Friends (for bereaved parents)
25 Kingsdown Parade
Bristol BS6 5UE                    Tel. 0272-47316

Cruse National Organization for Widows and their Children
Cruse House
126 Sheen Road
Richmond
Surrey                             Tel. 01-940-4818

Disabled Drivers' Association
Ashwellthorpe Hall
Ashwellthorpe
Norwich NR16 1EX                     Tel. 0508-41449

Disabled Living Foundation
346 Kensington High Street
London W14 8NS                       Tel. 01-602-2491

Ileostomy Association of Great Britain and Ireland
Drove Cottage
Fuzzy Drove
Kempshott
Basingstoke
Hants RG22 5LU                       Tel. 09905-8277

International Glaucoma Association
Kings' College Hospital
Denmark Hill
London SE5                   Tel. 01-274-6222 Ext. 2453

Invalids at Home
23 Farm Avenue
London NW2 2BJ                       Tel. 01-452-2074

Life (Anti-abortion organization)
35 Kenilworth Road
Leamington Spa
Warwickshire                         Tel. 0926-21587

Malcolm Sargent Cancer Fund for Children
6 Sydney Street
London SW3                           Tel. 01-352-6884

Marie Curie Memorial Foundation
124 Sloane Street
London SW1X 9BP                      Tel. 01-730-9157

Mastectomy Association of Great Britain
1 Colworth Road
Croydon
CR0 7AB                           Tel. 01-654-8643

National Association of Laryngectomy Clubs
30 Dorset Square
London NW1 6QL                    Tel. 01-402-6007

National Association for Mental Health
22 Harley Street
London W1N 2ED                    Tel. 01-637-0741

National Association for the Childless
318 Summer Lane
Birmingham B19 3RL                Tel. 021-359-4887

National Association for the Welfare of Children in Hospital
7 Exton Street
London SE1                        Tel. 01-261-1738

Patients' Association
11 Dartmouth Street
London SW1H 9BN                   Tel. 01-222-4992

Pregnancy Advisory Service
40 Margaret Street
London W1                         Tel. 01-409-0281

Renal Society
64 South Hill Park
London NW3                        Tel. 01-794-9479

The Royal Association for Disability and Rehabilitation
25 Mortimer Street
London W1N 8AB                    Tel. 01-637-5400

Royal National Institute for the Blind
224 Great Portland Street
London W1N 6AA                    Tel. 01-388-1266

Royal National Institute for the Deaf
105 Gower Street
London WC1E 6AH                Tel. 01-387-8033

Samaritans
17 Uxbridge Road
Slough
Berks                         Tel. 75-31011

Spinal Injuries Association
5 Crowndale Road
London NW1 1TU                Tel. 01-388-6849

Tenovus Cancer Information Centre
90 Cathedral Road
Cardiff CF1 9PG               Tel. 0222-48500

Urinary Conduit Association
36 York Road
Denton
Manchester                    Tel. 061-336-8818

Women's National Cancer Control Campaign
1 South Audley Street
London SW1H 5DQ               Tel. 01-499-7532

# Index